610.73

KT-500-233

Contexts of Nursing

Contexts of Nursing

An Introduction

Edited by

John Daly
RN BA BHSc(Nurs) MEd(Hons) PhD FINE FCN(NSW) FRCNA
Professor of Nursing & Head, School of Nursing, Family &
Community Health, College of Social & Health Sciences,
University of Western Sydney, Sydney, New South Wales.

Sandra Speedy
RN BA(Hons) DipEd MURP EdD MAPS FANZCMHN
Professor and Director, Graduate College of Management,
Southern Cross University, Lismore, New South Wales.

Debra Jackson
RN CommNursCert BHSc(Nurs) MNurs PhD STTI
Associate Professor of Nursing, School of Nursing, Family
& Community Health, College of Social & Health Sciences,
University of Western Sydney, Sydney, New South Wales.

Philip Darbyshire
RNMH RSCN DipN RNT MN PhD
Professor of Nursing & Head, Department of Nursing and
Midwifery Research & Practice Development, Women's and
Children's Hospital, University of South Australia and The
Flinders University of South Australia.

LIBRARY & INFORMATION SERVICE
STRAYSIDE EDUCATION CENTRE
STRAYSIDE WING
HARROGATE DISTRICT HOSPITAL
LANCASTER PARK ROAD
HARROGATE HG2 7SX

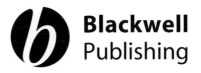

Blackwell
Publishing

© 2002 Blackwell Publishing Ltd
© Chapter 9 Professor Megan-Jane Johnstone 2002

Editorial Offices:
Osney Mead, Oxford OX2 0EL, UK
 Tel: +44 (0)1865 206206
108 Cowley Road, Oxford OX4 1JF, UK
 Tel: +44 (0)1865 791100
Blackwell Munksgaard, Nørre Søgade 35,
PO Box 2148, Copenhagen, DK-1016, Denmark
 Tel: +45 77 33 33 33
Blackwell Verlag, Kurfürstendamm 57,
10707 Berlin, Germany
 Tel: +49 (0)30 32 79 060
Blackwell Publishing, 10, rue Casimir Delavigne
75006 Paris, France
 Tel: +33 1 53 10 33 10

The right of the Author to be identified as
the Author of this Work has been asserted in
accordance with the Copyright, Designs and
Patents Act 1988.

All rights reserved. No part of this publication
may be reproduced, stored in a retrieval system,
or transmitted, in any form or by any means,
electronic, mechanical, photocopying, recording
or otherwise, except as permitted by the UK
Copyright, Designs and Patents Act 1988,
without the prior permission of the publisher.

First published 2002 by Blackwell Publishing
Adapted from Daly, Speedy and Jackson (2000)
Contexts of Nursing: An Introduction. MacLennan &
Petty, Australia.

A catalogue record for this title
is available from the British Library

ISBN 1-4051-0095-8

Set in 10/12 pt ITC Garamond Light by
Sparks Computer Solutions Ltd, Oxford, UK
http://www.sparks.co.uk
Printed and bound in Great Britain by
TJ International Ltd, Padstow

For further information on
Blackwell Publishing, visit our website:
www.blackwellpublishing.com

Contents

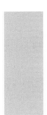

Contributors

Sally Borbasi RN CCNC BEd(Nurs) MA PhD
Associate Professor of Nursing, School of Nursing and Midwifery, Faculty of Health Sciences, The Flinders University of South Australia, Adelaide.

Angela Brown RN RM MA BSc(Hons) CertEd
Senior Lecturer in Nursing, School of Nursing and Midwifery, The University of Sheffield, Sheffield, UK.

Helen Caulfield
Solicitor and Health Policy Analyst, Policy Unit, Royal College of Nursing, London, UK.

Esther Chang RN CM BAppSc(AdvNurs) DipNEd MEdAdmin PhD
Professor of Nursing, School of Nursing, Family & Community Health, College of Social & Health Sciences, University of Western Sydney, Sydney.

Mary Chiarella RN ADipNEd LLB(Hons) PhD FCN(NSW)
Professor of Nursing in Corrections Health, Faculty of Nursing, Midwifery & Health, University of Technology, Sydney & Corrections Health Service, Sydney, Australia.

Judith Clare RN MA(Hons) PhD FRCNA FCNANZ
Professor of Nursing & Dean, School of Nursing & Midwifery, Faculty of Health Sciences, The Flinders University of South Australia, Adelaide.

Jane Conway RN BHSc BNursing(Hons) GradDip Further Education and Training, Grad CertHRM MEd
Lecturer, School of Nursing & Midwifery & Teaching Fellow, PROBLARC, The University of Newcastle, New South Wales.

Patrick Crookes RN RNT CertEd BSc(Nurs) PhD
Professor of Nursing & Head, Department of Nursing, Faculty of Health & Behavioural Sciences, The University of Wollongong, Wollongong, New South Wales.

John Daly RN BA BHSc(Nurs) MEd(Hons) PhD FINE FCN(NSW) FRCNA
Professor of Nursing & Foundation Head, School of Nursing, Family & Community Health, College of Social & Health Sciences, University of Western Sydney, Sydney, Australia.

Philip Darbyshire RNMH RSCN DipN RNT MN PhD
Professor of Nursing & Head, Department of Nursing and Midwifery Research & Practice Development, Women's and Children's Hospital, University of South Australia and The Flinders University of South Australia.

Steven Edwards RMN BA(Hons) MPhil PhD
Senior Lecturer, Centre for Philosophy and Health Care, University of Wales Swansea, UK.

Doug Elliott RN IntCareCert BAppSc(Nurs) MAppSc(Nurs) PhD MCN(NSW)
Professor of Nursing (Critical Care), Prince of Wales Hospital, Randwick & The Department of Clinical Nursing, The University of Sydney, Sydney, Australia.

Mary FitzGerald RN DipN CertEd MN PhD
Professor of Nursing, School of Nursing & Midwifery, The University of Newcastle, NSW & Central Coast Area Health Service.

Sally Glen RN MA PhD FRSA
Professor of Nursing Education & Dean, St Bartholomew School of Nursing & Midwifery, & Deputy Director of the Institute of Health Sciences, City University, London, UK.

Jennifer Greenwood RN CM DipN DipEd RNT MEd PhD FRCNA
Adjunct Professor of Nursing, School of Nursing, Family & Community Health, College of Social & Health Sciences University of Western Sydney, Sydney, Australia.

Rhonda Griffiths RN CM BEd(Nurs) MSc(Hons) DrPH FCN(NSW) FRCNA
Professor of Nursing, School of Nursing, Family & Community Health, College of Social & Health Sciences, University of Western Sydney, & Director, Centre for Applied Nursing Research, South Western Sydney Area Health Service, Sydney, Australia.

Debra Jackson RN CommNursCert BHSc(Nurs) MNurs PhD STTI
Associate Professor of Nursing, School of Nursing, Family & Community Health, College of Social & Health Sciences, University of Western Sydney, Sydney, Australia.

Martin Johnson RN PhD
Professor in Nursing, School of Nursing, University of Salford, Salford, UK.

Megan-Jane Johnstone RN BA PhD FCN(NSW) FRCNA
Professor of Nursing, Department of Nursing & Midwifery, Faculty of Biomedical & Health Sciences & Nursing, RMIT University, Melbourne, Australia.

Mark Jones RN MSc BSc(Hons) DipEd DipN
Lecturer in Nursing & Programme Leader-Adult Nursing, St Bartholomew School of Nursing & Midwifery, City University, London, UK.

Tina Koch RN BA PhD FRCNA
Director, Royal District Nursing Service Research Unit, Adelaide, South Australia, Adjunct Professor of Nursing, School of Nursing, Family & Community Health, College of Social & Health Sciences, University of Western Sydney, Sydney, Australia.

Christopher Maggs RN PhD
Professor of Nursing, School of Nursing, De Montfort University, Leicester, UK.

Judy Mannix RN ACNC BEd(Nurs) MNurs(Hons) MRCNA STTI
Lecturer, School of Nursing, Family & Community Health, College of Social & Health Sciences, University of Western Sydney, Sydney, Australia.

Margaret McMillan RN BA MCurrSt(Hons) PhD GradCert Mgt FRCNA
Professor of Nursing, Deputy Executive Dean, Faculty of Health, The University of Newcastle, New South Wales.

(I)Rena Papadopoulos RN PhD
Principal Lecturer & Head, Centre for Transcultural Studies in Health, Middlesex University, London, UK.

Judith M. Parker RN BA(Hons) PhD FRCNA
Professor of Nursing & Head, School of Postgraduate Nursing, The University of Melbourne, Australia.

Steve Parker RN RPN DipT(Nursing) BEd PhD
Lecturer, School of Nursing & Midwifery, The Flinders University of South Australia, Adelaide.

Elizabeth Plastow RMN RGN HV MSc PGDip(Ed)
Senior Lecturer, School of Nursing & Midwifery, University of Plymouth, Plymouth, UK.

Sandra Speedy RN BA(Hons) DipEd MURP EdD MAPS FANZCMHN
Professor and Director, Graduate College of Management, Southern Cross University, Lismore, New South Wales.

Irene Stein RN BA BHSc(Nurs) MA PhD FRCNA
Assistant Dean-Community Relations & Marketing & Professor of Nursing, Faculty of Health, University of Newcastle, NSW & Baptist Community Services (NSW & ACT), Australia.

David Thompson RN BSc MA MBA PhD FRCN FESC
Professor of Nursing, Department of Health Sciences, University of York, York, UK.

Jill White RN CM BEd MEd FCN(NSW) FRCNA
Professor of Nursing & Dean, Faculty of Nursing, Midwifery and Health, University of Technology, Sydney, Australia.

Foreword

Nursing textbooks have long been exported from the UK to Australia, but rarely the other way around, so it will be intriguing to see if this book originating 'down under' will make its mark on the British market for which it is primarily (although not exclusively) intended. The original version of *Contexts of Nursing* was published in Australia two years ago. The original editors – John Daly, Sandra Speedy and Debra Jackson (all from the University of Western Australia) – have been joined by Philip Darbyshire, a fellow Scot and one-time PhD student of mine, now working in the University of South Australia. The original publication had an all-Australian cast of contributors but, in this UK-published version, about a third of the chapters are contributed from the UK.

All of the contributors work in (or are associated with) a university-based School of Nursing, either in Australia or in the UK and so they know well (as they should do) how to write engagingly for nursing students who are the target readership for this book. The easy style and 'readability' of the book is one of its most pleasing features and the listing of learning objectives at the start of each chapter, and reflective questions at the end, give structure to the book as well as helping to engage its readers. Many of the writers are internationally-known nurse scholars and, in the main, they are writing here about 'contexts' which reflect closely their particular fields of interest and research. As a result, the individual chapters, on a stand-alone basis, are both interesting and authoritative. If student readers do engage actively throughout the book with the debates and discussions which unfold, then this text certainly will have achieved its aim of helping to inculcate the 'the language of nursing scholarship' in next-generation nurses.

In the UK, there is a tendency at the moment to shy away from using that sort of language, mindful of the criticisms which have been voiced about nursing education becoming 'too theoretical'. What is needed, we're being told, is a new generation of nurses who, first and foremost, are deemed to be 'fit for practice' and 'fit for purpose' in a health service which is under pressure and short of nurses. Those of us in academe well understand the rationale behind the stronger emphasis on 'practice' in the new pre-registration curriculum introduced under 'Fitness for Practice' (UKCC 1999). However, we also know – perhaps better, dare I suggest, than our service colleagues – just how vital it is that nursing students continue to have a strong theoretical grounding as well. We need to produce nurses for tomorrow who, as well as being clinically competent, also are thoughtful, critical and articulate about the many and complex issues which impact, both directly and indirectly, on contemporary nursing practice, on the re-design of health services and on the changing status and role of the users of health services.

It is precisely these issues which this book addresses as it travels across a range of contexts from a variety of perspectives: historical, definitional, philosophical, epistemological, ethical, legal, social and professional. It provides an ideal introduction for nursing students to current thinking on key issues in nursing culture and inquiry.

Contexts of Nursing is an ideal book for addition to reading lists for undergraduate nursing students in UK universities. It could be used particularly effectively as the reader for a tutorial course because, best of all, I think this *is* a book which will get nursing students thinking and talking and arguing about the profession they're joining, the patients they'll be nursing, and the problems and challenges which *their* generation must tackle intelligently over coming decades.

I will watch with interest to see how *Contexts of Nursing* fares in the UK. It also will be interesting to see if this book sparks off something of a trend in collaborative writing projects between Australia and the British Isles. As it happens, I am about to divide my time between the two countries over the coming few years so I will have plenty of opportunity to ponder whether there is special value in collaborative writing between these two countries. Or, perhaps, in the longer term, *Contexts of Nursing* might be coaxed into a more eclectic book for a wider international readership.

Alison J. Tierney
BSc, PhD, RGN, FRCN
Professor of Nursing Research
Department of Nursing Studies
The University of Edinburgh, Scotland, UK
From 1 October 2002:
Professor, Department of Clinical Nursing
University of Adelaide
South Australia

Preface

This text has been planned and developed to provide comprehensive coverage of key ideas underpinning the practice of contemporary nursing. The content is foundational from a theoretical and nursing practice perspective. Consequently the work introduces the student to the language of nursing scholarship. Each chapter addresses a major focal area in the undergraduate study of nursing. We have used the notion of 'contexts' to label what may be considered theoretical threads in the fabric of nursing knowledge. It will be clear to the professional reader that this book has been designed to deal with professional nursing, theory and knowledge.

The book has been written to reflect consideration of key ideas that underpin nursing in a global context, at least in the English-speaking world. The book is unusual in that it is a collaboration between Australian and British nurses. We believe that the topics selected for inclusion are highly relevant to nursing internationally. The content selected is a distillation of international nursing knowledge from an immense base of research and scholarly endeavour. This is provided in order to give a solid theoretical foundation for undergraduate students in nursing and demonstrates the commonality of key ideas in nursing culture and scholarship. We trust that this will enable readers to understand the parameters of global nursing knowledge, practice and related health care issues. The unique concerns and challenges confronting nursing are clarified as the process of professionalisation continues.

A number of individuals provided vital assistance in the preparation of this work. Special thanks go to Alison Sheppard of the University of Western Sydney for exceptional secretarial and administrative assistance, to Pamela Petty, Jenny Curtis and Debbie Lee of MacLennan & Petty in Sydney for encouragement and believing in the project. In addition special thanks are extended to Antonia Seymour and Guy Salkeld of Blackwell Science in the UK for supporting and encouraging the project. Finally thanks go to our copy-editor, Erika Sigvallius, for precise and careful work on the manuscript.

John Daly, Sydney
Sandra Speedy, Lismore
Debra Jackson, Sydney, and
Philip Darbyshire, Adelaide, Australia

1 So, You Want To Be a Nurse

Jill White, Mary Chiarella, Sally Glen and Mark Jones

LEARNING OBJECTIVES

Upon completion of this chapter the reader should have gained:

- an appreciation of the history of defining Western notions of nursing;
- an understanding of the complexity and difficulty of defining nursing;
- an appreciation of differences in the role definitions of registered nurses and health care assistants;
- insights into the development of nursing practice standards and codes in the United Kingdom (UK);
- an understanding of the differences between codes of conduct and codes of ethics in professional practice.

KEY WORDS

NURSING, PRACTICE, REGULATION, PROFESSIONAL, CODES, CONDUCT, ETHICS, STANDARDS, COMPETENCIES.

INTRODUCTION

So, you want to be a nurse? Isn't it interesting that everybody has an opinion on your choice and often that opinion is offered quite freely? Everyone has an image of nursing and has a response to your choice, coloured not only by their knowledge of you as a person but also by their presuppositions of nursing, what it is and what it isn't. Some may have romantic images of service, compassion and dedication, others of low pay, subservience and long hours. Still others have images of bedpans, or blood and other bodily discharges. One problem with belonging to one of the oldest and largest workforces in the world is that there are elements of historical and political 'truths' in each of these descriptions – but none captures the essence, the fun, the connectedness and the human and sociopolitical possibilities that are nursing.

According to the International Council of Nurses (ICN), education is a priority area in the development of nursing. Consequently, from the early 1990s, nursing education in many countries has been under development in order to educate nurses for health care that aims at offering accessible, affordable and ethically high quality care (Salvage & Heijnen 1997). Rarely is the public perception in the UK informed by these current developments. Rarely are we, as nurses, portrayed as belonging to a profession that is well educated, reasonably well paid and offering a career. A career that provides opportunities for specialisation and autonomy in a rich and diverse range of areas of practice. For example: in the independent sector and the NHS, working with people across the life span, in health and illness, in high technology environments and where the technology or therapy is the nurse herself or himself.

DEFINING NURSING

In her book *From Novice to Expert* Patricia Benner (1984) gives us a glimpse of the difficulty of attempts to define nursing in simple terms. In describing the corner-stone relationship of nursing practice she says 'the nurse–patient relationship is not a uniform, professionalised blueprint but rather a kaleidoscope of intimacy and distance in some of the most dramatic, poignant, and mundane moments of life' (p. xxii). Nursing is an international profession with a core that binds it as a single entity across nations. It is also a profession so diverse that its social status, remunera-tion, career patterns and work conditions can vary even from country to country. In the European Union nursing education is based on the European Commission laws (Directives 77/452/EU, 77/453/EU and 89/595/European Commission 1997). The purpose of these laws, subsequent reports and recommendations issued by the vari-ous European Union bodies have been to establish a commonly accepted education and qualifications framework for nurses across the Union (European Commission 1997). This chapter explores some aspects of nursing that bind us internationally and some aspects that set the parameters of our practice within the UK.

The International Council of Nurses (ICN) first provided a definition of the first level nurse (known as a registered or professional nurse) in 1969. This definition was revised in 1975.

> A nurse is a person who has completed a program of basic nursing education and is qualified and authorised in his/her country to practise nursing. Basic nursing education is a formally recognised program of study which provides a broad and sound founda-tion for the practice of nursing and for the post-basic education which develops specific competency. At the first level, the educational program prepares the nurse, through study of behavioural, life and nursing sciences and clinical experience, for effective practice and direction of nursing care and the leadership role. The first level nurse is responsible for planning, providing, and evaluating care in all settings for the promotion of health, prevention of illness, care of the sick and rehabilitation; and functions as a member of the health care team (p. 1).

This definition addresses the issues of how the nurse should be educated, what an educational programme should address and the responsibilities of the first level nurse. It expressly describes the nurse as a team member expected to plan, provide and evaluate care, but does not specifically address the question of what care is. This definition also addresses the duties, obligations and rights which nurses have.

An aspect of the UK Nursing and Midwifery Council (NMC) 'Code of Conduct' (UKCC 1992) that might be termed political is that they present a picture of what a nurse is, or should be. Payne (1988:174) says that the United Kingdom Central Council for Nursing, Midwifery and Health Visiting (UKCC) (The Nursing and Midwifery Council was established in April 2002) code of conduct points out 'the importance of particular patterns of thought, attitudes and forms of behaviour'. This code begins with a statement that:

> Each registered nurse, midwife and health visitor shall act at all times in such a manner as to justify public trust and confidence, to uphold and enhance the good standing and reputation of the profession, to serve the interests of society, and above all to safeguard the interest of individual patients and clients.
>
> UKCC (1992)

The UKCC code states that each practitioner is accountable for his or her practice. Payne (1988:174) argues that one of the features of the UKCC Code of Conduct is that it is an extended definition of professional accountability.

The most popular and most frequently reproduced definition of the nursing role is that developed by Virginia Henderson for the ICN in 1966. It is of particular value to nurses and nursing as it explicitly defines the unique function of the nurse both in relation to the patient and to other members of the health care team. It also provides an understanding of the nature of nursing care.

> The unique function of the nurse is to assist the individual, sick or well, in the performance of those activities contributing to health or its recovery (or to a peaceful death) that he [sic] would perform unaided if he had the necessary strength, will or knowledge. And to do this in such a way as to help him gain independence as rapidly as possible. This aspect of her [sic] work, this part of her function, she initiates and controls; of this she is master. In addition she helps the patient carry out the therapeutic plan as initiated by the physician. She also, as a member of a medical team, helps other members, as they in turn help her, to plan and carry out the total program whether it be for the improvement of health, or the recovery from illness or support in death.
>
> Henderson (1966:4)

So we know we have an international agreement that nurses assist individuals *sick and well*, that the areas in which we provide assistance are those the person would usually do for themselves if they had the necessary *strength, will or knowledge*. We have responsibilities in *health education* and in *doing for* the person those things that cannot be done by the person unaided. We work with the person in *health*, towards *recovery* and also, where inevitable, toward *a peaceful death*. In these aspects of care we act with authority and autonomy.

Explicit in Virginia Henderson's definition are the autonomous functions of the nurse as well as those delegated responsibilities initiated by the doctor but co-ordinated in action between the patient and the nurse, for example: intravenous therapy, medications and dressings. As we will see later in this chapter, there is not always harmony between the demands of the delegated medical responsibility, the clinical judgement of the nurse in the areas of autonomy and the caring or healing aspects of nursing practice.

REGULATING PRACTICE

Regulation of practice and registration of practitioners, whilst now taken for granted, has not been an uncontested issue. Those in favour of regulation and registration have seen its importance in both professional terms of enhancing the status of the profession and controlling conditions and payment for work, and in patient advocacy terms in providing standards for practice that safeguard the public. Those opposed to registration saw concern for the character, management and education of the nurse and the organisation of health care delivery as more important than professional status, and did not see these as being able to be controlled by a process of registration. Perhaps the most famous of the debates on registration took place in the 1890s between Florence Nightingale and Mrs Bedford-Fenwick, who was supported by the British Medical Association. Mrs Bedford-Fenwick was matron of St Bartholomew's Hospital, London and the editor of the *British Journal of Nursing* and fought a 20-year campaign for registration (see Wicks 1999:63 for discussion of this historic battle). The battle for registration in Britain culminated in the Nurses Registration Act of 1919.

In April 2002, the Nursing and Midwifery Council replaced the UKCC and the four National Boards, taking over both the maintenance of the registers of nurses, midwives and health visitors, and also the role of prescribing standards for education and fitness to practice. Its key objectives are to:

- treat the health and welfare of patients as paramount;
- collaborate and consult with key stakeholders;
- be open and proactive in accounting to the public and the professions for its work as well as reforming the regulatory structure and having 'explicit powers to link registration with evidence of continuing professional development'. The regulation of nursing as a profession has now progressed on from merely protecting the public against quacks and dangerous practitioners, to a position where registration is explicitly linked with constant improvement through lifelong learning.

LOYALTY AND OBEDIENCE

Before the late nineteenth century, nursing was closely allied with religion and religious orders so its practitioners followed the ethics developed within these religious contexts. With the social change accompanying industrialisation in England, nursing began to be practised by untrained and socially marginal individuals. Florence Nightingale (1820–1910), the founder of modern nursing, became famous for her organisational and training endeavour for nurses during the Crimean War and later, in 1860, opened the Nightingale Nursing School at St Thomas' Hospital, London. In a paper in 1893, she wrote that sick persons must be treated rather than the disease, that prevention is infinitely better than cure, that universal hospitalisation will not give positive health and that nursing must hold to its ideal but must change some of its methods (Bishop & Goldie 1962). Nightingale's concern was primarily with the character and behaviour of the individual nurse rather than a focus on the occupational group or profession. Appropriate nursing behaviour, she believed, would be achieved through education and role modelling. This understanding was embodied in the Nightingale pledge, which addressed the moral obligations nurses owed their patients and colleagues which countless nurses around the world have taken:

> I solemnly pledge myself before God and in the presence of this assembly to pass my life in purity and to practise my profession faithfully. I will abstain from what is deleterious and mischievous, and will not take or knowingly administer any harmful drug. I will do all in my power to elevate the standard of my profession, and will hold in confidence all personal matters committed to my keeping, and all family affairs coming to my knowl-edge in the practice of my calling. With loyalty will I endeavour to aid the physician in his work, and devote myself to the welfare of those committed to my care.

In the early twentieth century, a key goal was therefore a virtuous and obedient nurse. The need to follow the wishes of others was given priority over autonomous think-ing (Allmark 1995; Andrews & Hutchinson 1981; Fromer 1980; Johnston 1980; Vito 1983). Today the emphasis is on nurses' personal and professional moral autonomy (Benoliel 1983; Callery 1990; Cartwright *et al.* 1992; Cassells & Redman 1989; Hussey 1990; Johnston 1980; Kendrick 1994; Quinn 1990; Sellman 1996). Autonomy refers to accountability and responsibility in one's action (Callery 1990; Cartwright *et al.* 1992; Cassells & Redman 1989; Davis & Slater 1988; Fry 1989; Gaul 1989; Kendrick 1994; Quinn 1990; Thompson & Thompson 1989). Education should motivate students' moral autonomy (Hussey 1990). It should stimulate critical thinking and avoid both dogmatic value systems and ethical relativism (Johnston 1980).

As the government observed in *Making a Difference* (DoH 1999) public expec-tations have also changed. Users and carers expect to be actively involved in col-laborative decision making, rather than being passive recipients of care. Many are well-informed, and sometimes misinformed, by the wealth of health and treatment information available from the internet. The nurse's role as advocate, assisting users and carers to exercise their autonomy, becomes both more important and more technically difficult in such a context. Since 1999 there has been a number of other initiatives from the Department of Health (DoH) that aim to bring about very signifi-cant changes in the way the health service is managed and its integral linking with the social services provision (e.g. *Shifting The Balance*, DoH 2001). A significant part of this is the shift of purchasing power away from Health Authorities to primary care and therefore developing the localisation of decision making. The aim is to put users and carers at the centre of service delivery.

CODES OF CONDUCT AND CODES OF ETHICS: FLOORS OR CEILINGS?

A code spells out a commitment to a set of ideals. Insofar as they are open to revi-sion, they also provide the opportunity for signalling changes in policy (Hull 1981). The first code of nursing ethics was produced in Liberia in 1949 (Sawyer 1989). In 1950 the American Nurses Association published its first code; it was subsequently amended in 1976 and guidelines were issued to supplement it in 1980. The Inter-national Council of Nurses (ICN) published its first 'International Code of Nursing Ethics' in 1953, and amended it in 1965 and 1973. In 1973, clause 7, which required loyalty and obedience to the doctor, was deleted from the ICN Code at the instigation of a group of Canadian nursing students (Johnstone 1994). The American Nurses Association followed suit in 1976, replacing the requirement of loyalty to the doctor in its Code with loyalty to the patient. In theory, one would imagine that this would have solved the dual dilemma for nurses, as their sole duty (that to the patient) was now clear. One would imagine that finally, nurses would be clear about what they had to do. However, disciplinary and legal practices have demonstrated that this shift in allegiance has not been conveyed to the medical profession, the managers of health care or, indeed, the judiciary (Chiarella 1999).

In defining the nature of nursing the codes perform the function of distinguishing nursing from medical ethics. First, as Bandman and Bandman (1985) point out, a code reminds nurses and others of the status and importance of nursing in health care. Further, nursing is portrayed as having specific goals and values that may or may not coincide with those of the medical profession. When they do not, there is the possibility of conflict. The potential for conflict has been one of the grounds for criticism of codes for nurses. This problem can only be made worse, Hull (1980) argues, if groups in addition to doctors and nurses, such as pharmacists and physiotherapists, also have codes of conduct. Can it really be claimed that their existence is in the best interest of users and carers? This worry is lessened, however, if codes are seen, not as prescribing how individual members of the profession will behave, but as communicating the goals of the profession. The former UKCC (since April 2002 the NMC) developed its Code of Conduct for Nurses, Midwives and Health Visitors in 1983, and several sets of guidelines have been issued to assist in its implementation and comprehension. This UKCC Code was the first to describe itself as a code of conduct, rather than a code of ethics, although some codes did not declare themselves as either. Previously it was sometimes difficult to ascertain the intent of a code and its status – whether it was to be used as a 'ceiling' standard, or a 'floor', setting out the minimum standard for practice (Chiarella 1995).

Clearly, one function of codes is to uphold standards of competence 'even if the word competence is not specifically used in the code' (Klaidman & Beauchamp 1987) but they do more than that. In the UK, the code of conduct was a response to section 2(5) of the Nurses, Midwives and Health Visitors Act (1979), which states that the former UKCC and now the NMC should establish and improve standards of training and professional conduct. Thus, the law gave the council the power to determine what goes into the code of conduct, the contents of which may demand more of a nurse than conformity with the law of the land. Payne (1988:174), a professional officer of the UKCC, made it very clear that the UK code was designed, not only to provide advice to the profession 'on standards of professional conduct', but also to provide 'a backcloth against which allegations of professional misconduct can be judged'. A nurse may lose registration status as a result of a violation of the code of conduct, so we may see that it is not simply a guide, nor merely a political document, but also a means of regulating the profession.

STANDARDS AND QUALITY CONTROL IN THE UK

A code may be read by members of the public, whether or not they are patients. It may provide a means of reassuring them about quality control (Rumbold 1986) or of enhancing the public image of the nurse. In this function its role appears to be political.

Reg Payne describes the UKCC code of conduct as 'unashamedly political', in that it is a weapon which can be used by nurses to fight for improvements in standards. He suggests:

> the contents of this code quite deliberately challenge practitioners to become people who challenge. It challenges us to expose risk to patients, where such exists. It challenges us to make demands so that patients and clients receive the standards of care they both need and deserve. It challenges us, if necessary, to adopt a stance which might put us in conflict with people in authority.
>
> Payne (1988:174)

The above statement makes it quite clear that the code of conduct is designed to result in action, action that might sometimes be difficult for a nurse to take. It is not designed to be just a piece of window dressing for the purpose of reassuring the public. According to Swider *et al.* (1984) it is unclear how nurses respond to, and make decisions concerning ethical dilemmas, because of conflicting loyalties in bureaucratic health care environments. The code itself, however, requires positive action to report circumstances in which standards or safety may be compromised. Further guidance in *Guidelines for Professional Practice* (UKCC 1996) makes explicit the possible conflict between a professional obligation to speak out and a possible fear of losing one's job, emphasising the priority of professionalism. Furthermore, the significance of an orientation to professional values and ethics as objects of more serious study is very much heightened by the new problems of social ethics. The recognition of ethical problems requires that students engage in mentored practice in critical thinking and ethical decision making (Gold *et al.* 1995). Society has the right to require that nurses be educated people who can place health in its proper relationship to culture.

A CAREER FRAMEWORK

Since 1997, there have been numerous reports and directives from the government in the UK that steer the health and social care professions into new ways of working and therefore influence the educational programmes that support them. A new modern career framework (DoH 1999) has been developed by the government, NHS unions and professional organisations, which, when implemented, will allow career progress through four broadly flexible ranges (or stages). Progression is linked to responsibilities and the competencies needed for the job. A nurse's career can then move through the four stages:

(1) Health Care Assistant (HCA) and Nursing Cadets;
(2) Registered Practitioner;
(3) Senior Registered Practitioner;
(4) Consultant Practitioner.

The typical educational levels for each range would be that HCA and cadets would have completed National Vocational Qualifications (NVQ) levels 1, 2 or 3. The registered practitioner would have a higher education diploma or first level degree, hold professional registration and in some cases they would have specialist-specific professional qualifications. The senior registered practitioner would have a first or master's degree, hold professional registration and in many cased additional specific professional qualifications. The consultant practitioner would have a master's or doctorate degree, hold professional registration and additional specialist-specific professional qualifications recognised as a 'higher level of practice'. This framework provides an indication of the direction in which your career could move, however it does not illustrate the great diversity of posts and practice areas available to you during a career in nursing. It also permits those who undertake nursing activities, but are not registered nurses, i.e. health care assistants, to be part of and progress up the nursing career ladder.

Nursing's contribution to the health and the health care of society is yet to be fully realised. In 1860 Nightingale felt drawn to write:

> No system can endure that does not march, are we walking to the future or to the past? Are we progressing or are we stereotyping? We remember that we have scarcely crossed the threshold of uncivilised civilisation in nursing: there is still so much to do. Don't let us stereotype mediocrity. We are still on the threshold of nursing. In the future which I shall not see, for I am old, may a better way be opened! May the methods by which every infant, every human being will have the best chance of health, the methods by which every sick person will have the best chance of recovery, be learned and practised; hospitals are only an intermediate state of civilisation never intended, at all events, to take in the whole sick population.
>
> Nightingale (cited in Staunton 1997:7)

Nightingale's words have never been more relevant. With international trends in health care to decrease number of inpatient days for acutely ill people, the ageing of our society, and the differentiation of health status in our own and other countries between dominant culture and the indigenous peoples, nursing has major practice development, research, political and policy roles to play (White 1995). Many recent government initiatives have indicated very clearly that whilst there is a desire to put resources into areas of greatest need, this must be matched by local communities becoming involved in the decision-making processes in support of their local environment. There is therefore a need to rekindle the ideology of 'citizenship' where commitment, authority and responsibility come together, each member of the community playing its part for the greater good of that community. It is in this changing social context that we are now preparing the nurses of the future. There is a need for nurses to be competent, being an equal team member in developing and delivering contemporary health care; they also need to be politically aware of the social context in which they live and work and become involved in the wide aspects of their local community.

CONCLUSION

So you want to be a nurse? Well, you can look forward to joining a profession which now has well-defined competencies from entry to practice to advanced career opportunities as a nurse consultant. You can move laterally between clinical practice, research and education. To be a registered nurse you will follow either a 3-year or 4-year bachelor's degree or a 3-year diploma course at a university. For the Health Care Assistant (HCA) or Nursing Cadet, you will acquire National Vocational Qualifications and have the opportunity to progress to registration. You will have the opportunity to be well educated as a person and a nurse. You can work with people of all ages and in all kinds of settings, within well-defined parameters of both aspirational codes of conduct and minimum standards of acceptable practice. You will belong to an international professional community and can readily travel and practise within it. You can continue to study and specialise in any number of general or discrete areas. Most importantly, you can contribute to Nightingale's dream of having nursing fully engaged in providing health and illness services to all that need them. You can make a difference.

Wherever you work the connectedness you will feel with patients, friends, fellow nurses and other members of the health team will sustain you in the kaleidoscope of practice – those moments dramatic, poignant and mundane (Benner 1984). What a great choice! Good luck!

REFLECTIVE QUESTIONS

(1) Consider the definitions of the 'role of the nurse'. Do you agree with them? Is there anything lacking? How would you define the role of the nurse?
(2) In what way might the context in which the nurse works affect her or his practice? These contexts could include, for example, specialty area, geographic location, historical period.
(3) In what way do you imagine nursing practice changing in the next decade, and what may influence these changes?

RECOMMENDED READING

Benner, P. (1984) *From Novice to Expert: Excellence and Power in Clinical Nursing Practice.* Addison Wesley, Menlo Park.

Benner, P. & Wrubel, J. (1989) *The Primacy of Caring: Stress and Coping in Health and Illness.* Addison Wesley, Menlo Park.

Lawler, J. (1991) *Behind the Screens: Nursing, Somology and the Problem of the Body.* Churchill Livingstone, Melbourne.

Taylor, B. (1994) *Being Human: Ordinariness in Nursing.* Churchill Livingstone, Melbourne.

Wicks, D. (1999) *Nurses and Doctors at Work: Rethinking Professional Boundaries.* Allen & Unwin, Sydney.

REFERENCES

Allmark, P. (1995) Uncertainties in the teaching of ethics to students of nursing. *Journal of Advanced Nursing*, **22**, 374–378.

Andrews, S. & Hutchinson, S. (1981) Teaching nursing ethics: A practical approach. *Journal of Nursing Education*, **20**(1), 6–11.

Bandman, E.L. & Bandman, B. (1985) *Nursing Ethics in the Life Span*. Appleton, Century, Crofts, Norwalk, Connecticut.

Benner, P. (1984) *From Novice to Expert: Excellence and Power in Clinical Nursing Practice*. Addison Wesley, Menlo Park, California.

Benoliel, J. (1983) Ethics in nursing practice and education. *Nursing Outlook*, **31**(4), 210–215.

Bishop, N.J. & Goldie, S. (1962) *A Bio-bibliography of Florence Nightingale*. International Council of Nurses, London.

Callery, P. (1990) Moral learning in nursing education: A discussion of the usefulness of cognitive-developmental and social learning theories. *Journal of Advanced Nursing*, **15**, 324–328.

Cartwright, T., Davson-Galle, P. & Holden, R. (1992) Moral philosophy and nursing curricula: Indoctrination of the new breed. *Journal of Nursing Education*, **31**(5), 225–228.

Cassells, J. & Redman, B. (1989) Preparing students to be moral agents in clinical nursing practice: Report on a national study. *Nursing Clinics of North America*, **24**(2), 463–473.

Chiarella, M. (1995) Regulating mechanisms and standards: nurses' friends or foes? In: *Issues in Australian Nursing IV* (eds G. Gray & R. Pratt), pp. 61–74. Churchill Livingstone, London.

Chiarella, M. (1999) *The status of the registered nurse in law, society and scholarship*. Unpublished PhD Thesis, University of NSW.

Davis, A. & Slater, P. (1988) Ethics in nursing: implications for education and practice. *The Australian Nurses Journal*, **17**(8), 18–20.

Department of Health (1999) *Making a Difference*. Department of Health, London.

Department of Health (2001) *Shifting the Balance*. Department of Health, London.

European Commission (1997) Advisory committee on training in nursing. *Document XV/E/9432/7/96*. European Comission.

Fromer, M. (1980) Teaching ethics by case analysis. *Nursing Outlook*, **October**, 604–609.

Fry, S. (1989) Teaching ethics in nursing curricula. Traditional and contemporary models. *Nursing Clinics of North America*, **24**(2), 485–497.

Gaul, A. (1989) Ethics content in baccalaureate degree curricula. *Nursing Clinics of North America*, **24**(2), 475–483.

Gold, C., Chambers, J. & Dvorak, E. (1995) Ethical dilemmas in the lived experience of nursing practice. *Nursing Ethics*, **2**(2), 131–141.

Henderson, V. (1966) *The Nature of Nursing*. Collier Macmillan, London.

Hull, R.T. (1980) Codes or no codes. *Kansas Nurse*, **55**(10), 8, 18–19, 21.

Hull, R.T. (1981) The function of professional codes of ethics. *Westminster Institute Review*, **1**(3), 12–14.

Hussey, T. (1990) Nursing ethics and project 2000. *Journal of Advanced Nursing*, **15**, 1377–1382.

Johnston, T. (1980) Moral education for nursing. *Nursing Forum*, **19**(3), 284–299.

Johnstone, M.J. (1994) *Nursing and the Injustices of the Law.* WB Saunders/Baillière, Tindall, London.

Kendrick, K. (1994) Building bridges: Teaching ward-based ethics. *Nursing Ethics,* **1**(1), 35–41.

Klaidman, S. & Beauchamp, T.L. (1987) *The Virtuous Journalist.* Oxford University Press, Oxford.

Payne, R. (1988) On being accountable. *Health Visitor,* **61**, 173–175.

Quinn, C. (1990) A conceptual approach to the identification of essential ethics content for the undergraduate nursing curriculum. *Journal of Advanced Nursing,* **15**, 726–731.

Rumbold, G. (1986) *Ethics in Nursing Practice.* Baillière, Tindall, London.

Salvage, J. & Heijnen, S. (eds) (1997) *Nursing in Europe: A Resource for Better Health.* WHO Regional Publications, European Series, No. 74.

Sawyer, L.M. (1989) Nursing code of ethics: An international comparison. *International Nursing Review,* **36**(5), 145.

Sellman, D. (1996) Why teach ethics to nurses? *Nurse Education Today,* **16**, 440–448.

Staunton, P. (1997) Don't let us stereotype mediocrity. Forty fifth annual oration, New South Wales College of Nursing, Sydney, NSWCN.

Swider, S., McElmurry, B. & Yarling, R. (1984) Ethical decision making in a bureaucratic context by senior nursing students. *Nursing Research,* **34**(2), 108–112.

Thompson, J. & Thompson, H. (1989) Teaching ethics to nursing students. *Nursing Outlook,* **37**(2), 84–88.

United Kingdom Central Council for Nursing, Midwifery and Health Visiting (1992) *Code of Conduct.* UKCC, London.

United Kingdom Central Council for Nursing, Midwifery and Health Visiting (1996) *Guidelines for Professional Practice.* UKCC, London.

Vito, K. (1983) Moral development considerations in nursing curricula. *Journal of Nursing Education,* **22**(3), 108–113.

White, J. (1995) Patterns of knowing: review, critique and update. *Advances in Nursing Science,* **17**(4), 73–86.

Wicks, D. (1999) *Nurses and Doctors at Work: Rethinking Professional Boundaries.* Allen & Unwin, London.

2 Milestones in British Nursing

Christopher Maggs

LEARNING OBJECTIVES

Upon completion of this chapter, the reader should be able to:

- see how the historical narrative is highly selective and why this may be useful;
- understand the relationship between the development of modern nursing in the UK and the wider context of social change;
- understand the links between the development of nursing and the changing role of women in society;
- understand the role of reformers in developing the structures we recognise today as making up modern nursing.

KEY WORDS

HISTORY, REFORMERS, STANDARDISATION, NURSE EDUCATION, STATE REGISTRATION, REGULATION.

Facts relating to the past, when they are collected without art, are compilations; and compilations, no doubt, may be useful; but they are no more History than butter, eggs, salt and herbs are an omelette

Strachey (1931)

INTRODUCTION

Historical accounts are, by their nature, selective and owe as much to the author's judgement as to their relative importance. However, it is possible to write a historical account of the modern development of nursing in Britain that does acknowledge individual selectivity but points towards some general understandings that can be shared by many. This chapter sets out to do this by looking at some of the forces for historical change – the role of individuals, the state and the historical epoch – and their impact on the development of 'modern' nursing in Britain. It does not focus on specific aspects of that development, such as the movement of nurse education from hospital control to higher education, although some of these are dealt with as the discussion progresses. By taking this approach, it is hoped that the relevance of historical scholarship and understanding to modern practice might, at least, be hinted at. In so doing, it suggests specific but not exclusive milestones in nursing in Britain.

THE MODERN PERIOD

Any brief encounter with the prolific but generally unsophisticated literature of the history of nursing will show the average reader that there are claims for nursing's ancestry harking back to ancient times – Greek and Roman, if not Persian. Indeed, some historians of nursing, laying claim to the philosophical in nursing, suggest that nursing is a universal – it has always existed because caring for others as a human drive has always existed. It exists (existed?) in all cultures and societies except the base and is a consequence of humanness itself. To those who pursue this line, we might ask how they deal with nursing in the age and society of National Socialism or, indeed, more recently, in Rwanda. Since it is not integral to this discussion, we can reasonably leave such questions in the air. What concerns us here is how to date modern nursing.

Even those who posit an ancient tradition accept that nursing is different from doctoring – some label this caring and curing, without seeing the real contribution that the pursuit of true medicine plays in the care of an ill person. This dichotomy arose from a division of labour in illness that was industrial, urban and gendered. Thus, it is a product of a specific set of historical conditions that arose in Western society after the period of the French Revolution and which in the UK have come to be known as the Industrial Revolution.

Industrialisation, the emergence of the factory as the main method for production of goods with an obsession with mechanically structured and unnatural time, together with the understanding and embracing of the creation of wealth through the recreation of money itself, probably lasted for about a hundred years in Britain – the 1800s–1900s – and slightly less in France, Germany and the 'colonies' because of the lessons learnt from the pioneering economy. The potent and portentous symbol of that era – the factory – is mirrored and replicated in the design and processes of the hospital, the school and the prison.

A number of key elements constitute the 'factory' – a new account of time based on the visible clock, shift working, breakdown of complex production into essential elements, which are manufactured by individuals or groups separate from the whole, final product, employment of overseers or others to watch over the majority of workers engaged in the new form of production, and, most importantly, a new form of waged employment.

Importantly, the factory eventually generated a new form of living, the industrial town and city. The growth of existing towns and cities was accompanied by the emergence of new ones or the transformation of older, more rurally linked, ones into industrial centres. Urbanisation and industrialisation created, in turn, overcrowding, poor housing and poor public health. The industrial towns and cities became synonymous with disease, ill health and accidents.

Existing facilities for dealing with these exponentially increasing health problems were woefully inadequate and outmoded. Much 'ill-health' provision was based in neighbourhoods and met by a small number of medical men and sick nurses and midwives. Few hospitals with more than 10 beds existed and, of the few that did, the organisation of care and the practice of medicine lagged behind need.

The modern hospital was the reaction to these several, intertwined problems. The hospital provided in- and outpatient services, allowed medical education to develop and improve practice and enabled the embryonic hospital management system to start putting care on a formal, process-led basis.

Into these institutions came nursing, taking advantage of the opportunities to develop its own knowledge and skills base and of providing a growing workforce of female workers. It became a matter of some civic pride that every town and city had its 'infirmary' and even the Poor Law authorities began to invest in similar provision for the destitute.

The hospital, then, at least as it appears from the mid-nineteenth century onwards, marks an important milestone in the development of nursing. Even though domiciliary based nursing continued, provided for by charities and local authorities, especially in London and the great northern cities, the hospitals came to dominate the world of medicine. And the hospitals were a direct result of the fallout from processes of urbanisation and industrialisation. The number of general hospital beds grew from around 4000 in 1801 to over 28000 by the end of the century.

In 1861, the census recorded about 1000 nurses. By 1901, there were about 70000 nurses, of whom about 10% worked in hospitals of one kind or another. The majority of these nurses were 'new' – they had some sort of training, were paid annual salaries as employees rather than by the day or case.

It is of no great note to realise that 'nightingaleism' took place primarily and most effectively in the hospitals of the late nineteenth and early twentieth centuries. Nor that its core was not developments in the care of the sick but again primarily the organisation of the hospital as an institution. Perhaps the contribution that nightingaleism left to the profession was its over-keen sense of policing the nurse and the patient. It certainly led to the dominance of the hospital system of nursing, nurse education and nurse behaviours over other nursing systems such as domiciliary and Poor Law work.

WOMEN'S WORK AND THE DIVISION OF LABOUR

The second of our milestones recognises the characteristics of the nursing workforce and the consequences for the nature of nursing work in the historical period. Nursing is an occupation for women and is gendered – that is, it espouses values and systems associated with 'woman', which are constructed rather than biologically determined.

The proportion of women who were both single and within the economically active years of 20–34 rose over the nineteenth century at a higher rate than it did for men. More importantly, the proportion of men who did not marry, delayed the age of marriage or emigrated to the empire or the new world rose (Neff 1929). Consequently, more women were looking for paid employment than ever before and, especially, for paid work which did not carry the stigma of the factory. The new industries – commerce and the public services – were able to expand at relatively less cost than might have been the case because these 'surplus women' were available for employment.

It was from this pool of labour that the new nurses came. Few were from the middle classes, despite the rhetoric. Most came from families of the respectable, upper end of the working class, with fathers who were as likely to be foremen, clerks, shopkeepers and middling Irish tenant farmers. Many had some prior experience of employment, were educated to the leaving certificate standards of the day and were deliberating choosing nursing as a career. They came with the added advantage that they usually had no idea of the pre-industrial and often pre-urban world and hence shared none of its values that were seen as obstacles to the new order of work.

The cities and towns of the new industrialised nation acted as magnets for these women (and men) in search of new work opportunities. The more 'enlightened' hospitals recognised the fears of the migrant and their families and provided a safe environment, with nurses' homes, strict discipline and barriers between the nurses and the local environment.

Irrespective of the differences between medicine and nursing practice, the core distinction within the hospital was that between men and women. Within the hospitals, the division of labour based on contemporary male and female roles was seen in its most exaggerated form. Conventionally, the home, as the unit of social cohesion, held separate spheres for men and women. Man, the head of the household in law, economically and *de facto*, woman the helpmeet, wife/mother and companion. In the hospital, the man was the doctor and the woman the nurse. However, they were not 'married' to each other, although usually the doctor was a married man whilst the nurse was specifically prohibited from marriage if she wished to continue to work as a hospital nurse. Nightingale is said to have said, 'No woman can serve two hearths'; what she did write (with an untypical(?) disregard for the rules of evidence) was that '*married women (are) no longer attached to (their) work but to their husbands, and their patients are, more or less, neglected* (Seymer, cited in Baly 1986). Thus, an exact replication of the 'family' unit and its relationships could not exist within the hospital, so a distorted version emerged. That distortion or aberration sowed the seeds for a century (and more) of struggles around the boundaries of interprofessional rivalries (Gamarnikow 1978).

In contrast to the conventional family, the hospital and its wards were staffed by the unmarried and the widowed. The relationships between the female nurse and the medical man had to mimic not the husband/wife roles but the husband and unmarried female relatives' roles, with the arbiter role normally fulfilled by the supportive wife distorted into the inverted role of the matron.

In practical matters, doctors and nurses did different things that reflected the power relationships effected by gender and class as well as access to higher education and the professions. The training syllabuses for nursing made great pains to elaborate cleanliness as the science of hygiene, so that nursing could claim a scientific basis, like medicine. They also emphasised deference to authority, the male authority of the doctors and the hospital administrators, but also the devolved authority of the matron and the ward sister.

EDUCATION AND REGULATION

Interviewed by the matron, one prospective early twentieth-century probationer (student) nurse was surprised at the questions she was asked. Rather than being asked about her schooling, her standard of reading or her motive for wanting to become a nurse, the matron began a conversation about art and painting and music. This anecdote tells us much about nurse education and training. First, as we have noted, women were already educated to a good standard as a result of state inter-vention. Second, motive was assumed and not questioned. Third, the training of the nurse was not very challenging and hardly worth exploring at interview. It was more relevant to discover if the candidate had the mental or emotional capacity to fit in, to fit in with the enclosed world of the hospital and the nurses' home.

Forty years before, the matron of one of the largest 'new' provincial city infirmaries (Manchester) had her nurse training syllabus rejected by the hospital management board for failing to include sufficient anatomy and physiology, according to the medi-cal men on the board.

For much of the nineteenth and twentieth centuries, each training hospital had its own syllabus, although training institutions in the Poor Law (State sector) were work-ing hard at a common programme. And the length of the training varied between hospitals, from 2 to 4 years. Standardisation was anathema to contemporaries more concerned with emphasising the uniqueness of the individual institution rather than any common characteristics, in part to shore up their failing financial status as inde-pendents. Except, that is, in the twin respects of cleanliness and discipline where it became almost a matter of pride to establish the best hospitals for these qualities.

National attempts to influence the development of the syllabus through, for exam-ple, the burgeoning nursing press, met with little success. One reason, of course, is that the press was owned or controlled by a few energetic and polemical individuals like Ethel Manson (Mrs Fenwick). Individual matrons (*pace* the Manchester example, above) maintained control and stamped their values on training. Some movement be-came possible with the formation of groups such as the College (later Royal College) of Nursing and the Matrons' Council and with the sharing of experiences through international conferences attended by leading lights in the profession.

The idea of state intervention was hardly contemplated, although within the Greater London County Council area, local government did standardise to an extent. It may have been a consequence of the animosity between central government and local government, especially the monolithic Great London Council, which prompted the state eventually to intervene in nursing affairs after World War I.

Similarly, attempts to regulate nursing, to set down standards of entry to the profes-sion and to define the trained nurse met with firm resistance. The opening skirmishes of what became a war lasting over 40 years (1880–1920) were fought out between registrationists like Manson, antiregistrationists like Nightingale and Luckes, and regulationists like Burdett.

Registrationists, looking to medicine as a lead, wanted the state to back by statute standards of entry, training programmes and a register of nurses. They argued that this would protect the public, ensure that nursing developed as a discipline and would prevent untrained women from competing with trained nurses for work. The state was crucial because they wanted this to be regulated by statute rather than by consensus within the profession. A model for their campaign was State Registration of Midwives (1902).

Antiregistrationists rejected the involvement of the state in such matters as a mat-ter of course, in keeping with one side of contemporary politics. Acknowledging the right of the public to be protected from unsavoury or untrained characters, they argued that this would best be served by increasing the reputations of the best hos-pitals – and hence their nurses – through improving the practice of medicine.

Complicating matters were those who wished for some form of registration but not regulation, a public register which still permitted individual hospitals to maintain their individual status in the eyes of the public and the professions. Burdett, the principal but not only advocate of this line, wanted nurses to voluntarily register with an independent 'organisation', stating their training hospital. This could then be consulted by potential employers, whether an individual or another hospital. Burdett's case was somewhat hampered by suspicions about his motive – he had started a register of nurses using his pension fund scheme – and his bitter public and private rows with Ethel Manson, the arch pro-state registrationist.

The battles that followed were fought in the nursing, medical and national press and in both Houses of Parliament. Claim and counter-claims were made by all sides; appeals to the enlightened Nordic countries and to New Zealand, which had not only introduced a system of registration and regulation but were also further on towards female emancipation, and scaremongering abounded.

One reason for the long dispute was, as noted, a reluctance to support state interference in the economy in general and the failure of both sides to outflank their opponents' political supporters. Another was the almost total irrelevance of the struggle to the generality, concerned with imperial wars in Africa and looming conflict with Germanic expansion. Unlike the Crimean War, the Boer War did not highlight apparent deficiencies in caring for the wounded (civilians, especially in the concentration camps did not seem to matter). There was no scandal, no press revelations to force the government to look to reforms in nursing as a way out of another mess. Nor was there any charismatic character like Nightingale to galvanise public support, albeit at second hand through the war reporter.

The dispute also dragged on because there was little overt grassroots professional support either way – or at least, a clear split between two competing views. Whilst many rank and file nurses joined pressure groups in favour of registration, the protagonists failed to sell their case to the ordinary nurse and what it might actually mean to her. Registration would not rid the profession of the marriage bar or the tedium of daily work. It would not help recruitment or retention, problems not openly discussed but there below the surface as the economic prospects for women as workers improved. Such changes would come about only as part of a broader and more radical shift in the position of women in society and that had to wait for the end of World War I, the depression of the thirties and the effects of the women's movement.

Exasperated and faced with the wider demands to reward women, specifically VADs (women with a very short nurse training used to support the medical services for the armed services) in 1918 for their 'war work', government reluctantly caved in and passed the Nurses' Registration Act (1919). It was to be some years, however, before the General Nursing Council (GNC) was able to effect some degree of standardisation in the length of training, the syllabus and the kinds of institutions recognised for training. Since then, numerous reports, recommendations and reviews have been undertaken internally and externally to try to sort out the mess created by the Act and the GNC, perhaps still with little evidence of cohesion (see the recent 2000/2001 disputes about the title of the new Nursing and Midwifery Council to replace the UKCC).

PHILANTHROPISTS AND REFORMERS

Shown the awful conditions under which prisoners were kept in the prison hulks of Portsmouth and Chatham, Elizabeth Fry's Quaker conscience spurred her to campaign for reform. She and others found that it was not just prisoners who were treated with material and spiritual contempt; patients in the few hospitals of the early decades of the nineteenth century fared little better in what was a medical lottery or experiment.

Later, Dickens wrote of the casualties of industrialisation and urbanisation and the incomprehension of endemic contagious disease. In *Hard Times*, he attacked materialism and rationalism; in *Martin Chuzzlewit*, rationalism and medicine. Even later, Charles Booth, in the process of arguing for 'penal colonies' for the indigenous poor, suggested social opprobrium for those who were ill by self-neglect. The middle classes, supported by the wealth of the railways, decided quite correctly to live on the high ground above Swindon, one of the railway capitals of the mid century. They left the smallpox-ridden level, lower ground to the railway workers and their poorer families, allowing their drains to empty into the marshy ground around the station and its goods yards.

By the late nineteenth century, individual conscience and philanthropy had lost their way and their impact. The rawness of the touched sensibilities of the Victorians, faced with the evident success of capitalism but also its social consequences of poverty, disease and ignorance, resulted in organisations rather than campaigns, with the success of the Royal Society for the Prevention of Cruelty to Animals predating that for children. Philanthropy gave way to charity, conscience to co-ordination and efficiency.

Campaigns about disease and ill-health moved from the single cause politics, some of which had been very successful like the smallpox vaccination campaign, into the new phase of a co-ordinated attack on inefficiency and waste. Nursing and midwifery came under the spotlight as part of a wider concern with the consequences of the new industrial age. Those working to change nursing and midwifery were also involved in many other social issues, from prisons to housing for the working classes. They were thus able to enlist stronger support for their cause than the single-issue campaigners and were more likely of success.

For Burdett, reform of nursing was only part of his lifelong campaign against inefficiency. For him, the hospital was an unmanaged, wasteful institution that required reform in all its branches. He fought hard to develop the role and impact of the hospital administrator, putting them on a more formal and 'trained' basis. He was responsible for introducing a system of hospital accounting that could be used to root out inefficiencies.

One such inefficiency was nursing, particularly in the larger hospitals of London, Manchester, Leeds and Liverpool. He visited or was in contact with almost every hospital, large or small, across the country, collecting data on numbers of beds, length of stay, mortality and, of course, the numbers and conditions of employment of nurses. Published in his own journal, *The Hospital*, such figures could easily force individual hospital management boards to look to improve things; if they did not, there was a strong possibility that their income from subscriptions and from donations might fall. For many nurses, the drive for efficiency found itself expressed in the very work they did, where they were required to save on bandages and even on uneaten food in order to reduce costs. The drive to efficiency also gave legitimate authority to the matron and her assistants in all that they did connected with the nurses' lives.

It was not only the voluntary hospitals that came under scrutiny in this war on waste. The Poor Law authorities, local government bodies, were also driven to identify and eradicate waste in the interests of keeping the lid on spiralling local rates (taxes). Slow at first to open hospitals, eventually most local authorities had their own institution. Whilst training, to a large extent, their own workforce including nurses, they tried to import the 'discipline' of the voluntary sector through the employment of head nurses and matrons who had been trained in the larger voluntary hospitals. Trained nurses went from voluntary hospital to the Poor Law, not the other way round. Hence, the insidious promulgation of the values of the voluntary hospitals and their nursing systems permeated the hospital world, all in the interests of efficiency.

The state and the art of war

Social change in Britain is linked inexorably to war. As an example, the real shortage of fit men after so many had died in World War I to return to the old and new industries meant that, irrespective of any campaign to have women accepted as workers, women continued to find employment in almost all of the nonprofessional occupations. The sudden demobilisation of thousands of women who had trained (albeit usually for less than 6 months) and served in one or other of the emergency nursing organisations (the VADs, for example) and of whom many wished to continue to work as nurses caused panic among some nurse reformers. These women threatened to overturn the campaign to have nursing regulated as a profession with minimum entry requirements but a defined length of training of at least 3 years.

Pressure on government increased and, as we have noted, with reluctance a system of state registration was introduced. This did not have the immediate impact reformers had hoped for; they, anyway, were still divided about the way forward following the Act. Indeed, women continued to work as nurses without being entered on the register for almost a decade, until they disappeared by the slow attrition of retirement, death or leaving the profession.

It took World War I and the rise to real power of the Labour Party to bring about the socialisation of health care in Britain. With wartime experience of centralised control over hospitals and nursing, the state was able to construct a case for a single National Health Service for all as one of its four planks to combat social distress. In the face of fierce opposition, mainly but not exclusively from branches of the medical profession, the NHS came into being in 1947.

The GNC, the regulatory body for nursing, was one of several attempts over the following 50 years to organise the registration and regulation of entry to the nursing, midwifery and health-visiting professions. The latest in the long line of such bodies came into force in 2002, its own birth covered once again in controversy as the health-visiting profession fights to maintain its profile and role. Nurse education had had some presence in the universities, notably Manchester and Edinburgh, but it took almost as long for nurse education to be fully integrated into the higher education sector. Nurse education is still two-tiered in that some students follow a diploma programme whilst others the full 3-year honours degree mode. With no legal difference in professional status between the two, a possible explanation for this dichotomy might rest in the type of candidates and their educational achievements coming forward for training.

CONCLUSION

Britain makes strong claims for having the first universal National Health Service, free at the point of need. This has been a long time coming and, today, radical changes and alternatives to it are openly discussed. Nursing forms the core of that service, as it has for its predecessors – the voluntary and Poor Law medical services. Reforms in nursing have been painful and sometimes painfully slow to arrive. University education for nurses was, for example, an early (but quietly dropped) part of Ethel Manson's campaigns. Many have been watered down as compromises were sought in order for essential reforms to be put in place.

In this paper, a number of key factors in historical change have been touched on in order to provide an overview of some of the ways nursing has changed in the modern period. In order to understand that period in nursing's past, we must be aware of the key agents and agencies for change. Here, we have looked at the role of the state, the impact of reformers and the more general impact of the social context in which nursing sits. There can be no definite picture to emerge from such studies; we put into the mixing bowl our experiences and views and priorities. What emerges is one version of the milestones in the development of nursing in Britain in the modern period; if another person were mixing the omelette, perhaps another version would be found.

REFLECTIVE QUESTIONS

- With reference to the development of nursing in the modern period in Britain, how would you describe the historian's task?
- What relationships are there between the role of women in British society and the development of nursing?
- How did war impact on health care and the role of the nurse?
- Did the conflict between nursing reformers hold back or drive forward the development of nursing in Britain in the nineteenth and twentieth centuries?
- How would you describe the attitude of the state towards registration of nurses?

RECOMMENDED READING

Baly, M. (1986) *Florence Nightingale and the Nursing Legacy.* Heinemann, London.
Bynum, W.F. & Porter, R. (eds) (1993) *Companion Encyclopedia of the History of Medicine,* 2 Vols. Routledge, London.

Holcombe, L. (1973) *Victorian Ladies at Work.* David & Charles, Newton Abbot.
Smith, F.B. (1979) *The People's Health.* Croom Helm, London.

REFERENCES

Gamarnikow, E. (1978) The sexual division of labour: the case of nursing. In: *Feminism and Materialism* (eds A. Kuhn & A.M. Wolpe). Routledge, London.
Neff, W. (1929) *Victorian Working Women: An Historical and Literary Study of Women in British Industries and Professions 1832–1850.* pp. 11–12.
Seymer, L. (1986) In: *Florence Nightingale and the Nursing Legacy* (ed. M. Baly). Heinemann, London.
Strachey, L. (1931) *Portraits in Miniature and Other Essays.* Chatto & Windus, London.

3 The Art and Science of Nursing

Judith M. Parker

LEARNING OBJECTIVES

Upon completion of this chapter the reader should have gained:

- an understanding of the development of ideas about nursing as an art and a science within a historical context;
- an appreciation of the meaning of the art of nursing within the Florence Nightingale school of thought;
- an appreciation of debates about the art and science of nursing in the US context;
- an appreciation of emerging ideas about art and science and the relationships between them in the current context of health care;
- insight into the implications of these ideas for current nursing education, practice and research.

KEY WORDS

ART, SCIENCE, NURSING, GENDER, AESTHETICS, ENLIGHTENMENT, CONTEMPORARY.

INTRODUCTION

What is nursing? Is nursing an art? Is nursing a science? Is nursing both an art and a science? Is nursing neither an art nor a science? Over the years there has been extensive debate in the nursing literature about the art and science of nursing. Why are questions about the nature of nursing posed in these terms? What is it about how knowledge and practices are understood in our society that invites us to ask these questions about nursing? What are the implications of these perceptions for education, practice and research in nursing?

This chapter seeks to explore some of these questions. It considers some of the history of the development of ideas about modern nursing as an art and a science. More specifically, it examines the division between art and science and explores the impact that this separation has had upon ideas about nursing.

Two particular developments in the history of nursing ideas are discussed, one stemming from the United Kingdom, and the other from the United States. The first, often described as the Florence Nightingale school of thought, represents the first expression of nursing as an art in modern times. In this development, nursing as an art is conceived of in relation to the character of the nurse and the importance of character training in nursing education programmes.

The second is the impact of the development of nursing ideas within the university context of the United States. Of particular note in this discussion are the attempts to construct closed systems of thought through nursing theory development and the production of nursing science. It was in this context that tensions between nursing as an art and as a science began to be recognised and attempts made to reconcile the two.

The chapter then examines some of the implications of these ideas for nursing in the contemporary context where many of the binary divisions that occurred historically, including those between art and science, are collapsing. It concludes with a discussion of the art and science of nursing within the changing environments of health care delivery.

WHAT IS AN ART? WHAT IS A SCIENCE?

Many modern ideas about art and science have their origins in the scientific revolution of the seventeenth and the eighteenth century 'age of reason' that was generated by the philosophical movement known as the French Enlightenment.

The scientific revolution was a quest to understand, control and manipulate nature through rational, empirical means. As Capra pointed out in 1982:

> This development was brought about by revolutionary changes in physics and astronomy, culminating in the achievements of Copernicus, Galileo and Newton. The science of the seventeenth century was based on a new method of inquiry, advocated forcefully by Francis Bacon, which involved the mathematical description of nature and the analytical method of reasoning conceived by the genius of Descartes (p. 54).

The Enlightenment project had the aim of civilising all, of implementing its ideal of social betterment through the power of reason. It was based on beliefs in the universal superiority of the knowledge and values produced by Western science and culture. Those who believed in the democratic ideals of the Enlightenment sought to perfect humankind through reason and create a better world, a civilised and cultured one aided by the new knowledge produced by science (Parker & Gibbs 1998). Two ways of thinking about art can be linked to the Enlightenment, one concerning the cultural production of knowledge and the other the art of living.

A separation of the arts and the sciences occurred in the educational structures and processes that emerged in the wake of the Enlightenment period and with the rise of modern professions. Knowledge came to be packaged into the two domains of the sciences and the arts within university faculties, and a division emerged between those who were educated in the sciences and those who were educated in the arts (humanities). Each of these produced different ways of thinking and acting, and different types of knowledge. According to C.P. Snow (1964), writing of the United Kingdom, scientific training produces 'doers' and training in the arts produces 'thinkers' (intellectuals). He argued that by the 1950s, the science/art professional rift was so deep that the two groups worked completely independently of each other, a trend he saw as potentially dangerous for society.

Another way of thinking about art that emerged out of the Enlightenment concerns the art of living. The search for human perfectibility, which was a major plank of the Enlightenment, became linked to a philosophy of humanism, which, as Nelson (1995) points out, 'stresses the centrality of the human subject and sets freedom as the subject's destiny'. The human subject, however, was deemed to be male, and rationality was understood to be a masculine attribute. The art of living for men was linked to the pursuit of freedom through rationality, as 'doers' and 'thinkers'.

Women were seen as neither free nor rational. They were understood 'as an essential nature defined by purposeful organic functions' (Berriot-Salvadore 1993: 387). Medical discourse defined the feminine ideal in terms of natural determinism as 'the mother, the guardian of virtues and eternal values' (p. 388). Thus while men, defined as human subjects, were separated and freed from the constraints of nature via reason and culture, women, defined in relation to nature and the feminine, were not. Nature and culture merged in this understanding of the feminine, and women were defined in natural and moral terms. Good women exercised their womanly arts and civilised others through the exercise of these arts. By and large, women were excluded from education into the professions.

ART, SCIENCE AND MODERN NURSING

The nature of modern secular professional nursing as it has evolved since the days of Florence Nightingale has been influenced by some of these ideas. Of particular importance to this discussion is how the divisions that occurred between art and science were managed in nursing. These will be considered first in relation to the Florence Nightingale school of thought stemming from Britain and then in relation to university-based nursing in the United States.

The Florence Nightingale school of thought

The Florence Nightingale school of thought developed and was sustained within the nurse training schools that sprang up in hospitals, not only in Britain but also in Australia, New Zealand and other countries. I argue that within nursing education and practice, nursing as an art was seen to involve the character of the nurse in the exercise of feminine virtues, and the importance of character training in the development of nursing as a female profession/occupation. In this context, science was out of place: the scientific enterprise was a male one and, in the hospital and medical context, belonged to the doctor.

Nursing in nineteenth century industrial England was regarded as an inferior, undesirable occupation practised by morally suspect women. In *Martin Chuzzlewit*, Dickens epitomised the nineteenth century English nurse in the character of Sairey Gamp, writing that 'it was difficult to enjoy her company without being conscious of a smell of spirits' (1910:312–13). The contrast of Florence Nightingale's work in the Crimea, and the subsequent publicity, brought about her identification in the public mind as a 'ministering angel' (*The Times*, London, 20 November 1854). This image was instrumental in elevating secular nursing to the status of a female vocation based on Enlightenment ideals of the womanly virtues and the exercise of the womanly arts through the care of the sick. Indeed, Florence Nightingale described nursing as 'the finest of the fine arts' (Donahue 1996).

Enormous effort went into the attempts to position nursing as epitomising feminine ideals of the good woman. Nursing transgressed many prevailing ideas about the role of women in society and it was extremely difficult for nursing to gain acceptance as a legitimate and respectable occupation. Sairey Gamp and the 'bad woman' were never far beneath the surface; it is therefore not surprising that Florence Nightingale and her followers placed so much emphasis upon ensuring appropriate character formation among nurses in training (Parker 1990).

The first Florence Nightingale training school began at St Thomas' Hospital in London in 1860 and became the model for many training schools in Britain and its overseas territories in the latter half of the nineteenth century (Trembath & Hellier 1987). Student nurses were judged on their qualities of trustworthiness, neatness, quietness, sobriety, honesty and truthfulness (Smith 1982). Additionally, nurses were trained to ensure that they did not wish to usurp any of the doctor's functions. Isabella Rathie, the first trained matron of the Melbourne Hospital, noted, 'we are in a great measure the handmaid of the medical man and our function in this particular is to be obedient in every detail' (quoted in Trembath & Hellier 1987:19).

Thus, the division between art and science manifested within modern secular professional nursing of the Nightingale school of thought can be described as a gendered division. Nursing as a feminine art was developed through character training that resulted in nonassertiveness, obedience and compliance with medical directives. Specific nursing arts comprised procedures such as bathing, bed-making, positioning patients and comforting techniques. While some science content was included in nursing courses, '[t]here was minimal, if any, application of science content in nursing practice' (Peplau 1988:8). Nor were nurses educated in the arts subjects of the university, which produced the thinkers of society, for that belonged to the sphere of men. Rather they were instilled with womanly virtues.

Nursing education was a process of systematically inculcating a task orientation and the moulding of a set of appropriate attitudes within hospital training schools to produce nurses who exemplified the feminine ideal. Science belonged to the rational and objective world of men, of which medicine was one domain. Men were subjects (minds), women objects (bodies); nurses were therefore not positioned as rational subjects shaping the Enlightenment project and their own destinies, but rather as passive and compliant objects, subservient to medicine.

Hospital-based nurse training lasted for more than one hundred years in Australia and much longer in Britain. Many changes occurred over that time, including considerable strengthening of the science content, particularly from the 1950s onward. However, the gendering of nursing as a feminine art, developed in the restrictive environment of the hospital, placed limitations upon the possibilities for nursing to develop as a modern profession. It also limited the possibilities for nurses to develop knowledge, skills and attitudes in ways that would enable them to act as independent subjects. Nevertheless, it equipped them powerfully to work as moral agents engaged in socially significant work and to develop in-depth knowledge of the human condition in sickness and in suffering, although in an unarticulated, scientifically untested form.

Nursing in the university

In the United States a 4-year entry-to-practice programme had been established within a university by 1919. Within this system, it was possible to ensure the development of knowledge in a systematic and orderly way. By the late 1950s programmes for training nurse scientists had developed in a number of major universities, which stimulated interest in theoretical and scientific bases of practice. These developments were supported by a huge federal investment in nursing education during the 1960s and early 1970s (Gortner 1983). In the period from the late 1950s to the early 1980s, theories of nursing proliferated as nurse scholars sought to include in the concept of nursing an understanding of biological, behavioural, social and cultural factors in health and illness. Of particular note in this discussion were the attempts made to produce closed systems of thought through the development of nursing theory and the creation of nursing science.

This scientific orientation in nursing, however, came into conflict with ideas about the art of nursing. These stemmed not only from the Nightingale school of thought, but also from consideration of the art of nursing in relation to humanism and the nature of the human subject, by this time conceived of as including women. It is in this context that most of the debates about the art and science of nursing have occurred.

Nursing as a science

As has already been noted, a significant feature of the modern era has been the rise of professions, each clearly delineated by a separate body of knowledge. In the early modern era, nursing could not be regarded as a profession because it was seen to be subservient to and part of the medical tasks of diagnosis and treatment. With the location of nursing education within universities, and with the goal of securing professional status for nurses, a major task was to establish its own scientific base, separate from that of medicine.

One early nursing theorist, Johnson (1980), distinguished medicine from nursing by arguing that while the scientific basis of medical knowledge was biological systems, the scientific base of nursing was behavioural systems. She proposed a behavioural subsystem model of the person 'with behaviour understood as the sum total of physical, biological and social factors/behaviours' (Parker in Gray & Pratt 1995:334). These ideas were further developed by Roy (1980), who conceived of the person as an open adaptive system and nursing as the science and practice of promoting adaptation.

Other theorists, however, argued that these approaches did not sufficiently distinguish nursing from medicine. Like medical knowledge, the knowledge produced through study of systems was over-simplistic and mechanistic. Nursing, by contrast, needed to be conceptualised in much broader, more encompassing terms (e.g. Levine 1971). Ideas about nursing as a holistic science were developed by writers such as Rogers (1970) who conceived of the whole person as an energy field, coextensive with the environment, identified in terms of unified wholeness, openness, pattern, organisation and sentience.

Other writers further differentiated nursing science from medical science by emphasising nursing's caring function in opposition to medicine's curative function.

Watson, for example, pulled together two of the central ideas of the modern era by describing nursing as a humanistic science with caring the central unifying dimension of nursing (Cohen 1991).

Thus, with the shift of nursing education to universities in the United States, strong schools of nursing thought emerged. Each was developed in opposition to medicine, and understood nursing as a behavioural science, a holistic science or a caring science. These conceptual models for nursing practice were the work of a number of nursing intellectuals who had undertaken higher degree work in a range of disciplines, particularly in social sciences and education. Each model was designed to capture the complex dimensions of nursing although, naturally enough, each one tended to reflect the disciplinary base of its author.

Following the establishment of the basis for nursing science through these models, there were calls to test the models against practical experience and refine them. However, progress was slow as Flaskerud and Halloran pointed out in 1980 and Fawcett in 1984. There was also concern that the proliferation of models would weaken nursing's claims to be seen as a profession based in a single unique body of knowledge. Fawcett noted that '[t]he discipline of nursing will advance only through continuous and systematic development and testing of nursing knowledge' (p. 84). Nursing authors sought to concentrate on the common ground in nursing conceptual models. Fawcett, for example, proposed a 'metaparadigm' (an explanatory framework) for nursing built on the central concepts of the discipline – person, environment, health and nursing – and attempts were made to further unify nursing knowledge around these concepts.

Many nurses, however, rejected nursing theories altogether as a means of establishing a science base for nursing. Nursing administrators and clinicians were particularly vocal in their rejection of the theories following frustrating experiences of trying to implement them in practice. Nursing theories were seen to reinforce the splits between the theory and practice of nursing, between the education students received and the realities of providing health care service, and between nursing thinkers (academics in universities) and nursing doers (nursing administrators and clinicians). In their attempts to develop nursing science through the development of nursing theory, nursing theorists, not surprisingly, reproduced the binary modes of thought and practice of the general society.

While nursing theory was being elaborated, attempts were also being made to develop nursing science knowledge in ways that were linked more closely to practice. The nursing diagnosis movement attracted strong support following the First National Conference on the Classification of Nursing Diagnosis held in Missouri in 1973. Nursing diagnosis sought to identify and classify the phenomena of nursing, to develop a common language for nursing and to facilitate the development and testing of nursing concepts and techniques. However, by 1983 the first broad-scoped critical rejection of nursing diagnosis emerged (Kritek 1985).

This more practice-focused approach to developing nursing science suffered from the same fundamental problem as the theory-based approach. Once again, nursing was attempting to develop its science in opposition to medicine by identifying a discipline-specific scientific knowledge base that would legitimate nursing's claims as a separate profession. In doing this, nursing opened itself to some of the same critiques that were made of medicine. The development of a dedicated nursing language separated nursing not only from medicine but, more importantly, from patients. When viewed through the nursing diagnosis lens, the patients were reduced to objects of nursing diagnoses and treatments, a positioning that was contrary to nursing's understanding of the patient as a holistic subject.

Two broad approaches to the development of nursing science have been identified: one that focused on defining the domain of nursing theoretically and then testing propositions empirically; another that focused on the phenomena of nursing practice and on developing ways of defining and classifying them. Both approaches were consistent with prevailing philosophies of science. Neither appears to have been successful in providing a discipline-specific body of knowledge that would justify nursing's claims to professional autonomy and power.

Nursing as an art

Nursing's power seems to rest more in its moral claims than in its science base. Ideas that stem from the Nightingale school about the nature of nursing art as an expression of the essential goodness of feminine virtues persist in contemporary nursing practice. Peplau (1988), writing about the United States but presenting a view widely held internationally, points out that nursing has been called the conscience of the health care system, which 'suggests that nurses are major keepers of the morality, goodness, honesty, and ethics of client care' (p. 9). This positioning of nurses on the moral high ground in the battlefield of health care provision has been sustained by beliefs that nurses exemplify feminine ideals, and appears to have wide community support. It points to an ongoing belief in the Nightingale legacy, which presents nurses as good women. It also suggests that nurses and nursing organisations recognise and exploit the ways in which this characterisation of nursing serves wider political agendas and social functions. Additionally, it supports the idea of nursing as a caring and holistic art that sets itself in opposition to the rationality and reductive practices of scientific medicine and health care organisation. As Tanya Buchanan (1999) has noted: the 'Nightingale discourse generates myths about nursing that … appear to be eternal truths. We need to see past it' (p. 30).

And indeed, ideas that the art of nursing stems from essential female virtues have been challenged within the university setting. The essence of nursing has been claimed to lie in its humanistic philosophy and the artistic practice that flows from this philosophy. In a much-quoted paper, Munhall (1982) argued that nursing has identified itself as a humanistic discipline, adhering to a basic philosophy 'that focuses on individuality and the belief that the actions of men [sic] are in some sense free' (p. 176).

Munhall focuses attention on the extent to which university-based nursing education in the United States moved away from the Nightingale school of nursing thought based on female character training, and drew more upon a precisely set out philosophy of the discipline to provide the basis for artistic practice. However, this placed nursing philosophy in opposition to prevailing notions of nursing science. As Munhall pointed out, because nursing subscribed to a humanistic philosophy as well as a scientific research orientation 'incongruities, paradoxes, and conflicting ideologies resulted between philosophy and research'.

She also draws attention to the attempts made within nursing education to accommodate both a scientific and humanistic (arts) orientation. This suggests that professional university-based nursing education in the United States attempted to bridge the divide between the sciences and the arts that had been identified by C.P. Snow in the British higher education context. Nursing in the university aimed to produce practitioners who were both scientists in orientation as well as humanists in practice. However, in educational preparation, the aims and scope of science and the arts differ significantly, and the transfer of both scientific and humanistic orientations to the realities of practice is a complex process.

Many writers have noted that the differing orientations of art and science have resulted in problems for nursing practice. Peplau (1988), for example, notes that science and art are both essential for excellence in the performance of nursing's mission, but points out the difficulty for a discipline to accommodate these two forms of professional behaviour: 'Combining both the art and science of nursing, seeing and bringing to bear the distinctive characteristics of each form and of the relation between them, imposes a complexity in professional nursing that virtually defies description' (p. 9).

Holden (1991), an Australian nurse, argues that the split between the arts and the sciences seriously complicates the notion of nursing. She points out that the caring role in nursing pushes nursing into the domain of the arts while nursing that embraces high technology is pushed into the domain of science. Jennings (1986) suggests that it is not a matter of choosing *either* art *or* science, but rather of skilfully blending both for the betterment of nursing.

Peplau (1988) supports Jennings' view, pointing out that both science and art come together in practice, so that '[t]here is surely a seamless quality, a graceful and delicately balanced movement, between art and science portrayed by experienced expert nurses that transcends as it uses the differences between these forms' (p. 14). She suggests further that this transcending of the differing forms of art and science enables nursing to be practised not only as a helping art, but also as 'an enabling, empowering or transforming art'. People, she notes 'are touched (literally and figuratively) and sometimes changed at a very personal level by the art nurses practice' (p. 9).

The aesthetic dimension – the creative expression – of nursing has received increasing attention over the last two decades. It has built particularly upon the work of Carper, who noted in 1978 that the primary emphasis in the professional literature of the time was being placed on the development of the science of nursing. She pointed out:

> There is, nonetheless, what might be described as a tacit admission that nursing is, at least in part, an art. Not much effort is made to elaborate or to make explicit this aesthetic pattern of knowing in nursing – other than to vaguely associate the 'art' with the general category of manual and/or technical skills involved in nursing practice (p. 16).

Peggy Chinn and Jean Watson (1994) have been very influential in further developing ideas about aesthetics and nursing, drawing upon notions of nursing as a caring science. Later, Chinn *et al.* (1997) described the development of aesthetic enquiry in nursing and the conceptualisation that has emerged of nursing as an art form. Johnson undertook a philosophical analysis of conceptualisations of nursing art as a means of contributing to debate on the specific abilities required for artistic creation in nursing (1993, 1994, 1996a,b).

Despite these developments, other writers (e.g. Darbyshire 1994a,b; Lafferty 1997) suggest that science content is still emphasised in nursing curricula at the expense of humanities content and that, as a result, humanistic aspects of care believed to be essential to the artistic component of nursing are not being addressed sufficiently. Lafferty argues that nursing's dual identity as an art and a science requires a balance, and calls for the promotion of aesthetic knowledge and its acquisition by nursing students. She suggests that studying literature is a way of fostering this. Darbyshire makes a similar point, arguing that nursing as an art and a science is in danger of becoming a cliché unless attempts are made to reverse the marginalisation of arts and humanities within nursing curricula.

It can be seen that nursing as a contemporary secular profession has developed out of ideas about the essential nature of women, wherein nursing has been regarded as an art practised by virtuous women. This essentialist notion of nursing as a gender-based art may help account for the continuing failure to attract equal numbers of men into nursing. This view has also resulted in nurses sometimes regarding themselves, and being regarded by others, as the conscience of the health care system. Nursing as a gendered art is a continuing thread in professional nursing and appears to be a primary source of its moral claims.

However, this notion was challenged by the shift of nursing education into universities in the United States and by the attempts that have been made to discuss nursing as a science and a humanistic art. The literature explored indicates that nursing lies somewhat uneasily in the domains of both science and art, a division which stemmed from dividing practices in the cultural production of knowledge. Nursing developments, too, have replicated many of these dividing practices.

NURSING AND CONTEMPORARY HEALTH CARE

Many of the old divisions of the modern era are collapsing in both contemporary higher education and the health sector. This is certainly true in Australia, with implications for practices that sustained the conceptual, methodological and practical separations between art and science in nursing. The clear division between arts and sciences in higher education that reinforced the arts/sciences divide in knowledge development and the professions is clearly breaking down. It is becoming less possible for professions to define themselves in relation to discrete bodies of discipline-specific knowledge. The continuing knowledge explosion resulting in new fields of scientific enquiry and the development of information technologies have resulted in the proliferation of new professions that draw upon knowledge from a range of sources.

The nexus between professional knowledge and power is being subverted in a number of ways, not least through mass higher education and the access consumers now have to information enabling then to make their own decisions independently of professional advice. These changes are taking place in a wider context in which global market influences are strengthening and humanist principles are weakening. This is an era of market contestability, privatisation, accountability and competition. It is an era in which performance is measured and evaluated on the basis of outcomes.

The 'reinvention' of nursing

The health care sector is rapidly transforming in response to demands for identifiable, quantifiable indicators of cost-effective quality outcomes. Clinical areas are responding to the changes being wrought in diagnosis and treatment through the use of new investigative and surgical technologies. Nursing, like many other professions, is seeking to 'reinvent' itself to meet emerging challenges (Parker & Rickard 1999).

The reinvention of nursing, I would suggest, is occurring on several fronts, all of which have implications for the art and science of nursing. Measures are being undertaken in nursing education, research and practice to ensure that nurses have the necessary repertoire of knowledge and skills to play a part in the transformations currently under way that are aimed at cost-effective quality outcomes of health care. Efforts are being made to identify the nursing practices that positively influence health outcomes. Nurses are investigating traditional nursing practices to determine both their continuing appropriateness and the skill level necessary for their implementation.

Competencies for general, specialist and advanced practice are being refined to ensure greater accountability in relation to consumers, within the profession, in relation to other health professionals, and with regard to various contexts of practice (ANCI 1998). Nurses, in collaboration with other health professionals, are also contributing to the development, testing, implementation and evaluation of standardised clinical pathways. They are developing evidence-based nursing practices and contributing to developments in evidence-based health care. They are working with consumers of health services to satisfy their learning needs.

What is becoming clear in this aspect of its reinvention is that nursing is shifting away from attempts to define itself as an autonomous profession with its own discipline-specific body of knowledge. As it moves into an interdisciplinary, team-based and consumer-oriented approach to practice and research, it is drawing upon current science/technology and information systems and focusing upon nursing contributions to health outcomes and accountability for practices.

Nurses today need to draw substantially upon scientific knowledge to inform their practice, and scientific training needs to be a significant component of nursing education programmes. At the same time nurses can contribute to the development of scientific knowledge in interdisciplinary and nursing-specific research projects. Questions for – and about – nursing emerge out of what nurses ask about their practices and the people and communities that they serve.

But how is the art of nursing manifest in this reinvention of the discipline? In a multitude of ways, I would suggest. We live today in an era of diversity, multiplicity and hybrid practices. Nursing can be practised as a gendered art; as a humanistic, aesthetic endeavour; it can take fragments from both of these traditions and draw upon others as well. It can take up aspects of traditional art forms such as music, movement and touch, and incorporate them in diverse ways into repertoires of skilful practice.

In all of the multiplicity that is the art of nursing there is, however, a continuing thread, expressed as support of the sense of wholeness and integrity of individuals and communities rendered vulnerable through sickness and suffering.

CONCLUSION

In the current climate many nurses are expressing reservations about the market-driven approach and the economic ethic that underlie the health reforms. They are concerned that standardised approaches to care will compromise their ability to meet the demands of particular and unique situations. They are concerned that the increasing rationalisation of health services is causing fragmentation of services, despite the rhetoric of continuity of care. They are concerned that greater reliance upon advanced technologies is resulting in delivery of dehumanised services.

It is important that compliance with current health care reforms and resistance to them are not seen to be mutually exclusive endeavours. We can no longer claim that nursing is a holistic and artistic enterprise with humanistic and expressive concerns developed in opposition to the scientific, technical and instrumental dimensions of care (Parker 1995). The therapeutic tools and technologies of care we use are not separate from us: they are part of us and we are part of them. As they change, so we change. As we change, they change too. They are integral to our self-expression as nurses. The art of nursing, then, involves the perception and understanding of the inseparability of expression and technology.

Working within the framework of a standardised pathway does not prevent a nurse from recognising the individual and unique needs of particular patients. An aesthetic sensibility recognises the extent to which there is congruence between the standard (form) and the individual (content). Aesthetic integrity is responsive nursing in which standard and individual, form and content, become shaped into wholeness. An aesthetic sensibility facilitates expression of the art of nursing as part of the complex, ambiguous and technologically expressive milieus in which nurses work. An aesthetic sensibility responds to unified experiences both for recipients and providers of health care. It resists fragmented experience and can also 'empower people who are … sick, weak, vulnerable or disturbed to demand that attention is given to the particularities, complexities and ambiguities of their individual situation' (Parker 1995:2).

Nursing as art and/or science has been addressed somewhat differently at different times and in different contexts. A continuing thread nonetheless exists which demonstrates the significance that nursing has given as a discipline and a profession to both science and art and the nature of their relationship in nursing. Modern secular professional nursing since its beginnings in the nineteenth century has been and continues to be a complex set of practices that contains many anomalies and contradictions. The art and science of nursing manifests itself within a broader and changing social, cultural and political agenda. Nursing's social mandate acknowledges the art and science of nursing. The challenge for nurses in the contemporary health care context is to exercise that mandate judiciously and creatively.

REFLECTIVE QUESTIONS

(1) What do you think are the main reasons nursing has come to be viewed as an art?
(2) Why has nursing made consistent attempts to align itself with science?
(3) How do you think the art and science of nursing can interrelate in the current contexts of health care?

RECOMMENDED READING

Carper, B. (1978) Fundamental patterns of knowing in nursing. *Advances in Nursing Science,* **1**(1), 13–23.

Chinn, P.L., Maeve, M.K. & Bostick, C. (1997) Aesthetic inquiry and the art of nursing. *Scholarly Inquiry for Nursing Practice,* **11**(2), 83–100.

Johnson, J.L. (1994) A dialectical examination of nursing art. *Advances in Nursing Science,* **17**(1), 1–14.

Peplau, H. (1988) The art and science of nursing: Similarities, differences, and relations. *Nursing Science Quarterly,* **1**(1), 8–15.

Watson, J. (1985) *Nursing: Human Science and Human Care.* Appleton Century Crofts, Norwalk, Connecticut.

REFERENCES

Australian Nursing Council Inc (1998) *ANCI National Competency Standards for the Registered Nurse* 2nd edn. ANCI, Dickson ACT.

Berriot-Salvadore, E. (1993) The discourse of medicine and science. In: *A History of Women in the West: Vol. 3 Renaissance and Enlightenment Paradoxes* (eds N.Z. Davis & A. Farge). The Belknap Press of Harvard University Press, Cambridge, Massachusetts.

Buchanan, T. (1999) Nightingalism: Haunting nursing history. *Collegian,* **6**(2), 28–33.

Capra, F. (1982) *The Turning Point: Science, Society and the Rising Culture.* Simon & Schuster, New York.

Carper, B. (1978) Fundamental patterns of knowing in nursing. *Advances in Nursing Science,* **1**, 13–23.

Chinn, P.L. & Watson, J. (eds) (1994) *Art and Aesthetics in Nursing.* National League for Nursing, New York.

Chinn, P.L., Maeve, M.K. & Bostick, C. (1997) Aesthetic inquiry and the art of nursing. *Scholarly Inquiry for Nursing Practice,* **11**(2), 83–100.

Cohen, J.S. (1991) Two portraits of caring: A comparison of the artists, Leininger and Watson. *Journal of Advanced Nursing,* **16**, 899–909.

Darbyshire, P. (1994a) Understanding the life of illness: Learning through the art of Frida Kahlo. *Advances in Nursing Science,* **17**(1), 51–59.

Darbyshire, P. (1994b) Understanding caring through arts and humanities: A medical/nursing humanities approach to promoting alternate experiences of thinking and learning. *Journal of Advanced Nursing,* **19**(5), 856–863.

Dickens, C. (1910) *Martin Chuzzlewit.* McMillan Co, New York.

Donahue, P. (1996) *Nursing: The Finest Art.* Mosby, St Louis.

Fawcett, J. (1984) The metaparadigm of nursing: Present status and future refinements. *Image: The Journal of Nursing Scholarship,* **16**(3), 84–89.

Flaskerud, J.H. & Halloran, E.J. (1980) Areas of agreement in nursing theory development. *Advances in Nursing Science,* **3**(1), 1–7.

Gortner, S.R. (1983) The history and philosophy of nursing science and research. *Advances in Nursing Science,* **5**(2), 1–8.

Holden, R.J. (1991) In defence of Cartesian dualism and the hermeneutic horizon. *Journal of Advanced Nursing,* **16**(11), 1375–1381.

Jennings, B.M. (1986) Nursing science: More promise than threat. *Journal of Advanced Nursing,* **11**(5), 505–511.

Johnson, D.E. (1980) The behavioural system model for nursing. In: *Conceptual Models for Nursing Practice* (eds J.P. Riehl & C. Roy), 2nd edn. Appleton-Century-Crofts, New York.

Johnson, J.L. (1993) *Toward a clearer understanding of the art of nursing.* Unpublished PhD thesis, University of Alberta.

Johnson, J.L. (1994) A dialectical examination of nursing art. *Advances in Nursing Science,* **1**(1), 1–14.

Johnson, J.L. (1996a) The perceptual aspect of nursing art: Sources of accord and discord. *Scholarly Inquiry for Nursing Practice: An International Journal,* **10**(4), 307–327.

Johnson, J.L. (1996b) The art of nursing. *Image: Journal of Nursing Scholarship,* **28**, 169–175.

Kritek, P.B. (1985) Nursing diagnosis in perspective: Response to a critique. *Image: The Journal of Nursing Scholarship,* **17**(1), 3–8.

Lafferty, P.M. (1997) Balancing the curriculum: promoting aesthetic knowledge in nursing. *Nurse Education Today,* **17**, 281–286.

Levine, M. (1971) Holistic nursing. *Nursing Clinics of North America,* **6**(2), 253–263.

Munhall, P.L. (1982) Nursing philosophy and nursing research: In apposition or opposition? *Nursing Research,* **31**(3), 176–7, 181.

Nelson, S. (1995) Humanism in nursing: The emergence of light. *Nursing Inquiry,* **2**(1), 36–43.

Parker, J.M. (1995) Searching for the body in nursing. In: *Scholarship in the Discipline of Nursing,* (eds G. Gray & R. Pratt). Churchill Livingstone, Melbourne.

Parker, J.M. & Gibbs, M. (1998) Truth, virtue and beauty: Midwifery and philosophy. *Nursing Inquiry,* **5**(3), 146–153.

Parker, J.M. & Rickard, G. (1999) Nursing town and nursing gown: Time space and the re-invention of nursing through collaboration. *Clinical Excellence for Nurse Practitioners,* **3**(1), 36–42.

Parker, R. (1990) Nurses stories: The search for a relational ethic of care. *Advances in Nursing Science,* **13**(1), 31–40.

Peplau, H.E. (1988) The art and science of nursing: Similarities, differences, and relations. *Nursing Science Quarterly,* **1**(1), 8–15.

Rogers, M.E. (1970) *An Introduction to the Theoretical Basis of Nursing.* FA Davis, Philadelphia.

Roy, C. (1980) The Roy adaptation model. In: *Conceptual Models for Nursing Practice* (eds J.P. Riehl & C. Roy), 2nd edn. Appleton-Century-Crofts, New York.

Smith, F.B. (1982) *Florence Nightingale, reputation and power.* Croom Helm, London.

Snow, C.P. (1964) *The Two Cultures: And a Second Look.* The New American Library, New York.

Trembath, R. & Hellier, D. (1987) *All Care and Responsibility: A History of Nursing in Victoria 1850–1934.* Florence Nightingale Committee, Australia.

4 Heroines, Hookers and Harridans

Exploring Popular Images and Representations of Nurses and Nursing

Philip Darbyshire

LEARNING OBJECTIVES

After reading this chapter the reader will be able to:

- explain the importance of nursing's image for contemporary nursing;
- describe the various prevalent stereotypes of the nurse and nursing, and try to explain the persistence of these;
- debate the issue of whether nurses really wish to abandon the 'over-worked angel' image;
- explain the difficulties involved in proposing a 'realistic' portrayal of nurses and nursing;
- propose a strategy or small-scale project that could help promote alternative media representations of nurses and nursing.

KEY WORDS

IMAGES, ICONOGRAPHY, MEDIA, STEREOTYPES, PORTRAYAL, MYTHICAL, REALISM.

INTRODUCTION

Since the mid 1970s there has been a burgeoning interest in the study of popular images of nurses and nursing; it seems that every conceivable aspect of the image of nurses has been scrutinised. Writers have focused on images of nurses and nursing on television, in cinema, in novels and short stories, in news coverage and elsewhere. Why this fascination with the image of nurses? With the possible exception of doctors, why is there no comparable body of inquiry literature regarding the image of teachers, social workers, physiotherapists, accountants, occupational therapists or other professional groups?

In this chapter I will explore some of the early history and iconography of nurses and nursing in order to clarify the origins of many of the issues and 'images of nursing' which are so hotly contested and debated today. The 'so what?' question is important here. Why, when there are so many other pressing issues and concerns facing nursing and health care, should we worry about nursing's image? Delacour (1991:413) argues that:

> Certainly it is important that we analyse the process through which dysfunctional im-
> ages and discourses are maintained. Moreover, it is useful to regard reading media as
> a politically situated and critical activity for the nursing profession.

Developing a critical and questioning view of our historical and contemporary representations is thus important for every nurse's personal and professional development.
What we should strive for is to move beyond 'knee-jerk' response that this or that
image is good or bad, and to develop the critical thinking and analytic qualities that
help us understand both the production, meaning(s) and possible effects of popular
images of the nurse and nursing.

NURSING'S EARLY ICONOGRAPHY

Representations and images of nursing are as old as nursing and healing themselves.
By tracing the origins of modern nursing back to antiquity and to the earliest accounts
of babies, pregnant women, family and other members of early communities being
cared for, usually by women, we can see that, 'The nurse as saintly domestic is no
modern invention' (Kampen 1988:36). The earliest Greco-Roman depictions were
almost entirely of 'baby nurses' and the image of the 'modern' nurse as tender of the
sick or wounded was not to appear until the fourteenth century (Kampen 1988:16).

With the emergence of religious orders and associated charitable services came
a new iconography of nursing that showed women extending their care practices
from the immediate household and family arena to the care of strangers. This was
not always welcomed, however, and the Middle Ages in Europe especially saw the
slaughter of many 'wise women' who were burnt as witches (Darbyshire 1985). Com-
menting on fifteenth century depictions of 'nurses' working with the sick, Kampen
(1988:23) makes the significant observation that:

> Several features common to scenes of nursing sisters help to define the nature of their
> role: they nurse patients who are most often men lying in bed; they work in a distinctive
> location that does not look like a house; they wear distinctive costumes; their activities
> are domestic and religious rather than specifically medical; and most important, they
> are never subordinated to patients and doctors.

It is salutary to think that, with the exception of the last phrase, this description
would have fitted any typical Victorian infirmary almost 500 years later. So powerful
is this depiction of nurses as tenders of the prostrate sick, reinforced no doubt by the
iconographic imagery of Florence Nightingale wending her ethereal way through
the wards of Scutari Hospital during the Crimean War, that nursing has often been
seen in the public mind as being exclusively focused on this particular form of acute
care nursing. McCoppin and Gardner (1994:156) noted how this one-dimensional
view of nursing and nurses can occlude (obstruct) the view of all other forms and
areas of nursing, which can somehow be deemed to be 'less than' or 'other than' 'real

nursing', which of course was deemed to be practised exclusively at the bedsides of sick people:

> The stereotypical view of nurses as working only in acute care, high technology areas often portrayed in the media makes it very difficult to provide the alternative view of nurses working within the community which is more difficult to make 'attention grabbing'.

It is not only the various forms of community nursing which may be seen as less than 'real nursing' but also the myriad of other 'nursings', such as working in mental health, health promotion, school nursing, working with people with learning/intellectual disabilities and many others.

This masking of what, even in 1985, was more than half of the whole nursing workforce (Dunn 1985), is significant as it can help narrow and restrict students' and other nurses' perceptions of what nursing fundamentally 'is'. For example, in Kiger's study of student nurses in Scotland, she found that 'The picture of adult medical–surgical nursing as typical of real nursing persisted throughout (the students' concept of) "Working with people" ' (Kiger 1993). The 'real nurse as general nurse' is, however, only one of many distortions and misrepresentations that have plagued nursing since its inception. Why nursing should be such a fertile ground for image construction and manipulation is a hugely complex issue and one that has been discussed and argued over many years. One way of beginning to understand the heady brew of images, social constructions, myths and contradictions and 'realities' which form the image(s) of nurses and nursing is to look more carefully at the persistence and power of the major stereotypes of nurses which still exist in either blatant or more subtle forms even today.

Nursing's stereotypes

Perhaps it could be considered something of a backhanded compliment that there are so many stereotypes associated with nursing. At least we are not seen as bland and instantly forgettable! The problem is often, however, that the major stereotypes can be so unrelentingly negative in their connotations and so wholly untenable in their relationship to any notion of a 'reality' of nursing. (This notion of a single nursing reality is itself contentious and I shall return to this later.)

The problem with any stereotype is that it can become so pervasive that its effects become more than merely an annoyance. As Delacour (1991) observes:

> even stereotypes regarded as dubious may, after a measure of exposure, become internalized and naturalized; they are thereby metamorphosed into categories of the normal, the real, and the healthy and desirable (p. 413).

If the sole problem with nursing stereotypes was just that some get-well cards, tabloid newspaper stories or 'X-rated' films portrayed nurses as over-sexualised bimbos, then perhaps we could laugh it off, but when the effects of stereotyping are more serious, then there is more at stake than nursing's collective need to 'lighten up'.

The images and perceptions of nursing, both within the profession and in society in general are important for several reasons. We live in an era where image and the marketing of image has never been more important, and while we can certainly maintain that the 'core business' of nursing is caring for the health and well-being of people, we would be foolish to ignore the importance of nursing's image. If we are to attract creative, committed, intelligent and passionate people into nursing, then nursing needs to be seen as every bit as worthwhile and challenging a career as any other in the fields of health care or social service. The persistence of hackneyed old stereotypes does nothing to enhance the attractiveness of nursing as a career.

Muff (1982:211) has suggested six 'major nursing stereotypes': Angel of Mercy, Handmaiden to the Physician, Woman in White, Sex symbol/Idiot, Battleaxe, and Torturer, while Dunn (1985:2) credits the average tabloid newspaper with even less imagination, being interested in only three types of nurse: Angel, Battleaxe and Nymphomaniac.

Angels with pretty faces

If nursing iconography has an enduring stereotypic image, it must surely be the nurse as 'angel'. While much of the earliest artwork and imagery of nurses showed nurses ministering to the sick in various quasireligious ways and settings, nurses in Australia, even in the late 1800s, were 'redefining the image of nurses as motivated primarily by self-sacrifice' (Bashford 1997). However, it was Florence Nightingale's story that captured the public imagination and stimulated a swathe of hagiographic accounts (which critic Leslie Fiedler [1988:103] called 'shameless schlock'), and movies such as *The White Angel* and *The Lady with the Lamp* (Jones 1988; Kalisch & Kalisch 1983b). So powerful were these images of the angelic presence which lit up the wards of Scutari with her lamp, that Florence Nightingale has become easily identified as the soul or spirit of nursing and as the embodiment of selfless, devoted, compassionate care which borders on the saintly.

Despite some of the more recent, critical and balanced scholarship concerning the life and work of Florence Nightingale (e.g. Hektor 1994), the stereotype of the nurse as selfless angel is still prevalent, especially in the public imagination. There are several difficulties here. At first glance it may seem no bad thing to think that society views nurses as 'angels'. Who wouldn't like to be thought of in such a 'positive' light? Which nurse would not like to think that she was capable of such profound caring which could earn such adoration? Is this not just being held in high regard by society? Don't we feel good when opinion polls put nurses near the top of the list for perceived honesty, trustworthiness and hard work? Jane Salvage (1983:14) perceptively pointed out that nurses often collude in sustaining the 'selfless angel' stereotype while professing to scorn it. As she noted, 'The trouble is we are secretly flattered by the myths, especially those emphasising dedication and high-minded self-sacrifice'.

However, buying into the 'angels' stereotype may be a Faustian bargain, for there is a price to pay for this. 'Angels' may be saintly but such perfection is impossible for mere mortal nurses to achieve or maintain; nurses are, after all, only human. Nor do angels seem to require any education or experience, their sanctity being more of a divine gift. For real nurses, however, becoming a skilled and competent nurse is hard work. We may be born with particular dispositions and talents (although some would dispute even this), but we cannot be 'born nurses'. That will take more than an accident of birth. Such shafts of grace as we achieve are often hard won through our sustained engagement in the lives of those people who place their trust in us.

Doctors' handmaidens

If the 'angel' myth is a remnant of nursing's religious order origins, then the un-questioning obedience of the doctor's handmaiden owes much to nursing's military origins. This stereotype touts the image of the nurse as a kind of 'lady in waiting', or the doctor's 'right hand woman'. For decades this has been a hugely influential media view of nursing, that essentially the nurse is there to provide faithful and obedient service to the doctor and, like the 'angel' myth, this view has often been sustained by nurses themselves, who were flattered by the idea that 'their' doctors or 'their' consultant says that he or she couldn't manage without them. In her analysis of nurses' image in postwar Britain, Hallam (1998:37) noted also that 'Within the broadcasting environment, nursing's professional discourse of "service" was interpreted as service to medicine; nurses themselves did little to challenge the picture.'

In this sense, the 'handmaiden' stereotype may be less mythical than nursing would like to acknowledge. While nationally and internationally, particular nurses and nursing projects/initiatives have led health care advances (often in collaboration with medical colleagues), there are still many nurses who work with doctors who seem not to recognise nurses' ability and responsibility to make an equal contribution to care, and who assume that the nurse's role is to make coffee, not decisions. Despite claims of teamwork and 'multidisciplinary' co-operation, some nurses continue to work in 'teams' where teamwork is lots of people doing what one person says, and that one person is usually a doctor.

The battleaxe or monstrous figure

For images to be powerful and long lasting they must be capable of being both sus-tained and subverted. The battleaxe figure is in many ways a magnificent subversion of other stereotypes of the nurse, what Hunter (1988) calls in a slightly different con-text, the translocated ideal. Where the 'angel' is often portrayed as pretty, feminine, caucasian, slim, caring, white-clad for purity, fun, deferential and loved by patients, the battleaxe or matron figure was almost the exact opposite – tyrannical, fearsome, asexual, cruel, monstrously large, dark-clad, and set on crushing all fun and individu-ality. On a BBC radio programme that I compiled several years ago, I listened to a recording of a 1960s radio quiz show where one of the male panellists joked that the tragedy of nurses is that they were one day destined to become matrons. Matrons, like other nurses who refuse to fit the accepted stereotype of the pretty, kind, com-pliant nurse, are banished to the moral margins of societal acceptance where they become objects of fear or ridicule. Think here of 'bad' nurses like Charles Dickens' Sairey Gamp (Summers 1997), Ken Kesey's 'Big Nurse/Nurse Ratched' from *One Flew Over the Cuckoo's Nest* (Darbyshire 1995), Annie Wilkes from Stephen King's *Misery* and the more comic figures of Hattie Jacques from the *Carry On* film series or Matron Dorothy from Australia's 1990 television series, *Let the Blood Run Free* (Delacour 1991).

The 'battleaxe' stereotype cries out for a feminist analysis that reveals the fate of any nurse who does not comply with the mythical norms of the ideal nurse and who challenges male power (usually patients and doctors). Worse than this, perhaps, is that the battleaxe figure is a powerful woman who is unattracted to them (Darbyshire 1995), thus proving that she cannot be a 'real' nurse, as one of the most prevalent and damaging stereotypes is the nurse as an easily available sex bomb.

Naughty nurses and nymphomaniacs

When I was a lecturer in Scotland, I would discuss the question of nurses' image with the first year students who had just begun their course. I asked them what a common reaction would be at a party if they happened to mention that they were nurses. After the laughter and ribaldry had settled it was clear that a common, if not thankfully universal, reaction from some men was a 'knowing grin' and some suggestion that a night of unbridled sexual abandon might lie ahead. For this reason, many of the students said that they would make up an occupation rather than 'admit' to being a nurse.

Why is the 'naughty nurse' stereotype so prevalent? Why are there no 'naughty lawyer' sexual stereotypes? Why are there no pornographic films made about the adventures of a group of occupational therapy students? Why don't sex shops sell physiotherapist uniforms? What is it about nurses that makes them such a target?

This is a deep and complex issue but consider the following points in relation to Hunter's (1988) notion of a 'translocated ideal'. Nursing is utterly implicated in social power relations, between nurses and doctors, nurses and other nurses, nurses and patients, nurses and relatives, and more. When patients enter hospital, the traditional power relations are reversed and they find themselves vulnerable and dependent rather than strong and in control. At a societal level (for not every male patient will see his situation in this way) one way of redressing this balance is to metaphorically (or perhaps even practically) sexualise the encounters between nurses and patients.

We also know that nurses' practices in relation to patients' bodies are part of this process. Nurses are exceptionally privileged in that we are intimate body workers. Nurses have access to people's most private body areas and bodily functions (Lawler 1991). One of the most important practices that a nurse develops is the ability to work with patients' intimate body parts without sexualising the encounter. To transgress this boundary would be both embarrassing and dangerous. In an almost-too-painful-to-watch scene in Dennis Potter's television play, *The Singing Detective*, a nurse has to anoint with cream the genital areas of hero Philip Marlowe, as he has extremely debilitating psoriasis and cannot do this for himself. As the nurse applies his cream he becomes sexually aroused and, despite trying desperately to divert his thoughts, he develops an erection. The nurse, however, wants to get the procedure done and continues creaming, causing him to ejaculate and suffer an agony of humiliation.

Fagin and Diers (1983:117) are clear on the damaging implications of conflating sexualisation and intimate body work: 'Thanks to the worst of this kind of thinking, nursing is a metaphor for sex. Having seen and touched the bodies of strangers, nurses are perceived as willing and able sexual partners.'

The 'naughty nurse' stereotype also encourages the subversion of another ideal, that of the saintly purity of the nurse as 'angel'. Beneath the pristine white uniform, tightly bunched and restrained hair and sheepish obedience to authority lies the pornographer's win–win scenario. Either the nurse is really a 'sex-bomb' being barely held in check by the rules and regulations of the institution and awaiting the slightest excuse to release all of this pent-up passion, or she really is completely subservient to (male) authority, in which case she will willingly agree to every sexual demand.

If you think that these scenarios are far-fetched, consider a feature that ran several years ago in the UK tabloid newspaper, *The Sun*, which aroused furious opposition, and not only from nurses and their organisations. The feature had the headline: 'Calling All You Naughty Nurses' and read:

> Yes, we know you're out there. Lots and lots of people tell stories about those saucy times when temperatures soared in the wards. Who hasn't heard about the time the young nurse turned a bed bath into a saucy romp? And delighted male patients are always revealing how they got some very special medicine from the attractive sister when the screens were drawn. So come on folks. Let's hear from the naughty night nurses – and their happy patients – about the fun times in Britain's hospitals. We're opening our own special phone line between 10 AM and 6 PM today. Ring the number below and tell us your stories.

Such was the wave of protest from nursing organisations and others that the feature was withdrawn within days.

Nursing's image: blame the media?

For any nurse who wants to place the blame for the worst excesses and misrepresentations of nursing's image, then the media in general offer a clear if rather too easy target. Too easy perhaps because we assume that the media is almost automatically the most pervasive form of image transmission. Yet a study of 1155 people in the USA found that less than 10% of the respondents felt that they got their information from the media. Most said that their opinions came from first-hand impressions gained during visits to a hospital (Begany 1994). Delacour (1991:418) makes the important point that often it is not only the ways in which nursing is portrayed but, more than that, it is that nursing is 'symbolically annihilated by the mass media' and virtually ignored. To test this claim, it would be interesting to keep a local and a national newspaper for a month or two with a view to checking how many health stories included authoritative comments from nurses compared with doctors. Many nurses would say that they could confidently predict the results of such a survey well in advance.

Considerable research has been undertaken into the role of the media in constructing and shaping nursing's image. In the USA in particular, the team of Philip and Beatrice Kalisch in the 1980s produced numerous books and papers on many different aspects of this question (Kalisch *et al.* 1982, 1983; Kalisch & Kalisch 1983a,b, 1984, 1987). This criticism of the media in general continues to this day. Holmes (1997: 137), for example, advises that we should (perhaps) give up watching medical 'soaps' on television as they are 'anodyne and legitimating rather than transformative and critical'. While 'soaps' may well be 'anodyne', there are probably few viewers of *All Saints* or whatever, who bemoan that the show is no longer as 'transformative and critical' as it used to be. Blaming genres for not being what we would wish them to be is surely tilting at windmills. Simply to stop watching 'soaps' because we disagree with aspects of their portrayal of nurses and nursing is scarcely a mode of engagement. Nor is it particularly astute to imagine that the media exist to 'accurately' (or should it be positively/flatteringly?) depict nurses and their work. Much as we may dislike the notion, the mass media exists primarily as a profit-making business. It is not nursing's tame public relations machine.

There is also an argument to be made that criticisms of the portrayals of nurses often seem to misunderstand the different genres of representation. For example, criticising a film like *Carry on Nurse*, or a series like *Let the Blood Run Free* for giving a false image of nurses and nursing makes little sense. These are not documentaries and their purpose was never to represent the 'reality' of nursing. They are comedies, and they work by upsetting or translocating our understandings and expectations of nursing. Condemning a *Carry On* film for not being a true-to-life account of nursing is like criticising Thursday for not being the Blue Mountains.

While a 'blame the media' approach has a seductive simplicity, it is unlikely to achieve any significant results. However, working with the media in order to help create more 'realistic' portrayals of nursing's work has been reported to help (Buresh & Gordon 1995). In the early days of the filming of the medical soap *ER* there was virtually no consultation with nurses or ER departments. US emergency room nurses, however, did more than complain or stop watching – they became proactive and contacted the producers regularly with comments and criticisms, but also with offers of help, story line ideas, and the names of subspecialty ER nurses who were willing to help the show 'get it right'.

Nursing's image: depicting 'reality'?

In a news report, the warning of Joanne Rule, former head of the RCN (UK) public relations office was repeated, that 'if nursing were to succeed finally in shaking off the 'angel' image it so professes to hate, it might be replaced by an image that it hated even more' (Rule 1995). One of the significant difficulties in challenging potentially damaging images of nursing is that it is very difficult to give an agreed account of what a 'good portrayal' should look like. As Bashford (1997:74) noted in her study of how early Australian nurses challenged their systems:

> resistance was never straightforward. Often, rather than new discourses offering empowering new subject positions, they produced confusion, contradiction and insecurity. Women were asked to think about their work in religious terms in one moment and in one context, in scientific terms in another, and as a type of professionalism in another.

This historical dilemma will seem blindingly contemporary to today's nurses who are struggling with very similar issues around nurses' 'expanded role' and what this means for nursing's identity/identities. The other difficulty in looking for a 'realistic' image of nurses is that it would be a precious and narcissistic stance for nursing to adopt which stated that the only acceptable portrayals of nurses and nursing were those which were 'positive'. (And for 'acceptable', ask: Acceptable to whom? To me personally? To nurses at my hospital? To nursing in general?) It would be reassuring to think that nursing was a little more secure in its role and purpose than to require to be constantly flattered and inflated by an unrelenting diet of uncritical media comments and compliments. This quest for the 'positive' portrayal of nursing has been questioned by Hallam (1998:33) who argued that:

> This search for a positive image of nursing identity poses two crucial problems. On the one hand, it tends to presume a professional consensus in terms of what this image is or could be … the positive image approach can also be critiqued from the viewpoint of media reception; it conceptualises readers and viewers as uncritical receivers of messages who unquestioningly digest the authority of the image.

Similarly, Cheek (1995:239) has observed that 'the task is not to look for real and authentic representations of nursing, but rather to look for the speaking and representation that is done about nursing'.

This is not to say, however, that no 'positive' images and accounts of nurses and nursing can be found. For example, in his account of his serious injury and recovery, surgeon and rehabilitation specialist Tony Moore (1991:11) describes the artistic and technical expertise of the intensive care nurses who gave him a blanket bath:

> They worked like a ballet corps in slow motion, softly moving me forwards, to the side, sponging, touching, towelling with clean tenderness, and when one gently washed my genitals I felt nothing but the compassion of her care.

Richard Selzer (1993) was another surgeon who found himself a patient in intensive care following legionnaires' disease. He is hugely embarrassed by his dependency and incontinence, but again, his nurses are memorably skilled in what he calls 'the forgiveness of the flesh' (p. 56). Unlike the unfortunate Philip Marlowe in *The Singing Detective*, Selzer is spared by his nurses the embarrassment and pain that could so easily become part of his intimate body care. One nurse who makes such a profound difference to Selzer's care and recovery is Patrick, whom Selzer describes as being 'the sort of nurse who can draw the pus out of a carbuncle with his gaze alone, and turn it into a jewel' (p. 56). Selzer is quite emphatic that the power of skilled nurse caring is not merely 'nice to get' but that it is actually transformative. He describes his being carried back to bed by Patrick following a tub bath as the moment when his 'molecules rearranged themselves'. 'It is the true moment of cure', he says (p. 93).

Read these authors' accounts of their care and then consider that bathing patients is deemed by some to be basic nursing care – where for 'basic' read 'unimportant and thus able to be undertaken by virtually anyone'. There are many other 'positive' accounts in literature and popular culture of nurses and nursing that are valued, appreciated and have a markedly beneficial effect on the recipient. However, care is needed not to fall into the trap of 'collecting' these accounts as a kind of trophy for nursing. If we are to cultivate and develop our questioning and critical powers, then the positive accounts also need to be questioned and discussed.

Nursing's image: from affront to action

During the past two decades, there has been a plethora of research and discussion regarding nursing's image and the portrayals of nursing. We are now much more aware of the forces that shape and maintain many of popular culture's images of nurses and nursing. Perhaps the next two decades will see nurses moving from this position of greater awareness to one of more positive action. By this I mean that it is no longer enough to be outraged at the 'negative images' and stereotypes that we will continue to encounter. Indignation or 'refusing to watch' are not strategies for change. Nor will it be enough merely to call for negative images of nurses to be withdrawn or 'banned'. The most difficult task ahead is for nurses and nursing to use the media in a much more 'streetwise' way than we have in the past. If we do not like the images that are being presented, then we have a responsibility to provide alternatives. If we think that media reports and stories about nursing are inaccurate or inadequate, then we need to interest the media in alternatives. If we feel that the media completely ignores a particularly important programme, service or aspect of nursing, then why not alert them to this and highlight the importance of what it is that they are missing. No media like to feel that they are missing something interesting or important, especially in their local area.

Delacour (1991:419) lists excellent questions that we should ask about the images and representations of nurses and nursing:

> Who has speaking rights? Who says what? Which position? On behalf of whom? Who is silenced? What are the assumptions? What is privileged in the text? What is ignored, glossed over or marginalised? What is the target audience and how is the reading/viewing position constructed to promote a 'preferred' reading? Which genre and its codes and effects? What type of publication/programme and resultant status of discourse? How are power and knowledge articulated? How are gender, sexuality, roles and relationship, race, class, deviance and normality constructed? Which rhetorical devices? Which linguistic features?

These are questions which do not naively assume that there is a right or wrong image, but that begin the task of unpacking and exploring this complex yet highly revealing area wherein we can learn so much about both ourselves, our society and those whom we care for. To these questions we should add some others that will help us be more active in redressing nursing's image. Questions such as: what images would we want to see in the media? How can we show the positive power of nursing to local and national media? Why would/should the media be interested in this programme/innovation/nursing development? How can we 'sell' this idea or story to them in such a way that they can't ignore it? Whose expertise and support could we call upon to help us do this? (Clarke 1989; Monahan 1996; Strasen 1992).

CONCLUSION

We now know a great deal about representations of nurses and nursing in the various media and popular culture. As nurses, our task now is not simply to 'adapt' to, or merely observe and comment on future changes, but to get out there and make the changes happen.

REFLECTIVE QUESTIONS

(1) Discuss with a group of your peers the reactions that you have encountered, both favourable and unfavourable, when you have told
people that you are a nurse/student nurse and how you feel about
such reactions.

(2) Use Delacour's list of questions to assess and question some selected
images of nurses/nursing, e.g. a film, documentary, novel, medical
'soap', etc.

(3) Plan how you would go about creating your own media story about
nurses or nursing. What would you choose as the issue? Would it be a
nurse-led clinical initiative, an ethical dilemma, a particularly successful patient outcome, an exciting new approach in nursing education,
or a particular nurse who is doing something really special in an area?
How would you go about interesting the media in the story and how
would you present it?

RECOMMENDED READING

Davis, C. & Schaefer, J. (1995) *Between the Heartbeats: Poetry and Prose by Nurses.* University
of Iowa Press, Iowa City.

Jones, A. (ed.) (1988) *Images of Nurses: Perspectives from History, Art, and Literature.* University of Pennsylvania Press, Pennsylvania.

Donahue, M.P. & Donahue, P.M. (1996) *Nursing: The Finest Art.* Mosby Year-Book, St Louis.

McCoppin, B. & Gardner, H. (1994) *Tradition and Reality: Nursing and Politics in Australia.*
Churchill Livingstone, Melbourne.

Salvage, J. (1985) *The Politics of Nursing.* Heinemann, London.

REFERENCES

Bashford, A. (1997) Starch on the collar and sweat on the brow: Self sacrifice and the status
of work for nurses. *Journal of Australian Studies,* **67**, 74.

Begany, T. (1994) Your image is brighter than ever. *RN,* **57**, 28.

Buresh, B. & Gordon, S. (1995) Taking on the TV shows. *American Journal of Nursing,* **95**(11),
18–20.

Cheek, J. (1995) Nurses, nursing and representations: An exploration of the effect of viewing
positions on the textual portrayal of nursing. *Nursing Inquiry,* **2**, 235–240.

Clark, G. (1989) To be or not to be – it's time to market nursing's image. In: *Issues in Australian
Nursing 2* (eds G. Gray & R. Pratt), pp. 175–192. Churchill Livingstone, Melbourne.

Darbyshire, P. (1985) Bedpans or broomsticks? *Nursing Times,* **81**, 44–45.

Darbyshire, P. (1995) Reclaiming 'Big Nurse': A feminist critique of Ken Kesey's portrayal of
Nurse Ratched in One Flew Over the Cuckoo's Nest. *Nursing Inquiry,* **2**, 198–202.

Delacour, S. (1991) The construction of nursing: Ideology, discourse and representation. In:
Towards a Discipline of Nursing (eds G. Gray & R. Pratt), pp. 413–433. Churchill Livingstone, Melbourne.

Dunn, A. (1985) Images of nursing in the nursing and popular press. *Bulletin of the Royal College of Nursing (UK) History of Nursing Group*, **6**, 2–8.

Fagin, C. & Diers, D. (1983) Nursing as a metaphor. *The New England Journal of Medicine*, **309**, 116–117.

Fiedler, L. (1988) Images of the nurse in fiction and popular cultures. In: *Images of Nurses: Perspectives from History, Art, and Literature*, (ed. A. Jones), pp. 100–112. University of Pennsylvania Press, Pennsylvania.

Hallam, J. (1998) From angels to handmaidens: Changing constructions of nursing's public image in post-war Britain. *Nursing Inquiry*, **5**, 32–42.

Hektor, L. (1994) Florence Nightingale and the women's movement: Friend or foe? *Nursing Inquiry*, **1**, 38–45.

Holmes, C. (1997) Why we should wash our hands of medical soaps. *Nursing Inquiry*, **4**, 135–137.

Hunter, K. (1988) Nurses: the satiric image and the translocated ideal. In: *Images of Nurses: Perspectives from History, Art, and Literature* (ed. A. Jones), pp. 113–127. University of Pennsylvania Press, Pennsylvania.

Jones, A. (1988) *Images of Nurses: Perspectives from History, Art, and Literature*. University of Pennsylvania Press, Pennsylvania.

Kalisch, B. & Kalisch, P. (1983a) An analysis of the impact of authorship on the image of the nurse presented in novels. *Research in Nursing and Health*, **6**, 17–24.

Kalisch, B. & Kalisch, P. (1983b) Heroine out of focus: Media images of Florence Nightingale. Part 1: Popular biographies and stage productions. *Nursing & Health Care*, **4**, 181–187.

Kalisch, B. & Kalisch, P. (1984) An analysis of news coverage of maternal-child nurses. *Maternal-Child Nursing Journal*, **13**, 77–90.

Kalisch, P. & Kalisch, B. (1987) *The Changing Image of the Nurse*. Addison Wesley, Menlo Park, California.

Kalisch, B., Kalisch, P. & McHugh, M. (1982) The nurse as a sex object in motion pictures. *Research in Nursing & Health*, **5**, 147–154.

Kalisch, P., Kalisch, B. & Scobey, M. (1983) *Images of Nurses on Television*. Springer, New York.

Kampen, N. (1988) Before Florence Nightingale: A prehistory of nursing in painting and sculpture. In: *Images of Nurses: Perspectives from History, Art, and Literature* (ed. A. Jones), pp. 6–39. University of Pennsylvania Press, Pennsylvania.

Kiger, A. (1993) Accord and discord in students' images of nursing. *Journal of Nursing Education*, **32**, 309–317.

Lawler, J. (1991) *Behind the Screens: Nursing, Somology and the Problem of the Body*. Churchill Livingstone, Melbourne.

McCoppin, B. & Gardner, H. (1994) *Tradition & reality: Nursing and politics in Australia*. Churchill Livingstone, Melbourne.

Monahan, B.B. (1996) The nurses media handbook: A reference for nurses planning to meet the media. *Massachusetts Nurse*, **66**(5), 2, 6, 12.

Moore, T. (1991) *Cry of the Damaged Man*. Picador, Sydney.

Muff, J. (1982) Battle-axe, whore: An exploration into the fantasies, myths and stereotypes about nurses. In: *Socialization, Sexism and Stereotyping: Women's Issues In Nursing* (ed. J. Muff). CV Mosby, St Louis.

Rule, J. (1995) Nurses may live to regret the 'angel' image era has ended. (News item) *Nursing Management*, **2**(6), 5.

Salvage, J. (1983) Distorted images. *Nursing Times,* **79**, 13–15.

Selzer, R. (1993) *Raising the dead: A doctor's encounter with his own mortality.* Penguin, Harmondsworth.

Strasen, L. (1992) *The image of professional nursing: Strategies for action.* Lippincott, Philadelphia.

Summers, A. (1997) Sairey Gamp: Generating fact from fiction. *Nursing Inquiry,* **4**, 14–18.

5 Philosophy, Nursing and Knowledge

Steven Edwards

LEARNING OBJECTIVES

Having read and digested this chapter, the reader should be able to:

- think philosophically about the nature of nursing, in particular its ends and the means relevant to achievement of those ends;
- understand the difference between practical and propositional knowledge;
- understand the difference between knowledge and mere belief;
- appreciate the difficulty in knowing whether or not one is actually in possession of knowledge;
- understand the difficulty in obtaining knowledge of when the ends of nursing have been met.

KEY WORDS

KNOWLEDGE, BELIEF, ENDS, MEANS, SCIENTIFIC UNDERSTANDING.

INTRODUCTION

In recent years references to philosophical works in nursing scholarship have increased significantly (see e.g. Kikuchi & Simmons 1992, 1994). Some nurse theorists have even claimed to base their theory of nursing on the work of a particular philosopher or philosophical movement (e.g. Benner & Wrubel 1989; Parse 1998). And the past 15 years or so has seen a regular spate of conferences and publications specifically on what has come to be known as 'philosophy of nursing'. In 1989 an Institute for Philosophical Research in Nursing was established at the University of Alberta, Canada by Professor June Kikuchi and Dr Helen Simmons. More recently, a journal *Nursing Philosophy* has appeared with a specific remit to publish papers within the field known as 'philosophy of nursing'. So it is evident both that there is a good deal of interest in philosophy by nurses, and that a good deal of discussion of a philosophical nature about nursing is engaged in by nurses and non-nurses alike.

DOING PHILOSOPHY

But what is it to discuss or analyse something philosophically? Well, one of the major characteristics of philosophy is to pose and to try to answer the most fundamental and basic questions it is possible to pose. These include: 'what is a good life for a human being?', 'how ought we to live?', 'can I know anything?', 'do I exist?' and numerous others. So a concern with very general, fundamental questions is a key feature of philosophical questioning and inquiry.

Philosophy in nursing

It is natural to ask, now, 'Well, so what? In what way is this kind of questioning relevant to nursing?' Those who engage in discussion of a philosophical nature about nursing tend to pose very basic questions about the nature of nursing. Hence, they ask 'What is nursing? What kind of an activity is it?' (see Chapter 3 in this volume). What is a good nurse? They also ask 'What are the ends of nursing?' in other words, what is it that nurses are trying to do when they perform nursing actions? And it can also be asked what are the means by which nurses achieve the ends of nursing? How are these learned?

A first example: philosophical reflection on the **ends** of nursing

One obvious answer to the question 'What are the ends of nursing? (i.e. what is it that nurses try to do in their work?) is to say that nurses try to make patients 'better'. But thinking philosophically about the question would lead us to press other questions, such as, 'What does being "better" amount to?' Does this simply amount to being 'disease-free'? (Boorse 1975). That is, being in a state such that one's bodily system is purged of pathogenic micro-organisms or lesions?

This doesn't sound a very satisfactory answer since a patient might still complain of feeling ill even if 'disease-free'. Are we then obliged simply to send them packing, saying there is nothing that can be done for them? Also, of course, it is doubtful that anyone is 'disease-free'. We all harbour pathogens most of our lives even if they don't necessarily cause us to feel ill (e.g. one might be a 'carrier' of a virus without being affected or made to feel ill as a result of this).

Also one can ask 'Who is best placed to judge whether a patient is better?' The patient or the nurse? What if the nurse and patient have differing views on what is best for the patient?

Still focusing philosophically on the ends of nursing, one can ask whether it is possible to specify the ends of nursing in 'concrete' terms. For example, it may be claimed that the ends of nursing include the promotion of health, relief of suffering, promotion of well-being and quality of life. These seem plausible candidates for the ends of nursing. But they raise some deep and difficult questions. Just as we could ask who is best placed to judge whether or not a patient is better we can pose the same question in relation to any of the ideas just referred to. In fact it has been surprisingly difficult to articulate clear, widely agreed definitions of these key ideas (see Benner & Wrubel 1989; Fulford 1989; Nordenfelt 1995; Parse 1981; Seedhouse 1986). One is engaging in philosophy of nursing when one is engaged in trying to resolve these key problems.

A second example: reflection on **means**

These last questions have focused on what we have termed the *ends* of nursing, the whole *point* of nursing. But it is just as important to examine philosophically the *means* by which the ends of nursing can be brought about. Suppose it is agreed that the ends of nursing include the relief of suffering. It is then important to gain some view of how the relief of suffering is best achieved.

It seems natural to suggest that a nurse who becomes skilled at bringing about the ends of nursing (e.g. at relieving suffering, at making patients feel well) does so due to the possession and implementation of some kind of knowledge. And also, it seems reasonable to claim that the whole point of nurse education is to provide nursing students with those kinds of knowledge that they will need in order to nurse patients – i.e. to proliferate the ends of nursing. It is plausible to claim that among the things that distinguish the beginning nurse from the expert, experienced nurse, is that the latter possesses and can implement this knowledge and the former does not and cannot. This is of course a theme developed famously by Patricia Benner (1984).

Exactly what kinds of knowledge a nurse needs to possess in order to nurse adequately is an interesting and difficult question. The content of nursing curricula suggests agreement that some kinds of knowledge are essential, e.g. human anatomy and physiology, biology, sociology, psychology and so on. Hence knowledge of relevant aspects of these subject areas is judged necessary in order to be capable of nursing properly. Thus, it is widely held that possession of such knowledge forms part of the means by which the ends of nursing are achieved.

Given that nursing actions seem inevitably to raise *ethical* questions (see Chapter 9 in this volume) it has seemed plausible to some commentators to argue that nursing practice requires ethical knowledge. This is in addition to the empirical knowledge nurses acquire in learning human physiology, psychology, sociology, pathology and so on.

It is also evident that nursing practice requires the development of appropriate *practical* knowledge. Thus it is not enough for a nurse to be able to describe in words how to give an injection, or to dress a wound properly, it is necessary that the nurse can actually perform those activities. And of course it is reasonable to expect that the nurse's education will include opportunities to develop appropriate practical skills in the clinical setting under the supervision of appropriate experts.

In summary, it can be said that nursing practice requires the acquisition and development of at least two kinds of knowledge, propositional and practical. The first is the kind of knowledge learned from books and in the classroom. This is commonly termed 'propositional knowledge'. ('Proposition' is a technical term roughly equivalent to 'sentence'.) Thus in, for example, learning about the history of nursing (see e.g. Chapter 2 in this volume) one comes to learn certain facts that are conveyed in the form of propositions (sentences if you prefer). Clearly many of the kinds of knowledge that nurses need in order to practise can be conveyed and acquired in this manner. Indeed, this is presupposed by the use of textbooks in subjects such as anatomy, pharmacology for nurses, psychology for nurses and so on. So with regard to propositional knowledge, this can be obtained in the classroom, library or home via the reading of books and digesting of lectures, etc. Moreover, the extent to which students grasp appropriate levels of propositional knowledge can be tested in examinations and in discussions.

With regard to practical knowledge, as noted earlier, this cannot be learned simply by reading or by listening to lectures. Again as mentioned above, a person may be able to describe all the steps involved in the performance of a certain procedure and yet still not be able to perform that procedure. It has been argued persuasively, again by Benner (1984), that the kinds of practical knowledge that are necessary for nursing can only really be learned in the clinical context. Thus, even 'practical rooms' within nursing education establishments have a limited value since performing a task in the somewhat artificial environment of such rooms differs significantly from performing a task in the real clinical setting, with real patients watching, and with senior colleagues monitoring one's performance.

It is worth adding too that practical knowledge should not be considered simply to involve the performance of 'motor' tasks such as the giving of injections and dressing wounds in a sterile manner. Such knowledge extends to dealing with colleagues and patients, to being sensitive to the moods and feelings of such groups and to interacting with them appropriately. For example, one nurse may be particularly good at 'defusing' aggressive episodes and another less so. This may be the case even though both nurses are well aware of the relevant literature pertaining to that skill and can both demonstrate their knowledge of it in conversation.

There are some further features of practical knowledge to which it is worth drawing attention. We noted that in the case of propositional knowledge it is relatively easy to point to sources of this – i.e. books, articles, lectures, etc. Also, we noted that it is relatively easy to 'test' whether or not a person has acquired propositional knowledge. Can we identify similar sources and tests for the possession of practical knowledge? Well, as for sources, these will include the expert practitioners we spoke of earlier. By observing a good nurse, and by trying to emulate his or her practice, under the supervision of such a nurse, it is possible for students to develop practical knowledge. Tests for the acquisition of such can then take the form of practical assessments, e.g. can the student give an injection competently, can she or he dress a wound properly. Of course it is much more problematic to assess the kind of practical knowledge manifested in sensitivity to the moods and feelings of others, including moral sensitivity. But let this pass.

Having noted so far that nursing practice seems to presuppose the need for possession of at least two kinds of knowledge (propositional and practical) let us look more closely at the concept of knowledge itself.

KNOWLEDGE, BELIEF AND TRUTH

The idea of nursing knowledge is one that has received a tremendous amount of discussion within nursing scholarship (Benner 1984; Carper 1978; Kikuchi *et al.* 1996; Robinson & Vaughan 1992). There seem at least three reasons for this.

The first is that placing nursing practice on a basis of what is known seems preferable to basing nursing practice on what is merely believed or supposed. If preoperative counselling is known to aid postoperative recovery then nurses might justifiably devote their time to such counselling. But if it is merely believed or supposed that preoperative counselling aids postoperative recovery, then the justification for giving such counselling is weaker: perhaps the nurse's time could be better occupied with interventions that *are* known to help patients.

Relatedly, suppose it is known that a drug is therapeutically effective in relation to a specific illness. Suppose further that the drug has some moderately unpleasant side effects, in spite of its very considerable therapeutic efficacy. Given that the efficacy of the drug is known it is reasonable to judge that a patient suffering from the illness will be prepared to put up with the side effects of the drug, in the knowledge that it will cure her or him. But if the therapeutic efficacy of the drug is merely believed or supposed, then the patient may judge the justification for taking it and putting up with its unpleasant side effects to be much weaker.

So given a choice between basing nursing interventions upon knowledge or belief, it is reasonable to assert that nurses and patients would prefer such interventions to be based upon the former rather than the latter.

A second reason for the interest in nursing knowledge is the view that the articulation of a body of nursing knowledge will contribute very significantly to the articulation of the unique identity of nursing (Parse 1998). Such a body of knowledge might serve to individuate nursing in the way in which, say, astronomy is distinguishable from biology because of the body of knowledge within it.

Third, a further motivation for the focus upon nursing knowledge comes from the educational perspective. If a body of nursing knowledge can be described, then it is this that nursing students will be expected to learn during their nurse education.

But what is it that distinguishes knowledge from mere belief? Well, one answer to this question is that knowledge and belief have importantly differing relations to truth. In explanation of this, consider the following two statements:

(1) Smith knows that the nursing lecture begins at 10.00 am on 26th February 2001.
(2) Smith believes that the nursing lecture begins at 10.00 am on 26th February 2001.

For (1) to be true (i.e. for it to be the case that Smith knows the time of the lecture), it has to be the case that the lecture begins at 10.00 AM. In fact, for any proposition p which is known by someone, it is a necessary condition of their knowing that proposition p is true. (Here we follow the convention of using 'p' to stand for the proposition known or believed.) So the relationship between Smith and what is known is such that Smith only knows something if what Smith knows is in fact true.

Contrast this with (2). In relation to belief there is no such relationship between what is believed and Smith's believing it. It can be true that Smith *believes* the lecture begins at 10.00 AM whether or not it does actually begin then. In fact, it can be true that Smith believes anything, however bizarre, without it being the case that what Smith believes is true. Smith might believe pigs give birth to human babies, and though it may be true that Smith believes this, it does not follow that pigs do in fact give birth to human babies. But for it to be true that Smith *knows* that pigs give birth to human babies, it would have to be the case that they did.

Hopefully, then, the claim that knowledge is necessarily related to truth whilst belief is not is now understood. This helps account for a preference for knowledge over belief. For if we do genuinely know something, then what we know must be true. And for obvious reasons we would rather ground our decisions on what really is true rather than on what simply is believed to be true.

An important consequence

This view of the relationship between knowledge and truth has a rather important consequence, one that is of particular significance to the nursing context. Kikuchi *et al.* (1996:12) point with disapproval to the emergence within nursing of a specific view of the relationship between knowledge and truth in which knowledge and belief are conflated. In such a view, it is held that if a person believes something is the case, then what they believe is true. An important flaw in such views – in which belief is taken to be sufficient for knowledge – is worth setting out explicitly here.

Consider the two statements (3) and (4) below:

(3) Smith knows that the nursing lecture begins at 10.00 am on 26th February 2001.

(4) Jones knows that the nursing lecture begins at 10.30 am on 26th February 2001.

Assume Smith and Jones are thinking of the same lecture. Given the necessary relationship between knowledge and truth it follows that Smith and Jones cannot *both* know the time of the lecture. One of them (at least) must be mistaken. Either the lecture starts at 10.00 AM or 10.30 AM or some other time. What cannot be true is that the lecture both starts at 10.00 AM and also that it starts at 10.30 AM. For the truth of one of these logically excludes the possibility that the other is true. The reason why this truism is spelt out so pedantically here is as follows.

The trend in nursing scholarship to which Kikuchi and Simmons refer is one according to which believing that *p* is true, is sufficient for knowing that *p* is true. This leads to a position in which if A believes/knows the lecture begins at 10.00 AM then it is claimed to be 'true for A' that the lecture begins at 10.00 AM. Hence, if B believes/knows the lecture begins at 10.30 AM it is similarly claimed to be 'true for B' that the lecture begins at 10.30 AM.

It does not take long to see that such views are highly problematic, even untenable. For example how would communication be possible? One could never suppose any agreed standards or spatiotemporal co-ordinates. Suppose A and B decide to meet up for coffee. A says to B 'I'll meet you at 6.00 PM in the hospital café'. B is there promptly at 6.00 PM. A does not show up. B sees A the next day and asks why he didn't make their meeting. A responds: 'It may be true for you that I failed to show up, but it is true for me that I did and that you did not in fact turn up for our planned meeting'.

Such a response is legitimate in the view which conflates knowledge and belief. It would be possible to construct much more serious examples if the application of such a view of knowledge is applied to the nursing context. For example, it may be 'true for' nurse A that he has fed a patient, but 'true for' the patient that he has not been fed. So the general proposal is being made here that the position in which believing is sufficient for knowing is not in fact a very plausible one, and that its implementation in practice would have disastrous consequences.

Having made these observations concerning the differences between knowledge and belief, it is important to stress that it is extraordinarily problematic to discern whether or not one is in possession of knowledge or mere belief, especially with reference to scientific hypotheses and theories. I will give three examples to show this.

The first example is taken from the history of natural science. Prior to the fifteenth century it was generally believed that the earth was stationary and that the sun, moon and planets rotated around the earth. (The view can be found in Aristotle's *On the heavens*, bk. 2, ch. 12.) A rival Copernican system was proposed in the sixteenth century according to which the earth was not stationary but rotated around the sun. Adherents to the older Aristotelean view devised a 'test' situation. Defenders of the older view reasoned thus: if the earth really is in motion such that it completes a full rotation in 24 hours, then it must be moving pretty rapidly. Hence a stone dropped from a high tower will land some distance from the foot of the tower (since the tower will continue to move together with the surface of the earth). But since such a dropped stone is always found to fall at the foot of the tower from which it is dropped, defenders of the older view concluded that the newer Copernican view must be false. (See, e.g. Feyerabend 1975 for a discussion of the 'tower argument'.)

Thus defenders of the older view may continue to maintain (falsely) they know that the earth is stationary, having performed this test of the rival view. And of course they may simply point to 'common sense' as further evidence in support of the older view. Think to yourself, does it *really* seem likely that the earth on which you are currently sitting/standing is spinning around at thousands of miles per hour?

Of course, the view that the earth is spinning is now scientific orthodoxy. And this would likely be said to constitute scientific knowledge. But the history of science is one in which theories tend to be upheld for a time and then overturned. Each generation of scientists thinks their own theory is the correct one, only for this to be rejected later by later generations (see, e.g. Kuhn 1970).

A second example illustrating the same point as the 'tower argument' concerns a hypothesis regarding the cause of gastric ulcers. The hypothesis that such ulcers had a bacterial cause was resisted for years on the grounds that it conflicted with the (then) widely accepted view that the stomach is a sterile area within which such bacteria could not survive. But this view was later overturned and the hypothesis of a bacterial cause for gastric ulcers was later accepted (see Thagard 1998). So here a hypothesis (that ulcers have a bacterial cause) was rejected because it conflicted with a belief thought to amount to knowledge – that the stomach is a sterile area and therefore bacteria cannot survive in it long enough to cause ulceration.

A third and last example is from the nursing context. Apparently, it was widely believed that egg-white and oxygen applied four-hourly to pressure areas helps prevent pressure sores. A test situation for this would seem to involve not applying the egg-white and oxygen and observing the consequences of this. The patient is left unmoved and, sure enough, a pressure sore develops. Hence the 'egg-white and oxygen' hypothesis is confirmed. But of course the reasoning behind this 'test' is completely spurious. For it may be that the absence of pressure sores in patients subjected to the egg-white and oxygen regime is due to some other factor – such as the regular turning and massage of pressure areas during the process of application of the regime.

What these examples show is that hypotheses are tested against a background of other beliefs which are presumed erroneously to be true, to constitute knowledge. And a hypothesis might be rejected for spurious reasons. These examples suggest that we should regard beliefs we currently hold with a degree of modesty. For they may later turn out to be false. And we should be aware that test situations devised to confirm or falsify newer hypotheses may be rejected on spurious grounds. For the test situation we construct may simply 'load the dice' in favour of currently accepted theory (think of the tower argument again here). The examples also show us that it is difficult to know when we can be confident that we truly *know* something. For, especially with reference to scientific knowledge, this is subject to regular revision and change. Given what we said about the difference between knowledge and belief earlier we know it cannot be accurate to say that it is known both that the earth moves and that it is stationary. One (or both!?) of these must be false, must only have been believed and not known.

Ends again

The problems just identified concern the kind of knowledge recruited as part of the means to bring about the ends of nursing. The examples suggest we should not be overly confident about what we currently take to be knowledge. Hence we should be prepared to revise our view of specific knowledge claims currently considered necessary for achieving the ends of nursing. However, there are also problems in applying the idea of knowledge to the ends of nursing – especially scientific knowledge.

Philosopher Bryan Magee writes, 'To be publicly acknowledged source-material for a scientific understanding of anything, experiences need to be inter-subjectively available' (1997:486).

His point is roughly this. For any phenomena to be amenable to scientific study it is necessary that they be 'inter-subjectively available'; that is, they be accessible from the third person perspective. Hence, the colour of one's eyes, skin, one's weight, blood chemistry and so on all count as inter-subjectively available. But one's thoughts and feelings are not. They, it seems, are privately accessible. At least, they are accessible to each one of us in a way that differs fundamentally from the way in which they are accessible to anyone else. On Magee's view, it follows that they cannot be studied scientifically.

Magee's view presents something of a challenge to the view that we can know when the ends of nursing have been met. For in nursing we are most concerned to relieve pain, suffering, promote well-being and so on. All these states have a 'private' inner aspect to them which is not 'inter-subjectively available'.

Of course, it may be argued that certain inter-subjectively available states can be correlated with these private states, such as pain and suffering. For example, it may be noted that increased blood pressure, pulse rate and certain neuronal changes correlate with intense pain. But of course the blood pressure, the pulse rate, the neuronal changes are not the pain. That remains only privately accessible. So in correlating physical changes with mental experiences such as pain it is not clear that we are subjecting pain to scientific study.

So Magee would be correct to claim that the mental experiences *themselves* are not inter-subjectively available. As such it seems difficult to be sure we have knowledge that the ends of nursing have been met. Of course, though, we can make judgements about this. And good sources of evidence would seem to be the patient's own opinion, and the patient's 'outer' appearance (is the patient grimacing, looking anxious, etc.). Thus although Magee's claim gives us grounds to be cautious about the extent to which we can claim to know whether or not the ends of nursing have been met, there are sources of evidence we can resort to in order to make informed judgements about this.

CONCLUSION

In this very short chapter it is only possible to give a brief snapshot of what is involved in bringing philosophical reflection to bear on nursing. In the early part of the chapter we saw something of the flavour of philosophical questioning: it is questioning directed at very basic presuppositions. We then began to apply such questioning more systematically to nursing. This involved focusing on ends and means. Since the means by which nurses achieve the ends of nursing includes at least two forms of knowledge, propositional and practical, we looked briefly at the distinction between them. Then we focused more narrowly on the ideas of knowledge, belief and truth. In doing so we noted difficulties that can arise in being sure that one is actually in possession of knowledge rather than belief. And we highlighted the danger in not giving newer hypotheses (knowledge claims) a fair chance due to their conflicting with beliefs we assume to have the status of knowledge. Finally, we returned briefly to reconsider the ends of nursing and we noted the difficulty of subjecting these to scientific scrutiny.

REFLECTIVE QUESTIONS

(1) What is it to think philosophically about nursing?
(2) What is the difference (if any) between knowledge and belief?
(3) How can I know whether or not I know anything?

RECOMMENDED READING

Edwards, S.D. (ed.) (1998) *Philosophical Issues in Nursing.* Macmillan, London.
Edwards, S.D. (2001) *Philosophy of Nursing: An Introduction.* Palgrave, Basingstoke.
Reed J. & Ground, I. (1997) *Philosophy for Nursing.* Arnold, London.
Polifroni, E.C. & Welch, M. (eds) (1999) *Perspectives on Philosophy of Science in Nursing.* Lippincott, New York.
Seedhouse, D. (2001) *Practical Nursing Philosophy.* Wiley, Chichester.

REFERENCES

Benner, P. (1984) *From Novice to Expert: Excellence and Power in Clinical Nursing Practice.* Addison-Wesley, Menlo Park, California.
Benner, P. & Wrubel J. (1989) *The Primacy of Caring: Stress and Coping in Health and Illness.* Addison-Wesley, Menlo Park, California.
Boorse, C. (1975) On the distinction between disease and illness. *Philosophy and Public Affair,* **5**(1), 49–68.

Carper, B.A. (1978) Fundamental patterns of knowing in nursing. *Advances in Nursing Science*, **1**(1), 13–23.

Feyerabend, P. (1975) *Against Method*. Verso, London.

Fulford, K.W.M. (1989) *Moral Theory and Medical Practice*. Cambridge University Press, Cambridge.

Kikuchi, J.F. & Simmons, H. (eds) (1992) *Philosophic Inquiry in Nursing*. Sage, London.

Kikuchi, J.F. & Simmons, H. (eds) (1994) *Developing a Philosophy of Nursing*. Sage, London.

Kikuchi, J.F., Simmons, H. & Romyn, D. (eds) (1996) *Truth in Nursing Inquiry*. Sage, London.

Kuhn, T.S. (1970) *The Structure of Scientific Revolutions*, 2nd edn. University of Chicago Press, Chicago.

Magee, B. (1997) *Confessions of a Philosopher*. Phoenix, London.

Nordenfelt, L. (1995) *On the Nature of Health: An Action Theoretic Approach*. Kluwer, Dordrecht.

Parse, R.R. (1981) *Man-Living-Health: A Theory of Nursing*. Wiley, New York.

Parse, R.R. (1998) *The Human Becoming School of Thought*. Sage, London.

Robinson, K. & Vaughan, B. (eds) (1992) *Knowledge for Nursing Practice*. Butterworth-Heinemann, Oxford.

Seedhouse, D. (1986) *Health: The Foundations for Achievement*. Wiley, Chichester.

Thagard, P. (1998) Ulcers and bacteria I: Discovery and acceptance. *Studies in History, Biology and Biomedical Science*, **29**(1), 107–136.

6 The Caring Conundrum
Should Caring be the Basis of Nursing Practice and Scholarship?

Debra Jackson and Sally Borbasi

LEARNING OBJECTIVES

This chapter will:

- introduce caring as a professional concept;
- differentiate professional and informal caring;
- explore issues related to care and cure;
- discuss perceptions of nurse caring behaviours from the perspective of patients and nurses;
- explore some problems that might occur if caring formed the basis of the discipline of nursing;
- contemplate threats to nurse caring.

KEY WORDS

CARING, CARE CURE DEBATE, WHOLISM, TECHNICAL COMPETENCE, INFORMAL CARING, PROFESSIONAL CARING.

INTRODUCTION

Contemporary nursing has increasingly identified the concept of caring as central to the theory and practice of nurses. At the theoretical level the concept is considered a major one in the worldview (nursing ontology) of the profession. In nursing knowledge development processes (nursing epistemology) caring is also held to be a core concept and concern. Caring is proposed as the characteristic that distinguishes nursing, and sets it apart from other health-related activities, and the desire to 'care', or help people remains a strong motivator for choosing a nursing career (Caffrey & Caffrey 1994; Sullivan & Deane 1994; Wilkes & Wallis 1993). Although it may be argued a caring perspective is not unique to nursing (Caffrey & Caffrey 1994; Peter & Gallop 1994), it is almost universally accepted within the profession that nursing has an imperative to care for the health of individuals, families and communities, and many believe the care given by nurses has the potential to restore health (Benner *et al.* 1999; Williams 1997; Wolf *et al.* 1994).

Indeed, the caring imperative of nursing is reflected in the many definitions and perspectives of nursing that proclaim caring as inherent and central to the nursing role (see for example: Benner 1984; Leininger 1984; Rawnsley 1990; Swanson 1993; Watson 1988). Swanson (1993:352–357), for example, proposes nursing as 'informed caring for the well-being of others'. Yet caring remains a nebulous concept (Astrom *et al.* 1995; Morse *et al.* 1990), although it has been defined in broad or general (i.e. generic) terms. *The Macquarie Dictionary* (Delbridge *et al.* 1991:274) defines caring as 'worry, attention, concern, serious attention, solicitude, protection, charge, [to be] the object of concern or attention, [to be] troubled or affected emotionally, [to be] concerned or solicitous, [to have a] fondness or affection for …'. Caring then, would seem to be a personal, and potentially intimate activity, which would, at first glance, seem to be difficult to achieve within a professional context where, as Taylor (1994: 234) suggests, 'nurses and patients are thrown together in random couplings'. However, when used professionally, care cannot be oversimplified. Caring is a complex, multidimensional concept (i.e. one comprised of many facets), and 'has been postulated to be a philosophy and science, an ethic, an interactive set of client expectations and nursing behaviours, expert nursing practice, the hidden work of nursing and a synonym for nursing itself' (Rawnsley 1990:42).

DEFINING NURSE CARING

According to Sullivan and Deane (1994), nurse caring prizes human relationships, and is informed by principles of sharing, sincerity, concern and moderation. Wolf *et al.* (1994:107) propose that nurse caring has several tangible dimensions, including 'respectful deference to others, assurance of human presence, positive connectedness, professional knowledge and skill, and attentiveness to the other's experience'. Pepin (1992) suggests caring may be considered to have two dimensions – love and labour. Love is said to consist of affective (that is, pertaining to feelings) concepts such as altruism, compassion, emotion, presence, connectedness, nurturance and comfort, and it is this aspect of caring that has dominated the nursing literature (Pepin 1992). Labour refers to the element of care related to toil and service and encompasses roles, functions, knowledge and tasks. This dimension of caring has received much less attention in the nursing literature (Pepin 1992).

Several theories of nursing have been developed from the standpoint of defining and describing caring practices. Leininger (1986) believes caring is the essence of nursing but dismisses the idea of nurses' care motivated by a sense of duty. Rather, she considers caring as learned because it is an integral part of cultural life. However, factors within various cultures may either curtail or facilitate the use of care knowledge by nurses. Watson (1985) writes of a science (and practice) of caring, and draws upon phenomenological, existential and spiritual concepts to ground these theories. Along with Astrom *et al.* (1995), Watson (1985) sees caring as the ethical and moral ideal of nursing that has humanistic and interpersonal qualities, and believes nursing as art is 'lived, expressed and co-created in the caring moment' (1994:xvii). Walters (1994:3) also links caring with art – he sees caring as an 'aesthetic activity', that is, activity associated with the artistic aspects of nursing (and its creative expression), something that is not easily captured in words.

Pearson (1991:199) describes the broad, global human concept of caring as 'investing oneself in the experience of another sufficiently enough to become a participant in that person's experience', and goes on to discuss the historical imperatives that have seen care devalued. He urges nurses to reclaim caring as a central concept that does make a difference to outcomes for patients. Wolf *et al.* (1994) propose caring as an aspect of nursing work that is invisible and may not be recognised except when the actions and attitudes that compose caring are not in evidence.

In a content analysis of nursing literature, Morse *et al.* (1990) identify five main views on the nature of caring. These, they propose, are 'caring as a human trait, caring as a moral imperative or ideal, caring as an affect, caring as an interpersonal relationship, and caring as a therapeutic intervention' (Morse *et al.* 1990:3). Additionally, they found some nurses described caring from an outcomes perspective, and these were described as: caring as a subjective (patient) experience, and caring as a physical (patient) response (Morse *et al.* 1990). These authors conclude the concept of caring is ill-defined, and suggest if nursing is to continue to propose caring as the essence and philosophical base of nursing, further exploration of caring as a concept is required.

Feminist and nurse, Falk Rafael (1996:3–17), suggests caring may be considered either 'ordered caring', 'assimilated caring', or 'empowered caring' (p. 4). Ordered caring she proposes as problematic for nurses because is about merely following orders; 'it allows only a severely limited scope of caring, one that is devoid of knowledge, power or ethics' (Falk Rafael 1996:11). To illustrate this point, she draws on the example of the kindness and gentleness shown by nurses toward psychiatric patients as they were led towards the Nazi gas chambers. Assimilated caring is described as a form of caring in which the feminine construct of caring is grounded in (male) scientific discourses. This appropriation of a male construct is proposed as giving legitimacy to the essentially female activity of caring. Empowered caring, Falk Rafael positions as the most desirable and effective form of caring. This form of caring is grounded within a feminist perspective, and involves the use of power, knowledge and ethics. Falk Rafael (1996) proposes the acronym of CARE (Credentials, Association, Research, Expertise) to encapsulate the elements of this empowered caring.

Williams (1997) names holistic caring as a form of nurse caring, and proposes this as a global concept with four dimensions. These she calls physical caring, interpretive caring, spiritual caring and sensitive caring (Williams 1997). Holism is of course viewed as a concept crucial to the effective practice of nursing, and is the term used to describe the belief a 'patient is a person with social, physical, mental, and spiritual components' (Williams 1997:61–62). Holism is positioned as central to notions of professional caring, and is so intrinsic to this, it is often taken for granted – viewed as a 'given', and therefore often not described or examined in discussions on professional caring. The use of a holistic perspective is said to facilitate an ethos that recognises the uniqueness and value inherent in individuals, and allows for the provision of individualised nursing care.

Differentiating professional and informal caring

The importance placed on the concept of caring has seen many attempts by nurses to construct the notion of 'professional caring' – to turn what is essentially a subjective, intimate and personal construct into one which is professional, objective and able to be readily achieved between strangers. For no matter how desirable it may be to position caring as the essence of nursing, there is an inherent difficulty with reconstructing caring so as to make it a professional characteristic somehow unique to nursing and nurses, rather than an attribute intrinsic to human existence, and therefore not unique to, or especially connected with, nursing (Morse *et al.* 1990; Rawnsley 1990; Webb 1996).

Of course, to support the assertion caring is the essence of nursing, nursing needs to be able to reconstruct caring as a professional characteristic, that is somehow different and superior to amateur, or informal caring, and this has remained a challenge for nurses. In an exploration of women's caring in personal and family situations, Wuest (1997) interviewed 21 women from diverse social backgrounds, all of whom were involved in one form or another of informal caring. Wuest found that, for these women, caring behaviour consisted of 'connectedness, availability and responsibility', and 'caring connections were maintained through acts of nurturance, attending and being with' (Wuest 1997:51). These findings have similarities to the constructions of professional caring held by nurses (see, for example, Swanson 1993), suggesting that caring in and of itself is not unique to nurses. Rather, as suggested by Falk Raphael (1996), the knowledge and particular skills held by nurses permits a particular type of caring that complements and supports the informal caring given by carers in the community, who have a personal relationship with recipients of care.

Nurse caring behaviours

Defining caring as a concept central to nursing is not only important for the profession but is relevant to patients, yet patients are rarely included in these discussions (Webb 1996). Nevertheless, if nurses claim they are caring professionals, they are obliged to find out what nurse caring means to patients, and how nurses can demonstrate care for patients (Larsson *et al.* 1998). A review of the literature reveals patients' views of professional caring may be very different from those proposed by nurses, with nurses often (but not always) embracing psychosocial models of caring, while studies of patients often (but not always) suggest that patients value caring that is more technical or task-orientated in nature.

However, findings from a phenomenological study that explored patients' experiences of being nursed, suggest nurses can deliver care in a manner described as 'detachment' or 'engagement' with the recipients of that care (Kralik *et al.* 1997). The theme of engagement captured psychosocial qualities such as compassion, kindness, cheerfulness, availability, gentleness and friendliness, while detachment reflected negative characteristics such as feeling depersonalised by nurses and being treated roughly by nurses. Findings of this study are particularly interesting because, though nursing is examined from the perspective of patients, it shows consistencies between patients' views and ideas about nurse caring, and those held by nurses. In a pilot study, Dyson (1996) aimed to elicit constructions of behaviours and attitudes that embody caring, from the perspectives of registered nurses. Findings revealed nurses in the study conceptualised caring as essentially an interpersonal construct. They identified attributes such as kindness, friendliness, sensitivity, consideration, giving of self, honesty, sincerity, and expertise as evidence of caring attitudes and behaviours (Dyson 1996). Similarly, Wolf (1986) describes nurse-identified caring behaviours as attentive listening, comforting, honesty and so on. A study of patients and nurses, aimed at exploring their perceptions of the importance of caring behaviours, revealed significant differences between the views of patients and nurses, with nurses placing a higher value on the emotional affective aspects of caring (Larsson *et al.* 1998).

Greenhalgh *et al.* (1998) explored caring behaviours with hospital nurses and found physical caring behaviours such as 'monitoring' were ranked much higher than aspects of caring such as 'trusting relationships', which could be considered to be affective or psychosocial in nature. Webb (1996) describes studies in which nurses and patients' perceptions of caring were sought. Again, nurses judged the interpersonal aspects of their work as more caring, and yet the patients valued technical know-how and clinical competence above interpersonal dimensions of caring. From these studies it was concluded, because their physical needs had primacy, patients could not focus on aspects other than physical/technical care, whereas for the nurses, clinical competence was taken for granted. Webb's (1996) review indicated that patients consistently value care that is technically competent and tangible in nature; she cautions nurses against placing too much emphasis on the psychological elements of care, and neglecting physical or technical aspects of care.

The differences in perceptions of caring between nurses and patients warrant consideration. In Western industrialised societies, technological skills and expertise are viewed as high status, and the domain of 'professionals'. In times of vulnerability, such as when people are ill, they like to be assured they are in the care of competent health professionals, and perhaps view technological proficiency as evidence of such competence and expertise. The interpersonal aspects of caring so highly idealised by nurses may be viewed by patients as 'nonprofessional' caring – the type of caring available to them within their own social worlds, and not something they necessarily seek within a context of professional caring. As Pepin (1992) states, the caring that occurs at home, differs from that occurring in institutions (such as hospitals), and is mainly affective. Similarly, from the perspective of nurses, it has been suggested nurses perceive clinical competence as a given, and thus do not regard it as an indicator of nurse caring (Webb 1996).

CARE AND CURE

Rapid developments in medical science, nursing knowledge and related health technologies have acted to improve dramatically patient outcomes. In most parts of the world, these same technologies have radically and permanently changed the face of nursing (Jackson 1995; Pepin 1992; Sandelowski 1997), and this has been the catalyst for a discussion in nursing and health, that has become known as the 'care/cure' debate (see for example: Johnston & Cooper 1997; King & Norsen 1994; Leftwich 1993; Webb 1996). Johnston and Cooper (1997) suggest the health care system in the United States was designed to cure illness and disease, rather than care for people and their health. This is the case for many Western health care systems, and provides a challenge for those whose main imperative is to care.

Clearly, caring alone will not meet all the health needs patients have but, as Webb (1996) points out, curing strategies may be insufficient unless accompanied by a caring dimension. Similarly, Morse *et al.* (1990:11) pose the question, 'can a cure be realised without caring?' Williams (1997) also suggests caring is, in itself, essential to cure. She proposes that caring nurse behaviours have been demonstrated to have positive effects in terms of patients' wellness and, conversely, noncaring behaviours by nurses have been shown to negatively affect patient well-being and recovery.

Notions of care and cure have been constructed as binary and oppositional, however, it is the contention of several scholars that these two concepts are not truly antagonistic (see for example: King & Norsen 1994; Leftwich 1993). The differences between the roles of nurse and physician are often centred around ideas of the nurse as caring and the physician as curing. Sullivan and Deane (1994; similarly, Caffrey & Caffrey 1994) suggest caring (as nursing) is viewed as a traditionally feminine activity, and has not been conferred the power and status of male-defined activities, to which the physician/curer may more easily lay claim.

Florence Nightingale may well have rejected the idea nurses have an essential curing role. In her book *Notes on Nursing* (1859/1946:74), she states 'nature alone cures', but goes on to say 'what nursing has to do is to put the patient in the best position for nature to act upon him [sic]' (Nightingale 1859/1946:75). More recently, in defining professional caring, nurses identify elements of both caring and curing, and certain science-based skills and knowledge are highly valued as essential to caring (Beare & Meyers 1994; Carper 1978; Wolf *et al.* 1994). Furthermore, patients themselves expect nurses to have a high level of professional proficiency and technical skill, which are associated with 'cure', and as previously discussed, these are constructed as key aspects of professional caring (Borbasi 1996; Ray 1987; Wolf *et al.* 1994).

King and Norsen (1994) contend that notions of 'care/cure' as solely the domain of either nurse (care) or physician (cure) are not helpful nor acceptable, as nurses and physicians have both curing and caring dimensions to their practice areas (similarly Leftwich 1993). Holden (1991) also takes issue with nursing's propensity to distinguish between the caring role of the nurse and the curing role of the doctor, believing each encompasses aspects of the other. In a similar vein, Webb (1996) urges nurses to overcome the cure/care dichotomy between medicine and nursing and argues it is no longer important to distinguish the care given by specific professional groups but to focus instead on establishing clear goals of care. Rather than regarding notions of care and cure as being polarised or at opposite extremes then, it is more accurate to say the notions of care/cure are compatible and complementary. Both are acknowledged and accepted as key aspects of nursing's agenda, and both are reflected in the theories of professional caring constructed by nurses (Beare & Meyers 1994; Wolf *et al.* 1994).

CARING AS THE BASIS OF THE DISCIPLINE OF NURSING

Far from being a simple concept, caring is revealed as complex and multidimensional. It is also controversial, for amongst members of the profession, the debate continues about the centrality of caring to nursing (Dyson 1996). There are conflicting trains of thought and these challenge the relevance of caring as a foundational aspect of nursing. Lea *et al.* (1998:663) suggest that the difficulty in defining the relationship between caring and nursing arises (in part) because 'caring and nursing [both] defy precise description'. In a philosophical critique, Walker (1995) discusses the problem of nurses' attempts to represent nursing as both a discourse of science and a discourse of caring in contemporary thought. Macdonald (1993) suggests that concepts of caring as they now stand are unrealistic, as carers are unable to maintain the level of caring expected from such theories. Moreover, the question of whether caring is actually consistent with the issue/s of power and/or professionalisation in nursing is increasingly being addressed. Although caring is universally acknowledged as necessary and beneficial, it is in conflict with notions of autonomy. Because caring is considered central to their practice, and is perceived as inconsistent with notions of power, nurses as women have been reluctant to acknowledge that power is productive. Though attempts have been made to combine the two (Benner 1984), there exists some natural friction between the concepts of power and caring (Falk Rafael 1996).

Tensions between the concepts of caring and empowerment in relationships between patients and nurses are especially salient. For example, how does the caring professional avoid the cries of paternalism that come with clinical decisions about what is 'best' for the patient (Malin & Teasdale 1991)? Altruism is associated with caring (Pepin 1992) and it is also problematic because it implies self-sacrifice. Searching for a way to forge a link between altruism and autonomy, Reverby (1987: 10) contends that nurses seek to be allowed to have 'caring with autonomy'. Kitson (1987) argues that if nurses choose to align themselves with care rather than cure, with the nurturing processes rather than with technology and treatment, then they will need to identify how to organise and put into operation those skills they possess. Successful execution of the caring role is, she believes, 'intimately bound up with having the necessary space to practice, sufficient room to manoeuvre and to be able to explore new areas of knowledge and expertise' (p. 324). Dunlop (1986) questions whether a science of caring is possible and resolves that, if it is, it will have to take a hermeneutical form (i.e. based on hermeneutics) – a 'form that in many ways does violence to our traditional ideas of science', but one that 'challenges the male hegemony of science' (p. 669).

The emergence of differing perspectives about the nature of nursing has not been without debate, and there are nurses who believe that an emphasis on alliance to concepts such as caring and holism, with their attendant rejection of the natural sciences, will do more harm than good to nursing's attempts to become a credible academic discipline, and to the process of professionalisation. Meeting the demands of the caring imperative concerned with cure requires that nurses have considerable specialist knowledge of a range of scientific disciplines such as pharmacology, anatomy, physiology, biochemistry, immunology, microbiology and physics. A sound scientific knowledge base is undeniably essential for nursing, given the need for continued development of the discipline and the need to meet the demands of increasingly technological societies; none would argue that competency in the scientific disciplines is not an essential aspect of nursing knowledge and integral to the caring imperative claimed by nursing.

THREATS TO CARING

The concept of caring is inherently incompatible with the underlying objectives of many of the organisational structures in which nurses find themselves. In many parts of the (Western) world, health care is not intrinsically altruistic; nor is it based on any real system of equity (Duffield & Lumby 1994). Rather, health care tends to be resourced on a fee-for-service basis, and access to health care services is therefore linked very strongly with an individual's ability to pay for such services. In many instances health care is looked at with entrepreneurial, rather than philanthropic eyes. To investors, provision of health care services may represent an opportunity for profit, and even 'whilst appropriating the language and images of nursing for business purposes, many entrepreneurs treat professional nursing care as a commodity to be whittled away until it becomes impotent' (Jackson & Raftos 1997:38). This positioning of the wealth of an individual as a major indicator for allocation of (increasingly scarce) health resources is, by its very nature, incompatible with nursing's caring imperative, which places a high value on the individual (Chinn 1989; Morse *et al.* 1990; Williams 1997).

Indeed, faced with a future health care system which 'not only cares more about economics than health but which is structured in such a way as to reflect social inequalities' (Kenway & Watkins 1994:44), nursing has undoubtedly much exploration and debate still ahead of it in terms of the epistemological tenets it will use to ground its efforts to gain equal footing with other professionals in the health care arena. Furthermore, care is likely viewed by nurses as a resource to be allocated on the basis of need rather than ability to pay. These tensions are inherent to the working life of many nurses, and compromise the ability of nurses to provide care in the way idealised by the profession.

Although nurses undoubtedly comprise the largest occupational/professional group within the health care system, the system itself is based on a set of values that directly challenge and compromise the very essence of nursing. The health care system is shaped by economic influences such as cost containment and profit margins, and this economic impetus has been the catalyst for re-examining the whole concept of 'patient care'. Attempts have been made to reconceptualise traditional care delivery, to come up with ways of doing more with less resources (Caplan & Brown 1997; Johnston & Cooper 1997; Ray 1989). These new approaches in provision of care are sometimes presented as strategies to improve patient care but, as Williams (1997) suggests, frequently they are more concerned with institutional cost-saving, than on quality patient care (similarly Duffield & Lumby 1994).

This key philosophical difference between nursing's caring imperative and the underlying ethos of many (Western) health care systems, throws nurses and health administrators into a permanent state of possible conflict, and has the potential to become a source of professional tension for nurses (Jackson & Raftos 1997; Johnston & Cooper 1997; Kralik *et al.* 1997). Large, impersonal institutions may, by their very nature, devalue caring by providing little incentive or opportunity for nurses to demonstrate behaviours associated with caring, or failing to provide an environment where caring can be expressed (Morse *et al.* 1990). Ray (1989) has attempted to reconcile the seemingly irreconcilable by proposing a theory of caring compatible with the bureaucratic cultures existing within large organisations. She suggests it is essential the discipline of nursing come to terms with the corporatisation of health care, and goes on to indicate that a failure to do this would be disastrous for nursing.

> The transformation of American and other western health care systems to corporate enterprises emphasizing competitive management and economic gain seriously challenges nursing's humanistic philosophies and theories and nursing's administrative and clinical practices. The recent refocusing of nursing as a human science and the art and science of human caring places nursing in a vulnerable position. When pitted against the new goal of corporate advancement in health care delivery, nursing faces a loss of self-identity and an increased risk of alienation and confusion in this competitive arena.
>
> Ray (1989:31)

Using a grounded theory approach, Ray generated a 'theory of the dynamic structure of caring in a complex organization' (Ray 1989:31), and proposes this as a means by which nurses can practise within bureaucratic health structures without compromising nursing's caring imperative. This theory proposes several 'structural caring categories', which Ray names as political, economic, legal, technological/physiological, educational, social, spiritual/religious, and ethical (Ray 1989). However, Caffrey and Caffrey (1994) suggest that caring will never be accommodated as a core value while profit remains a primary motive of health care systems.

The truth of this statement is evident in a paper exploring the experience of whistle-blowers, registered nurses who attempted to challenge managerial practices that severely compromised the standard of care provided to residents of a long-term care institution (Jackson & Raftos 1997). These nurses described the struggle to maintain their professional integrity by ensuring adequate levels of care, and how they were thwarted in these attempts by the management. The nurses were prevented from providing adequate care by forces external to nursing – forces driven by an economic (rather than a caring) agenda. This suggests that, certainly in some settings, nurses have not yet achieved the level of autonomy necessary for the provision of acceptable and approved standards of professional care.

CONCLUSION

Caring is proclaimed and understood as the basis of modern nursing, and nurses have produced vast amounts of literature on aspects of care and caring, and how they may be applied in a nursing context. However, while the concept of professional caring is difficult to articulate, it is recognised as being a complex concept involving the development of a range of knowledge, skills and expertise. Professional caring has similarities with nonprofessional, or informal caring and applies knowledge derived from various discipline areas to promote the health and well-being of people.

The major perspectives of caring recognise the importance of various types of knowledge and, with few exceptions, all allude to the expressive, artistic and scientific perspectives said to construct nursing. Other common themes that characterise the constructions of caring adopted by nurses are holism, compassion, empathy and communication. Evidence suggests that patients too, view caring as a perceptible concept, and highly value it as an essential and healing aspect of their professional encounters with nurses. However, in contrast to the ways nurses view caring, reflection on what is known about patients' attitudes to nurse caring suggests that, above all, patients want a nurse who demonstrates caring through clinical and technical competence, as well as through interpersonal skills.

Accepting caring as the basis of nursing practice and scholarship is not without problems. Issues of autonomy and power are ill at ease with the concept of caring. Servitude and altruism are intrinsically linked to caring, and these do not sit well with nursing's move to professionalism. Many nurses work within organisational structures whose primary motivation lies with the cost containment or the accumulation of wealth rather than a mandate to heal – these economic factors may compromise or even be antithetical to nursing's imperative to care. The caring imperative, therefore, represents a potential source of stress and occupational conflict for nurses. While it is argued that the need for nursing to place caring as a central concept has never been greater, there are concerns that the caring components of nursing are deemed unsophisticated and hence inferior to the therapeutic interventions of medicine and other allied health service providers.

Despite the many creative theories of nurse caring, the tasks of establishing coherent and clear connections between caring and notions such as professionalism, scholarship and autonomy remain incomplete. Nurses are left with many issues to consider and debate. The conundrum of caring as the basis of nursing practice and scholarship will no doubt continue to captivate and confound nurses for many years to come.

REFLECTIVE QUESTIONS

(1) What challenges does a concept like caring present to the discipline of nursing?
(2) Consider the differences in the ways nurses and patients perceive nurse caring. What are some of the ways in which these two perspectives may be more closely linked?
(3) In nursing, how could the concept of caring be reconciled with professional constructs such as power and autonomy?

RECOMMENDED READING

Brykczynska, G. (ed.) (1997) *Caring: The Compassion and Wisdom of Nursing.* Arnold Books, London.

Dunlop, M. (1986) Is a science of caring possible? *Journal of Advanced Nursing,* **11**(3), 661–670.

Morse, J., Solberg, S., Neander, W., Bottorf, J. & Johnson, J. (1990) Concepts of caring and caring as a concept. *Advances in Nursing Science,* **13**(1), 1–14.

Walters, A.J. (1994) *Caring as a Theoretical Construct, Monograph.* University of New England Press, Armidale.

Webb, C. (1996) Caring, curing, coping: Towards an integrated model. *Journal of Advanced Nursing,* **23**, 960–968.

REFERENCES

Astrom, G., Norberg, A. & Hallberg, I.R. (1995) Skilled nurses' experience of caring. *Journal of Professional Nursing*, **11**(2), 110–118.

Beare, P. & Meyers, J. (1994) *Principles and practice of adult health nursing*. Mosby, St Louis.

Benner, P. (1984) *From Novice to Expert: Excellence and Power in Clinical Nursing*. Addison-Wesley, Menlo Park, California.

Benner, P., Hooper-Kyriakidis, P. & Stannard, D. (1999) *Clinical wisdom and interventions in critical care: A thinking-in-action approach*. WB Saunders, Philadelphia.

Borbasi, S.-A. (1996) Living the experience of being nursed: A phenomenological text. *International Journal of Nursing Practice*, **2**(4), 222–228.

Caffrey, R. & Caffrey, P. (1994) Nursing: Caring or codependent? *Nursing Forum*, **29**(1), 12–17.

Caplan, G. & Brown, A. (1997) Post acute care: Can hospitals do better with less? *Australian Health Review*, **20**(2), 43–52.

Carper, B. (1978) Fundamental patterns of knowing in nursing. *Advances in Nursing Science*, **1**(1), 13–23.

Chinn, P. (1989) Awake, awake. *Advances in Nursing Science*, **11**(2), 1.

Delbridge, A., Bernard, J., Blair, D., Peters, P. & Butler, S. (eds) (1991) *The Macquarie Dictionary*, 2nd edn. The Macquarie Library, Macquarie University, Sydney.

Dunlop, M. (1986) Is a science of caring possible? *Journal of Advanced Nursing*, **11**(3), 661–670.

Duffield, C. & Lumby, J. (1994) Caring nurses: The dilemma of balancing costs and quality. *Australian Health Review*, **17**(2), 72–83.

Dyson, J. (1996) Nurses' conceptualizations of caring attitudes and behaviours. *Journal of Advanced Nursing*, **23**, 1263–1269.

Falk Rafael, A. (1996) Power and caring: A dialectic in nursing. *Advances in Nursing Science*, **19**(1), 3–17.

Greenhalgh, J., Vanhanen, L. & Kyngas, H. (1998) Nurse caring behaviours. *Journal of Advanced Nursing*, **27**(5), 927–932.

Holden, R.J. (1991) In defence of Cartesian dualism and the hermeneutic horizon. *Journal of Advanced Nursing*, **16**, 1375–1381.

Jackson, D. (1995) Constructing nursing practice: Country of origin, culture and competency. *International Journal of Nursing Practice*, **1**(1), 32–36.

Jackson, D. & Raftos, M. (1997) In uncharted waters: Confronting the culture of silence in a residential care institution. *International Journal of Nursing Practice*, **3**(1), 34–39.

Johnston, C. & Cooper, P. (1997) Patient-focused care: What is it? *Holistic Nursing Practice*, **11**(3), 1–7.

Kenway, J. & Watkins, P. (1994) *Nurses, power politics and post-modernity: A Monograph*. University of New England Press, Armidale.

King, K. & Norsen, L. (1994) The care/cure, nurse/physician dichotomy doesn't do it anymore. *Image: Journal of Nursing Scholarship*, **26**(2), 89.

Kitson, A.L. (1987) Raising standards of clinical practice – the fundamental issue of effective nursing practice. *Journal of Advanced Nursing*, **12**(3), 321–329.

Kralik, D., Koch, T. & Wootton, K. (1997) Engagement and detachment: Understanding patients' experiences with nursing. *Journal of Advanced Nursing*, **26**(2), 399–407.

Larsson, G., Peterson, V., Lampic, C., von Essen, L. & Sjoden, P. (1998) Cancer patients and staff ratings of the importance of caring behaviours and their relations to patient anxiety and depression. *Journal of Advanced Nursing*, **27**(4), 855–864.

Lea, A., Watson, R. & Dreary, I. (1998) Caring in nursing: A multivariate analysis. *Journal of Advanced Nursing*, **28**(3), 662–671.

Leftwich, R. (1993) Care and cure as healing processes in nursing. *Nursing Forum*, **28**(3), 13–17.

Leininger, M. (1984) *Care: The Essence of Nursing and Health.* Slack Books, New Jersey.

Leininger, M. (1986) Care facilitation and resistance factors in the culture of nursing. *Topics in Clinical Nursing*, **8**(2), 1–12.

Macdonald, J. (1993) The caring imperative: A must? *The Australian Journal of Advanced Nursing*, **11**(1), 26–30.

Malin, N. & Teasdale, K. (1991) Caring versus empowerment: Considerations for nursing practice. *Journal of Advanced Nursing*, **16**, 657–662.

Morse, J., Solberg, S., Neander, W., Bottorf, J. & Johnson, J. (1990) Concepts of caring and caring as a concept. *Advances in Nursing Science*, **13**(1), 1–14.

Nightingale, F. (1859/1946) *Notes on Nursing.* Harrison Book Company, London.

Pearson, A. (1991) Taking up the challenge: The future for therapeutic nursing. In: *Nursing as Therapy* (eds R. McMahon & A. Pearson). Chapman & Hall, London.

Pepin, J. (1992) Family caring and caring in nursing. *Image: Journal of Nursing Scholarship*, **24**(2), 127–131.

Peter, E. & Gallop, R. (1994) The ethic of care: A comparison of nursing and medical students. *Image: Journal of Nursing Scholarship*, **26**(1), 47–51.

Rawnsley, M. (1990) Of human bonding: The context of nursing as caring. *Advances in Nursing Science*, **13**(1), 41–48.

Ray, M. (1987) Technological caring: A new model in critical care. *Dimensions in Critical Care Nursing*, **6**(3), 173–177.

Ray, M. (1989) The theory of bureaucratic caring for nursing practice in the organizational structure. *Nursing Science Quarterly*, **13**(2), 31–42.

Reverby, S. (1987) A caring dilemma: Womanhood and nursing in historical perspective. *Nursing Research*, **36**(1), 5–11.

Sandelowski, M. (1997) (Ir)reconcilable differences? The debate concerning nursing and technology. *Image: Journal of Nursing Scholarship*, **29**(2), 169–174.

Sullivan, J. & Deane, D. (1994) Caring: Reappropriating our tradition. *Nursing Forum*, **29**(2), 5–9.

Swanson, K. (1993) Nursing as informed caring for the well-being of others. *Image: Journal of Nursing Scholarship*, **25**(4), 352–357.

Taylor, B. (1994) *Being Human: Ordinariness in nursing.* Churchill Livingstone, Melbourne.

Walker, K. (1995) Courting competency: Nursing and the politics of performance in practice. *Nursing Inquiry*, **2**(2), 90–99.

Walters, A.J. (1994) *Caring as a theoretical construct.* University of New England Press, Armidale.

Watson, J. (1985) *Nursing: The Philosophy and Science of Caring.* Colorado Associated University Press, Boulder.

Watson, J. (1988) *Nursing: Human science and human care: A theory of nursing.* National League for Nursing, New York.

Webb, C. (1996) Caring, curing, coping: Towards an integrated model. *Journal of Advanced Nursing,* **23**, 960–968.

Wilkes, L. & Wallis, M. (1993) The five Cs of caring: The lived experience of student nurses. *The Australian Journal of Advanced Nursing,* **11**(1), 19–25.

Williams, S. (1997) Caring in patient-focused care: The relationship of patients' perceptions of holistic nurse care to their levels of anxiety. *Holistic Nursing Practice,* **11**(3), 61–68.

Wolf, Z.R. (1986) The caring concept and nurse identified caring behaviours. *Topics in Clinical Nursing,* **8**(2), 84–93.

Wolf, Z., Giardino, E., Osborne, P. & Ambrose, M. (1994) Dimensions of nurse caring. *Image: Journal of Nursing Scholarship,* **26**(2), 107–111.

Wuest, J. (1997) Illuminating environmental influences on women's caring. *Journal of Advanced Nursing,* **26**, 49–58.

7 Nursing Theory
Its Nature and Purposes

Jennifer Greenwood

LEARNING OBJECTIVES

Having read and 'digested' this chapter the reader will:

- understand that all nursing practice is underpinned by 'theories', whether the nurse practising is aware of them or not;
- be able to describe how nursing theories that are research-based or 'scientifically derived' and those that are derived from 'experience' are constructed and tested;
- be able to distinguish between levels of theory;
- be able to articulate nursing's central or 'domain' concepts;
- be able to articulate the purposes of nursing theory.

KEY WORDS

RELATIONSHIPS, EMPIRICAL, METAPHOR, CONCEPTS, REASONING, PARADIGM.

INTRODUCTION

It is true to say that 'nursing theory' is among the least-loved subjects in the undergraduate curriculum, and this for (at least) three reasons. Firstly, nurse academics often find nursing theory difficult to teach and resort to describing various 'models' of nursing to nursing undergraduates, who often find them boring and apparently irrelevant to their everyday clinical activities. Secondly, the remnants in clinical colleagues' minds of an anti-intellectual attitude towards all things 'theoretical' reinforces undergraduates' perceptions of the irrelevance of nursing theory. Thirdly, because nursing theory and nursing practice are taught by different instructors, the apparent divisions between nursing theory and nursing practice are reinforced. Undergraduates believe that nursing theory is learned only from nurse academics and nursing literature, whereas nursing practice, or clinical nursing skills, are learned only 'by experience' while working alongside more experienced clinical colleagues. That's not quite right, you know! Nursing theory is also learned 'by experience' while working with senior clinical colleagues – it is just that the 'theory' that is learned is different from that taught in universities. Likewise, insights into clinical nursing skills are derived from nursing theory (the type taught in universities) even if these insights apply to procedures as routine as sterile dressings.

The point I am making here is that nursing practice is *inevitably* informed by theory, and in this chapter I will try to explain why. In order to do this, the discussion will focus on:

- the nature and development of nursing theory;
- the purposes of nursing theory;
- the relationship of nursing theory to practice and research.

It will also focus on types of theory and levels of theory to provide a comprehensive introduction to the subject. The author hopes that these discussions will enhance your understanding of, and increase your interest – even enjoyment – in studying nursing theory as your course progresses.

WHAT IS NURSING THEORY?

Nursing theory is a blanket term that generally refers to all the insights derived from nursing research, be it conceptual research or empirical research. 'Conceptual research' means the research that goes on primarily in the researcher's head; philosophy, of course, is the best example of a conceptual discipline. In nursing, the results of conceptual research are nursing's 'grand theories' or models, which will be discussed later. 'Empirical research' means research which, although conceived (as it has to be) in the researcher's head, is generated and tested primarily in the real world. 'Science' as it is generally (if a little simplistically) construed is the best example of an empirical discipline. In nursing, the results of empirical research – e.g. what interventions (practices) are most effective and under what conditions – are the basis for 'evidence-based practice'. That is, the results of empirical research inform nurses what they should do, why they should do it, for whom they should do it, when and where and how they should do it and how they will know they have done it well. In short, such results inform their practice theories (which will be discussed in some detail later).

THE NATURE OF NURSING THEORY

According to Chinn and Kramer (1995), theory is 'a systematic abstraction of reality that serves some purpose' (p. 62); to Watson (1985) it is 'an imaginative grouping of knowledge, ideas and experience that are represented symbolically and seek to illuminate a given phenomena' (sic) (p. 1); to Dickoff and James (1968) a theory is a conceptual system or framework invented to some purpose. Whilst all of these definitions are correct, they may not be immediately intelligible to undergraduate nurses!

Stevens Barnum (1994:1), following Visintainer (1986), uses the metaphor of a map to explain what a theory is and what it does:

A theory is like a map of a territory as opposed to an aerial photograph. The map does not display the full terrain (buildings, moving vehicles, or grazing livestock); instead it picks out those parts that are important for its purpose. If its aim is to guide travellers, the map will highlight the roads; if its purpose is to describe the physical terrain, it shows mountains, plains and rivers.

Visintainer (1986:33) puts it somewhat differently:

> The maps of a discipline operate in a way similar to that of maps of a geographic region. They provide a framework for selecting and organising information from the environment. In studying a discipline, one learns the maps and through mastery of the maps learns what to ask about, what to observe, what to focus on, what to think about.

My preferred metaphor for theory is 'a net'. A theory is a net of concepts ('symbolic abstractions') that people construct ('invent') to render their experiences meaningful and manageable ('to some purpose'). Each knot in the net represents a concept and the strings between knots represent the relationships between concepts. Thus, concepts can be at the same level of generality, e.g. wing, beak and claw, or at differing levels of generality, e.g. feather, wing and bird. The more complete and accurate such theoretical nets are, the more meaningful and manageable human experiences (including clinical nursing experiences) become.

CONCEPTS AND THEORIES

A concept is a mental image (Hardy 1974; Walker & Avant 1988) constructed in the mind in response to both 'objects' of experience – both inanimate (a chair) and animate (a dog), situations, events, actions – and the person's subjective experiences of such 'objects' (e.g. fear, love). The concept 'dog', for instance, is constructed in response to the experience of or exposure to a variety of different dogs. It is through exposure to different *individual* dogs that people construct concepts of *typical* dogs. It is important that concepts represent typical features of 'objects' of experiences (dogs!) because concepts of 'typical' dogs allow people to recognise individual instances of dogs when they encounter them. Recognition of individual instances of a type (e.g. a typical dog) allows people to render their experiences meaningful. To recognise something as a dog reflects an underlying interpretive act which allows people to recognise that this stimulus means 'dog' and this, quite literally, renders it meaningful.

Knowing how to respond to such experiential objects is also a function of concepts that are constructed through experience – that is, through the planning and executing of responses (actions). It is through the planning and execution of appropriate responses that experiences become manageable because, quite literally, they demonstrate that people know what to do in certain situations. Knowing what to do is also reflective of an interpretive act, but one which allows people to recognise that they should do X. The appropriateness of their response (action) is signalled through the feedback it elicits. The action may elicit positive feedback, which will ensure its repetition in future similar situations, or negative feedback, which will discourage its repetition. (Consider the different sorts of feedback you might elicit from a labrador or pitbull terrier when attempting to stroke them.)

To summarise thus far, let us return to the 'net' metaphor: theories are collections of concepts of objects, situations, events and actions and their subjective experiences (the knots) joined together, in different combinations, or levels of generality (the strings), to make significant aspects of our lives meaningful and manageable.

The construction of concepts and theories

Concepts are constructed in two ways: deliberately and consciously, or incidentally and relatively unconsciously (Tomlinson 1995). Those constructed consciously are often done so as a result of teaching, reading, researching, etc. They may also be constructed as a result of problem-solving, i.e. when a person constructs a new concept to deal with a problem arising from an unfamiliar, unusual situation. Concepts constructed incidentally and relatively unconsciously are rather different. They are constructed simply in response to repeated, everyday situations. They differ in other respects, too.

Firstly, they differ – or potentially differ – with respect to accuracy and adequacy. Concepts constructed as a result of effort, from teachers, literature and research, tend to be 'clear cut' (Howard 1987), i.e. they state precisely what the concept includes. What clear-cut concepts include is often presented in feature lists because they are well defined and important to remember. Thus, a feature list for nurses to learn concerning concepts might be:

- that they are constructed automatically in response to 'experience';
- that they can be constructed consciously and unconsciously;
- that consciously constructed concepts tend to be clear cut, and so on.

That such concepts are clear cut and can be presented in feature lists reflects the care and attention that went into their initial construction. Most of what is taught in universities is the result of painstaking and systematic conceptual and/or empirical research and, because of this, it is termed 'scientifically derived'. Scientists, including nurse scientists (researchers), take great pains to ensure that the concepts they construct are the most adequate and accurate (or valid) representations of the realities they seek to render meaningful and manageable. They ensure this by carefully seeking empirical evidence and linking concepts logically and consistently, i.e. in theories. Generally speaking, whenever scholars and scientists refer to 'theory' they are referring to concepts and theories developed in this way. They tend not to recognise as 'theory' concepts developed in any other way (hence the mistaken belief that practice can be 'atheoretical').

Incidentally and relatively unconsciously constructed concepts tend not to be clear cut, and therefore cannot be presented in feature lists. Such concepts tend to be 'fuzzy' (Howard 1987) because what they include is not clearly delineated and they tend to be constructed pictorially (that is, in images) and holistically. For example, toddlers and young children learn holistically and experientially – primarily from their caregivers – how certain objects are named in their parent culture, how they are valued and how they should be responded to, i.e. how to interpret certain stimuli and respond to them. Thus, when a mother puts a kitten in her toddler's lap and says,

'... kitty, Toby ...'
'nice kitty, Toby ...'
'Toby cuddle kitty ...'

the child learns from this one experience that:

- this stimulus means kitty;
- it is a nice kitty, i.e. how it is valued in his parent culture;
- it should be cuddled, i.e. how it should be responded to.

This is precisely how many of nurses' everyday practice concepts and theories are constructed. Through experience, they learn what certain 'objects' in clinical settings mean, how they are valued and how they should be treated (Greenwood 1996a,b). Such objects include different kinds of patients, other health care professionals, clinical procedures and protocols, power relationships, etc.

Unconsciously constructed fuzzy concepts and theories can be problematic in terms of adequacy and accuracy, too. For if a nurse is unaware of having constructed them, she or he will be unaware of what they are. This means that the nurse will also be unable to surface them, articulate them and examine them against the realities they were meant to render meaningful and manageable (Greenwood 1996a,b).

Patients can be subjected to very poor nursing care when inappropriate, unconscious 'fuzzies' form the basis of nurses' practice. At its most general, when nursing is conceptualised as a series of tasks to be performed in order to get through the workload and fit into the ward team, patient care is skimped, rushed and depersonalising (cf. Greenwood 1993; Madjar *et al.* 1997; Melia 1987).

It is worth emphasising yet again that practice is inevitably informed by theories, be they scientifically derived (clear-cut, consciously held, tested carefully for accuracy) or experientially derived (fuzzy, relatively unconscious, not tested carefully for accuracy). This is because practice, by definition, is purposeful; nurses practise to some purpose. The purpose behind nursing practice is the protection or improvement of individual and community health status. Purposeful activity (practice) therefore presupposes some idea (concept, representation) of what is to be done, to whom, why, where, how, when and with what.

Given this, it is extremely important that nurses ensure that the theories which inform their practice are as adequate and as accurate as they can make them. The next section offers some suggestions to assist in this.

The relationship of clear-cut and fuzzy concepts and theories

As previously stated, fuzzy concepts are largely unconscious but deeply embedded in everyday nursing activities; this means that their surfacing (or identification) could be difficult. Nurses will frequently require the sensitive assistance of peers and tutorial colleagues to help them surface inappropriate 'fuzzies'. Once surfaced, however, they can be examined for adequacy and accuracy against the realities they are supposed to render meaningful and manageable, i.e. represent.

For instance, there is a commonly held view ('fuzzy') that babies and very young children do not experience pain in the same way or to the same extent as adults. This 'fuzzy' can be tested by examining carefully the reaction of babies and very young children to painful clinical procedures. The second way to examine the validity of this 'fuzzy' is to search the relevant 'scientifically derived' literature. You should know that there is no evidence at all that the very young do not experience pain, and a great deal which suggests that they do (Nagy 1995).

Both of these point to further and critically important functions of the study, development, evaluation and critique of nursing theory. These intellectual activities help to develop nurses' analytic and critical skills, clarify their values and assumptions and determine the purposes of nursing practice, education and research (Marriner-Toomey 1994).

TYPES OF THEORY

Theories, in general, may be categorised according to level (e.g. Dickoff & James 1968) or purpose (e.g. Chinn & Kramer 1995). According to Dickoff and James (1968), there are four levels of theory, viz: factor-isolating, factor-relating, situation-relating and situation-producing theories. The most complex of these four levels is situation-producing theory, because it presupposes the existence of theory at the three first, more primitive levels. In contrast, Chinn and Kramer (1995) suggest that theory is either theory generating or theory testing.

Theory, we have established, is invented to some purpose, i.e. to render experiences meaningful and manageable. The first step in rendering any object of experience meaningful is to label it – to isolate it by naming it. Dickoff and James (1968) refer to objects of experience as 'factors'. Thus, in rendering their clinical experiences meaningful, nurses need to isolate or name the factors (or variables) in them. The second step in rendering experiences meaningful is to *relate* concepts of experiential factors or variables; this enables people to broaden their understanding of their worlds. For instance, nurses relate wound hotness, redness, pain, and loss of function to infection. Having related these factors or variables, the nurse can then make predictions based upon the expectancy of their co-occurrence. If the wound is hot and red, then it will probably be painful; if it is hot, swollen and red it is probably infected. As nurses' theorising with respect to their clinical experiences becomes more sophisticated, so too does their understanding of them.

Situation-producing or control theories (Argyris & Schön 1977) are the most sophisticated theories a person can construct because, as noted earlier, their construction presupposes the construction of other theories at more primitive levels. Situation-producing theories are action theories (Greenwood 1994); they tell a person what to do, when to do it, where to do it, to whom and/or with whom to do it, how to do it and why to do it. Clearly, this level of theorising is not possible without knowing which factors in a situation are important (salient) and how they relate to others.

Chinn and Kramer (1995) describe theory-generating research as that designed to 'discover and describe relationships' (p. 143), while they consider that the role of theory-testing research is to ascertain how accurately the theory 'depicts phenomena and their relationships' (p. 145). The former, they suggest, is developed through a process of inductive reasoning, the latter through deductive or hypothetico-deductive reasoning (these terms are described below).

It is often helpful to remember that reasoning is merely the process human beings use to progress from their existing state of knowledge to an enhanced or increased state of knowledge (Anderson 1995). Thus, for instance, if your dog barks when the doorbell rings, you can reason that if the bell rings, the dog will bark.

Reasoning takes two forms: (1) from specific instances to more general conclusions, and (2) from more general conclusions to specific instances (Hockey 1986). An example may help: a nurse notices that wound redness, hotness and swelling tend to occur together and, when they do, a diagnosis of wound infection is made. The nurse induces, therefore, that wound redness, hotness and swelling indicates wound infection (*inductive reasoning*). This enables the nurse, in future, when told that a certain patient's wound is infected, to deduce that it will be hot, red and swollen *(deductive reasoning)*. And because deductions of this kind are often couched in 'if ... then' statements ('if this wound is infected, then it will be hot, red, swollen ...') they are sometimes termed *hypothetico-deductions*. Hypotheses are merely informed guesses that *if* certain antecedent conditions exist, *then* certain consequences will follow.

Another way of distinguishing levels of theory – and this, again, is related to purpose – is simply to classify them as 'descriptive' and 'explanatory'. A *descriptive theory* describes factors, variables, events, etc., and their interrelationships. It does not describe why these factors are as they are, how they relate to each other, or how they affect each other (Stevens Barnum 1994). By way of contrast, an *explanatory theory* does exactly what its name implies it should; it explains why and how different concepts relate to each other. Explanatory theory deals with cause and effect relationships and, because of this, might also be termed *predictive theory*. This is because an understanding of precise causes of certain effects allows scientists to predict that if certain 'causes' are present, then certain effects will follow. Thus, if every time ice is heated to 30°C it melts, scientists may reasonably predict that when ice is heated to 30°C, it will melt.

When predictive theory is used to generate specific outcomes – that is, when certain antecedent conditions are deliberately generated to cause certain outcomes – the theory is described as *prescriptive* or *situation-producing*. For instance, when a nurse wishes to allay the fears of an anxious preoperative patient, the nurse will inform him or her, in language that will be understood, of the procedure, the required preparation for it, its benefits and so on.

THEORY AND RESEARCH

It will be clear from the above account that research – the 'careful search or enquiry, a course of critical investigation' (Sykes 1976 cited in Roberts & Taylor 1998) or 'a process of systematic scientific enquiry' (Macleod-Clarke & Hockey 1989) – attempts to generate the most adequate and accurate concepts and theories to enable people to render their experiences meaningful and manageable.

As stated above, concepts and theories can be factor-isolating, factor-relating, situation-relating and situation-producing. They are generated through inductive processes and tested through deductive processes.

More particularly for nurses, nursing research aims to invent and test concepts and theories representing variables in nursing situations, and their interrelationships. Such concepts and theories enable nurses to interpret their clinical realities accurately ('... this stimulus means X ...') and plan and execute an appropriate response ('... therefore I should do Y ...'). When most of the insights (concepts and theories) that inform nursing practice are constructed through research, then nursing will be a research or evidence-based profession (Kitson 1997).

Research and the scientifically derived theories it produces are important in enhancing nursing's professionalism and political power because it enables the articulation of nursing's knowledge base and care rationales. Professionalism is enhanced when theory guides practice, education and research; similarly, political power is persuasive when nurses can justify their activities and positions by drawing on theory when challenged.

Levels of theory development

Walker and Avant (1988) suggest that there are four levels of theory development in nursing: metatheory, grand theory, middle-range theory and practice theory.

Metatheory in nursing is actually a theory of nursing theories (!); it focuses on broad issues related to nursing theories. Such issues include the analysis of the kind of theory required in nursing, the critique of the methods used in theory development in nursing, and how theory in nursing should be evaluated.

Grand theories in nursing often refer to what many nurses know as 'nursing models'. They articulate different theorists' views on what nursing could or should be (not necessarily what nursing is) in terms of the goals and structure of nursing practice. They are constructed carefully by nurse theorists to ensure that the concepts they include relate logically and consistently. Because of this they are 'scientifically derived' although, generally speaking, they are entirely conceptually constructed and not empirically tested or verified. Fawcett (1984:84) identified four areas of conceptual commonality (common ground) that exist in all of nursing's grand theories, and she termed these nursing's 'meta-paradigm'. Each grand theory, in one way or another, addresses the central concepts of the discipline, i.e. person, environment, health and nursing. Somewhat differently, Meleis (1985:184) identifies what she terms 'domain concepts'; these are nursing client (patient), transitions, interaction, nursing process (see Glossary), environment, nursing therapeutics and health. Nursing's grand theories describe the interrelationship of these central or domain concepts. For instance, they suggest how nursing therapeutics may influence the health status of recipients of nursing (patients) in certain physical and social environments. Meleis would also see nursing therapeutics being expressed in nursing process and as assisting people to transit from one health status to another. So although nursing's grand theories may differ in detail with respect to these central concepts, they all address them, more or less explicitly (Greenwood 1996a,b).

Nursing's grand theories or conceptual models fall into two categories: totality paradigm models and simultaneity paradigm models. *Totality paradigm models* view the person as a total summative organism (hence the name) whose uniqueness or individuality is a function of biopsychosocial and spiritual features. These models see the environment as something in which people live and interact and which is experienced by them as a series of internal and external stimuli (or experiential 'objects').

Totality paradigm models can be classified into five groups (Salvage & Kershaw 1986):

(1) developmental, e.g. Peplau (1952);
(2) systems, e.g. Johnson (1980), King (1981);
(3) interactionist, e.g. Reihl (1974);
(4) self care, e.g. Orem (1991);
(5) activities of daily living, e.g. Roper *et al.* (1990).

Simultaneity paradigm models view the person quite differently. They view the person as being in 'mutual process' with the environment rather than merely 'experiencing' it. The person and environment exist as one and change mutually. Rogers (1970) and Parse (1995, 1998) are nursing's main simultaneity paradigm theorists.

The breadth and scope of grand nursing theories makes them extremely difficult to test (against the realities they are meant to render meaningful and manageable). Indeed, two scholars (Fawcett & Downs 1986) go so far as to suggest that grand theories cannot be tested directly; they contend that only theories of lesser generality which are derived from them – those that Walker and Avant (1988) termed 'middle-range' – can be tested.

Middle-range theories contain a limited number of variables, which makes them testable, but they are sufficiently general to be scientifically interesting. Middle-range theories, derived from nursing's grand theories, are hypothetico-deductively constructed and tested, e.g. if a person expresses her uniqueness through her activities of daily living (as activities of daily living models suggest she does), then allowing her maximum choice with respect to these will enhance her sense of personhood. And this is testable empirically (even if we simply ask her how increased choice affects her sense of 'self').

Practice theory is a result of nursing's metatheorising (about what sort of theory nursing theory should be, and what should be its purposes). Practice theory identifies a desired goal and the prescriptions for action to achieve the goal. My view is that practice theories are action theories or situation-producing theories (see above).

You should note that 'conceptual models' and 'theories' differ only in the extent to which what they propose or claim (in statements of relationship, i.e. propositions) is tentative, and the degree to which they are supported by empirical evidence. In addition, they differ in the extent to which they are accepted as true or valid by the community of scholars in the discipline to which they relate (Keck 1994). Those propositions that are heavily supported by empirical evidence and are accepted as true or valid by the relevant community of scholars are considered to be 'theories'. Those that are supported by little empirical evidence and which are considered speculative by the relevant community of scholars are viewed as 'conceptual models'.

CONCLUSION

Grand and middle-range theories appear to enjoy rather more status among many nursing scholars than do action theories, although this is changing, especially in Australia. Scope of theory clearly has more value than utility of theory, even for some scholars in a practice discipline like nursing. This seems to be mistaken. For nurses can theorise interminably but, unless they *act* to change the health status of individuals or communities, they will be failing to fulfil the mission of a practice discipline, which is to bring about change (Langford 1973).

The linkages between levels of theory development are clear. Metatheory clarifies what grand theories and other theories should include or address; grand theories guide or fuel the development and testing, through empirical nursing research, of middle-range and/or practice theories. Importantly, however, testing of practice and middle-range theories informs the ongoing refinement and elaboration of grand theory and metatheory.

Scientifically derived nursing theories articulate nursing's knowledge base and care rationales. They are critically important, therefore, in enhancing nursing's professionalism and political power. In addition, the careful examination of both scientifically and experientially derived theories for adequacy and accuracy assists in the development of nurses' analytic and critical skills.

REFLECTIVE QUESTIONS

(1) What 'experientially derived' theories of nursing informed your decision to become a nurse? How did you acquire them?

(2) Health care reflects the sexism, racism and ageism that occur more generally in the society in which the health care is being practised. Consider how these 'experientially derived' -isms could affect the language and behaviour of nurses.

(3) You are about to help an elderly patient onto a commode. What psychological, physiological and nursing theoretical insights will you draw on?

RECOMMENDED READING

Chinn, P.L. & Kramer, M.K. (1995) *Theory and Nursing: A Systematic Approach*, 4th edn. Mosby, St Louis.

Greenwood, J. (ed.) (2000) *Nursing Theory in Australia: Development and Application*, 2nd edn. Prentice Hall Health, Sydney.

Marriner-Toomey, A. (ed.) (1998) *Nursing Theorists and their Work*, 4th edn. Mosby, St Louis.

Pearson, A., Vaughan, B. & FitzGerald, M. (1996) *Nursing Models for Practice*, 2nd edn. Butterworth Heinemann, Oxford.

Roper, N., Logan, W. & Tierney, A. (2000) *The Roper-Logan-Tierney Model of Nursing: Based on Activities of Living*. Churchill Livingstone, Edinburgh.

REFERENCES

Anderson, J.R. (1995) *Cognitive psychology and its implications*, 4th edn. Freeman, New York.

Argyris, C. & Schön, D. (1977) *Theory in practice*. Jossey Bass, San Francisco.

Chinn, P.L. & Kramer, M.K. (1995) *Theory and Nursing: A Systematic Approach*, 4th edn. Mosby, St Louis.

Dickoff, J. & James, P. (1968) Theory in practice discipline: Part I. *Nursing Research*, **17**(5), 415–435.

Fawcett, J. (1984) The metaparadigm of nursing: Present status and future refinements. *Image: The Journal of Nursing Scholarship,* **16**(3), 84–89.

Fawcett, J. & Downs, F. (1986) *The relationship of theory and research*. Appleton-Century-Crofts, Norwalk, Connecticut.

Greenwood, J. (1993) The apparent desensitisation of student nurses during their professional socialisation: A cognitive perspective. *Journal of Advanced Nursing*, **18**, 1471–1479.

Greenwood, J. (1994) Action research: A few details, a caution and something new. *Journal of Advanced Nursing*, **20**(1), 13–18.

Greenwood, J. (1996a) Nursing research and nursing theory. In: *Nursing Theory in Australia: Development and Application* (ed. J. Greenwood), pp. 16–30. Harper Educational, Sydney.

Greenwood, J. (1996b) Nursing theories: An introduction to their development and application. In: *Nursing Theory in Australia: Development and Application* (ed. J. Greenwood), pp. 1–14. Harper Educational, Sydney.

Hardy, M.E. (1974) Theories: Components, development, evaluation. *Nursing Research*, **23**, 100–107.

Hockey, L. (1986) The nature and purpose of research. In: *The Research Process in Nursing* (ed. D.F.S. Cormack). pp. 3–13. Blackwell Scientific, Oxford.

Howard, R.W. (1987) *Concepts and Schemata: An Introduction*. Cassell Education, London.

Johnson, D.E. (1980) The behavioural system model for nursing. In: *Conceptual Models for Nursing Practice* (eds J.P. Riehl & C. Roy), 2nd edn. Appleton-Century-Crofts, New York.

Keck, J.F. (1994) Terminology of theory development. In: *Nursing Theorists and their Work* (ed. A. Marriner-Toomey). Mosby, St Louis.

King, M. (1981) *A Theory for Nursing: Systems, Concepts Process*. Wiley, New York.

Kitson, A.L. (1997) Using evidence to demonstrate the value of nursing. *Nursing Standard*, **2**(11), 34–39.

Langford, G. (1973) The concept of education. In: *Essays in the Philosophy of Education* (eds G. Langford & D.J. O'Connor), pp. 3–32. Routledge & Kegan Paul, London.

Macleod-Clarke, J. & Hockey, L. (1989) *Further Research for Nursing*. Scutari Press, London.

Madjar, I., McMillan, M., Sharkey, R. & Cadd, A. (1997) *Project to review and examine expectations of beginning registered nurses in the workforce*. NSW Nurses Registration Board, Sydney.

Marriner-Toomey, A. (1994) Introduction to analysis of nursing theory. In: *Nursing Theorists and their Work* (ed. A. Marriner-Toomey), pp. 3–16. Mosby, St Louis.

Meleis, A.I. (ed.) (1985) *Theoretical nursing: Development and progress*. Lippincott, Philadelphia.

Melia, K.M. (1987) *Learning and Working: The Occupational Socialisation of Nurses*. Tavistock, London.

Nagy, S. (1995) *The reactions of nurses to the pain of their patients: A personal construct analysis.* Unpublished PhD thesis, University of Wollongong.

Orem, D.E. (1991) *Nursing: Concepts of Practice,* 4th edn. Mosby, St Louis.

Parse, R.R. (ed.) (1995) *Illuminations: The human becoming in practice and research.* Pub. No. 15–2670. National League for Nursing, New York.

Parse, R.R. (1998) *The Human Becoming School of Thought: A Perspective for Nurses and other Health Professionals.* Sage, Thousand Oaks, California.

Peplau, H.E. (1952) *Interpersonal Relations in Nursing.* Putman, New York.

Reihl, J.P. (1974) Application of interaction theory. In: *Conceptual Models for Nursing Practice* (eds J.P. Riehl & C. Roy), 2nd edn. Appleton-Century-Crofts, New York.

Roberts, K. & Taylor, B. (1998) *Nursing Research Processes: An Australian Perspective.* Nelson ITP, Melbourne.

Rogers, M.E. (1970) *An Introduction to the Theoretical Basis of Nursing.* Davis, Philadelphia.

Roper, N., Logan, W. & Tierney, A. (1990) *The Elements of Nursing,* 3rd edn. Churchill Livingstone, Edinburgh.

Salvage, J. & Kershaw, B. (eds) (1986) *Models for Nursing.* John Wiley & Sons, Chichester.

Stevens Barnum, B.J. (1994) *Nursing Theory: Analysis, Application, Evaluation,* 4th edn. Lippincott, Philadelphia.

Sykes, J. (ed.) (1976) *Concise Oxford English Dictionary.* Oxford University Press, Oxford.

Tomlinson, P.D. (1995) *Understanding Mentoring.* Open University Press, Buckingham.

Visintainer, M.A. (1986) The nature of knowledge and theory in nursing. *Image,* **2**, 32–38.

Walker, L.O. & Avant, K.C. (1988) *Strategies for Theory Construction in Nursing,* 2nd edn. Appleton & Lange, Norwalk, Connecticut.

Watson, J. (1985) *Nursing: Human Science and Human Care.* Appleton Century Crofts, Norwalk, Connecticut.

8 Research in Nursing
Concepts and Processes

David Thompson, John Daly, Doug Elliott
and Esther Chang

LEARNING OBJECTIVES

Upon completion of this chapter the reader should have gained:

- an understanding of the role of research in the development of contemporary nursing;
- an appreciation of the need for a range of approaches to research in nursing;
- basic knowledge and understanding of research processes in nursing;
- an appreciation of the contribution of research to the development of knowledge and clinical practice standards in nursing;
- an understanding of research critique and research dissemination processes in nursing.

KEY WORDS

PROCESSES, RESEARCH, TRADITIONS, QUANTITATIVE, QUALITATIVE, DISSEMINATION, CRITIQUE, EVIDENCE.

INTRODUCTION

This chapter introduces the reader to basic concepts and processes of research in nursing. Research has assumed a position of great importance in British nursing but, while there has been a dramatic increase in nursing research activity, this research culture remains in an early stage of development. History tells us that the concept of research in nursing is not new, at least in the Western world (D'Antonio 1997; Mulhall 1995). In Britain, Florence Nightingale was a research pioneer in nursing in the nineteenth century, though it was not until 1940 that further progress with nursing research activity occurred and it was 1963 before the first government-funded post to facilitate research in nursing was established in the Ministry of Health (Mulhall 1995). However, it was 1972 before a research base for nursing practice was recommended in a government report (Briggs 1972). Two decades later a research and development strategy for the National Health Service was launched (DoH 1991) with the prime objective of seeing that research and development becomes an integral part of health care. The taskforce for a strategy for research in nursing, midwifery and health visiting (DoH 1993) chose to integrate nursing research within this overall health research agenda.

It is only since the late 1990s that the academic discipline of nursing has established a significant presence in universities in the UK. Consequently, there is still a shortage of appropriately prepared nurse researchers who can provide research leadership and contribute to the ongoing professionalisation of nursing in the UK. This situation will change significantly as more nurses pursue research training opportunities through higher degrees. The important role that research will play in the continued development of nursing as a practice discipline with a research-based body of knowledge has been emphasised (DoH 1993, 1999). The recent national strategy for nursing, midwifery and health visiting signals a commitment to develop a strategy to influence the research and development agenda, to strengthen the capacity to undertake research, and to use research to support practice (DoH 1999). Despite considerable progress in recent years the nursing contribution to research and development fails to be maximised. In some cases this is due to a lack of professional confidence and co-ordination, but in others nurses have encountered institutional barriers that have constrained development of both capacity and capability. In essence, there are too few nurse researchers and too few nurses in practice who are sufficiently research-aware. Also, though the production, dissemination and implementation of research is important, it is of no use to nurses if they do not, or cannot, gain access to it. A coherent and sustained strategy is needed to ensure that the nursing contribution to key health priorities is properly researched, evaluated and supported by robust evidence, and that the research and development agenda is properly informed by nursing expertise (DoH 2000).

WHAT IS RESEARCH?

Research is a rigorous process of inquiry designed to provide answers to questions about phenomena of concern in an academic discipline or profession. In the Oxford Dictionary research is defined as 'careful study and investigation, especially in order to discover new facts or investigation'.

Research is a complex subject and field comprising a number of well established but diverse traditions. In a chapter such as this it is possible to present only broad brushstrokes to familiarise the reader with key underpinning ideas about research processes in nursing. To develop in-depth knowledge and understanding of any one or a range of research traditions, processes and/or methods, further study and reading from a variety of sources will be necessary.

Research traditions can be investigated in relation to their philosophical underpinnings, and in the course of your reading of research you will encounter a number of essentially different paradigms. A research paradigm is an overarching framework that is based on values, beliefs and assumptions. This framework contains theory about the nature of reality and guidelines for the methods to be used in carrying out research using (or within) the paradigm. In addition, the ideas within the paradigm have implications for the type of knowledge being sought in a research study, the way in which the study will be carried out and the way in which outcomes from the work will be used.

As nursing is a complex field, researchers use a range of research paradigms. Quality research is labour, skill and resource intensive, therefore a number of important decisions need to be made before embarking upon a research project. Not least, all research must be ethical, and this means adhering to strict guidelines and obtaining the necessary approval from institutional ethics committees. Recently, the Department of Health (2001) has produced a research governance framework for health and social care. This makes explicit that the dignity, rights, safety and well-being of participants must be the primary consideration in any research study.

Research has the potential to serve a number of purposes in a practice-based discipline such as nursing. Research in nursing is necessary to:

- test commonly held assumptions;
- widen understanding of a subject;
- stimulate self-action/study;
- develop best practice (i.e. research-based practice);
- explain behaviours;
- allow predictions;
- assist in the formation of a body of nursing knowledge.

The four As of research (Crookes & Davies 1998:xi) are:

(1) awareness (including access);
(2) appreciation;
(3) application;
(4) ability.

The aim of the first three As of research is not to produce research workers but to cultivate and nurture nurses to:

- accept research as a normal and integral aspect of nursing practice;
- read and understand research reports;
- apply research findings to clinical practice (i.e. evidence-based practice);
- influence colleagues on the use of research data;
- accept responsibility for their own professional development.

TYPES OF NURSING RESEARCH

Nursing research has traditionally been described as using either 'quantitative' or 'qualitative' approaches. Oakley (2000:42) notes that 'the 'quantitative-qualitative' dichotomy functions chiefly as a gendered way of knowing. The 'qualitative' is the soft, the unreliable, the feminine, the private – the world of the 'subjective' experience. The 'quantitative' and the experimental are hard, reliable, masculine, public: they are about 'objectivity'. As Oakley points out, the two terms are relative: much 'quantitative' research measures quality and numbers frequently occur in qualitative research. The use of such terminology is artificial and unhelpful as a technical guide to research methods. Although nursing would be better off without this terminology an overview of the two traditions is provided below.

Quantitative research

The term 'quantitative research' refers to studies that seek to measure some concept or phenomenon of interest, for example blood pressure, pain, or student attitudes to learning about research. The quantitative research paradigm is also called positivist, reductionist, or empirical. Quantitative reasoning is termed deductive, which means the thinking leads from a known principle to an unknown and is used to test a particular research hypothesis.

Quantitative research encompasses a range of research designs and associated methods; the most common designs used in health care research are listed in Table 8.1. Selection of an appropriate design relates to the research question being posed (Sackett & Wennberg 1997). The topic of interest may be framed as a question, objective, or research hypothesis. Each design incorporates a number of variations; readers are directed to any number of nursing research texts for amplification of the designs (e.g. Burns & Grove 1998; Crookes & Davies 1998; Martin & Thompson 2000).

Quantitative studies rely on sampling a smaller group of individuals who have similar characteristics to the overall population of interest. Inclusion and/or exclusion criteria (defined in Table 8.2) are developed that guide the selection of subjects. In experimental studies, the independent variable (an intervention) is manipulated by randomly assigning subjects to a treatment or control group while the (dependent) variable of interest is measured and other related variables are controlled, e.g. randomised controlled trial (RCT).

Measurement of the concepts of interest are conducted using single or multiple 'measuring instruments' (also called tools); these can be physiological (e.g. heart rate monitor; blood glucometer) or psychological/psychometric (e.g. anxiety scales; functional status; quality of life). Ideally, an instrument should exhibit characteristics that are valid, reliable and responsive. Well-developed instruments generally have had the above characteristics rigorously tested over time, and have been accepted as a useful research tool. Development of new instruments is time-consuming and resource-intensive as the validity, reliability and responsiveness must be tested, and

Table 8.1 Common quantitative research designs.

Design	Purpose
Descriptive	Examines characteristics of a single sample; clarifies concepts; generates questions about potential relationships between variables (e.g. case study, cross-sectional analysis)
Correlation	Examines (describes, predicts or tests) relationships between two or more variables, but does not imply a cause-and-effect relationship
Quasi-experiment	Tests a cause-and-effect relationship, but without control or randomisation (e.g. case control, cohort)
Experiment	Tests a cause-and-effect relationship using randomisation, manipulation of an intervention and control of other variables (e.g. randomised controlled trial [RCT], laboratory experiment)

Table 8.2 Glossary of common quantitative research terms.

Term	Meaning
Descriptive statistics	Description of characteristics (e.g. frequency, percentages) but no implication of relationships between variables
Exclusion criteria	A list of characteristics that exclude an individual from being recruited into a study (e.g. less than 24 hours' admission in hospital; presence of other illnesses that may influence patient outcomes)
Explanatory variable	Independent variable; the intervention being manipulated to exhibit a change in the outcome variable
Inclusion criteria	A list of the characteristics required for a subject to be included in a study (e.g. patients admitted for cardiac surgery: 16 years or older; English language skills [reading and writing] sufficient to complete the study questionnaires)
Inferential statistics	Statistical procedures used to test a hypothesis about the relationships between two or more variables (e.g. t-tests, analysis of variance, regression modelling) and the application of study findings to the population being studied (generalisability)
Measuring instrument	The tool used to measure the concept of interest (e.g. questionnaire; biochemical test)
Normal distribution	Distribution of scores for a particular variable follow a bell-shape pattern around the mean score for the sample
Outcome variable	Dependent variable; measurement of the concept being studied
Primary research	Original research conducted on subjects
Sample	A selected group of subjects that have similar characteristics to the population from which they were drawn (i.e. representative); allows for generalisation of results from the study sample to the wider population
Secondary research	A study where data from previous primary research studies are reinvestigated (e.g. systematic review; clinical practice guidelines)

modification of items (questions) may be required to improve the performance of the instrument.

Instrument validity refers to whether the instrument actually measures what it is intended to measure. There are numerous subforms of validity that have been used to describe increasing rigour for testing an instrument's performance, for example:

- face (on the face of it, appears to measure the concept);
- content (appears to include all major elements of the concept; often assessed by an expert panel of relevant professionals);
- criterion-related (examines the instrument against another or the 'gold-stand-ard' criteria);
- construct.

The aim is for an instrument to have appropriate construct validity, which is the extent that an instrument accurately measures a theoretical construct or trait that is established over time, following repeated use and testing of the instrument in various studies. With any instrument there is the possibility of measurement error. The aim of a good study or instrument is to minimise the chance of that error.

Reliability relates to the accuracy with which the instrument measures the concept being investigated, and which can be tested in terms of stability (test–retest: similar scores on repeated testing for a stable trait), homogeneity (internal consistency: all parts of the instrument measure the same characteristics), and equivalence (inter-rater reliability: consistency between observers using the same instrument with the same subjects). There are a number of statistical tests for reliability, which are commonly expressed as a correlation coefficient, ranging from 0.0 to 1.0. A reliability of 0.80 is considered the minimal acceptable coefficient for a developed instrument.

Responsiveness is the ability of an instrument to detect clinically important changes in the variable of interest with a patient (study subject) (Harris & Warren 1995). This is the opposite characteristic to stability, and relates to the precision of measurement for the instrument. Unfortunately, assessment of this performance characteristic has been minimal when compared to reliability and validity testing (Deyo & Carter 1992).

In addition to the Glossary at the end of this book, Table 8.2 explains some common quantitative research terms used in this chapter. More detailed glossaries are available in specific nursing research texts (e.g. Crookes & Davies 1998; Martin & Thompson 2000).

Quantitative studies collect numerical data to answer the questions or objectives posed. Therefore, all variable information is transformed to numbers prior to data management and analysis. Data analysis procedures can be descriptive or inferential, depending on the design and the levels of measurement for each variable, i.e. nominal, ordinal, interval, ratio. The categories must be mutually exclusive and collectively exhaustive:

- *Nominal.* Assigns values to classify characteristics into nonordered categories, e.g. sex, religion, diagnosis. The assigned numbers do not convey any relative order or weight between the values, e.g. 1 = male, 2 = female; in this instance there is no implication that '1' is ordered higher than '2' or that '2' is twice the score of '1'.
- *Ordinal.* Values are ordered in a logical way in providing a relative ranking; e.g. pain; levels of mobility; self-care; use of Likert Scales – 'Strongly Agree', 'Agree', 'Undecided', 'Disagree', 'Strongly Disagree'.
- *Interval.* Values exhibit a rank ordering with equal distance between values, e.g. temperature; scores on a linear analogue scale (from 1 to 10).
- *Ratio.* Values have the above characteristics plus a meaningful baseline (absolute zero), e.g. weight, height, heart rate.

Data management and analysis are commonly undertaken using software packages (e.g. MS Excel™ spreadsheet software can undertake certain statistical analysis procedures; Statistical Package for the Social Sciences [SPSS] is a comprehensive analysis package). Study designs and methods that provide findings using inferential statistics

Table 8.3 Statistical purposes and related parametric and nonparametric tests. (Adapted from Burns & Grove 1998; Greenhalgh 1997.)

Statistical purpose	Parametric test	Nonparametric test
Compares *mean scores* for two independent samples	Two sample (unpaired) t-test *[interval/ratio data]*	Mann–Whitney U-test *[ordinal data]*
Compares *mean scores* for two sets of observations from the same sample	Paired t-test *[interval/ratio data]*	Wilcoxon matched pairs test *[ordinal data]*
Compares *mean scores* for three or more sets of observations	One-way Analysis of Variance (ANOVA)	Kruskall–Wallis ANOVA by ranks
Compares *proportions* from two samples	Chi-square (χ^2) test	Fisher's exact test
Compares *proportions* from a paired sample	McNemar's test	No equivalent
Assesses strength of straight line *association* between two variables	Product moment correlation coefficient (Pearson's r)	Spearman's rank correlation coefficient (r^s)
Describes *relationship* between two variables, allowing one to be *predicted* from the other	Simple linear regression	Nonparametric regression
Describes *relationship* between a dependent variable and several predictor variables	Multiple regression	Nonparametric regression

allow the researcher to 'infer' that the results from this sample of subjects (e.g. patients) can be applied to the wider population being investigated. Inferential statistics are further categorised into parametric or nonparametric procedures. Parametric tests are used when the following assumptions are met: the sample was drawn from a normal distribution; random sampling was used; and data were measured at least at interval level.

As beginning research consumers, students must consider the objectives of the study and the related purposes for the statistical tests performed. Table 8.3 can be used to critique papers for consistency between the purpose, the level of measurement, and actual tests that are appropriate to answer those questions. More in-depth information regarding the actual statistical tests is beyond the scope of this chapter, but can be found in comprehensive research texts.

Qualitative research

Qualitative research includes a range of research designs and methods. This field of research has its roots in philosophy, anthropology, history and sociology (Denzin

& Lincoln 1994). Qualitative research refers to research that is focused on human experience, including accounts of subjective realities; it is conducted in naturalistic settings involving close, often sustained contact between the researcher and research participants (Oiler Boyd 1993). Naturalistic research is often referred to as field research (Polit & Hungler 1995) because it is conducted in the 'field'. This label may be applied to a range of contexts, for example a community health centre or an intensive care unit.

The qualitative researcher approaches the research project with a different set of values and beliefs to the purely quantitative researcher. These differences relate to the world view (ontology) of the researcher, notions about epistemology (ways of knowing) and research methodology. For example, in the positivist paradigm, concepts such as control, precision, objectivity, testing, one truth, prediction and cause–effect are valued and individual perceptions are not considered. In the qualitative or interpretive paradigm the opposite applies and value is placed on subjectivity, multiple truths may be accommodated, and individuals who participate in this type of research are regarded as research participants, not research subjects as with the positivist approaches. Variables, hypotheses, cause–effect relationships and randomisation are not considered in qualitative approaches. This type of research takes the 'emic' perspective, the insider's point of view (Holloway & Wheeler 1996). Consequently, sampling approaches in qualitative research often deliberately seek people who have lived the experience under investigation. Reasoning in qualitative research is inductive but may involve a process of induction–deduction.

Qualitative research methods are mostly descriptive in nature and allow exploration of a range of human experiences that are of interest in a discipline such as nursing; for example, the experience of suffering for people living with terminal cancer, the characteristics of cultural groups, including their health beliefs, or the question 'What is comfort for recipients of nursing?' It may be possible to study these phenomena using a quantitative approach, but this could be very limiting. The advantage of using a qualitative approach is that the phenomenon may be studied more holistically taking account of shared human reality (Oiler Boyd 1993), there is a focus on human experience, research participants are valued and treated as equals by the researcher, and it is possible to develop a rich description of the experience under investigation with implications for nursing knowledge and often nursing practice. Qualitative research, then, involves

> broadly stated questions about human experiences and realities, studied through sustained contact with persons in their natural environments producing rich, descriptive data that help us to understand those persons' experiences. The emphasis (here) is on achieving understanding that will in turn, open up new options for action and new perspectives that can change people's worlds.
>
> Oiler Boyd (1993:69–70)

Qualitative studies are commonly carried out on small numbers of research participants and involve in-depth inquiry into the phenomenon of concern. The data in qualitative research are presented in the form of words rather than numbers as in quantitative research (Miles & Huberman 1994:1). For example, in many approaches to qualitative research work the researcher may interview the research participants and audio-tape the conversation, which is later transcribed for data analysis. In this way narrative text is often assembled by the researcher in working with the research participants. This text can be analysed and broken down into themes to reflect core ideas or recurring features in the data (Miles & Huberman 1994). This process involves intensive reflection on the part of the researcher. The qualitative paradigm is often referred to as the interpretive paradigm because it centres on interpretation and creation of meaning by human beings, and their subjective reality. Researchers must understand the socially constructed nature of the world and realise that values and interests become part of the research process (Holloway & Wheeler 1996).

The qualitative researcher can choose from a range of research approaches and this selection will be linked to the aims or purposes of the study. Each approach incorporates a way of structuring the study, selecting the research participants, collecting and analysing the data. Some examples are provided below. Readers are directed to any number of nursing research texts for amplification of the approaches to qualitative research described below (Denzin & Lincoln 1994; Holloway & Wheeler 1996; Munhall & Oiler Boyd 1993).

Phenomenology is a philosophy and a descriptive research method designed to uncover the essence and meaning of lived experiences, for example suffering or grieving. 'The focus of phenomenological inquiry ... is what people experience regarding some phenomena and how they interpret those experiences' (Polit & Hungler 1995:197).

Ethnography is a qualitative research approach that is applied to study of the culture of a group. Culture may 'be broadly defined as the learned social behavior or the way of life of a particular group of people. Ethnography provides knowledge (theory) that can be used to help us understand our own culture(s) and those of others' (Germain 1993:237). The ethnographer sets out to uncover insiders' (emic) view of the culture under study as opposed to the outsiders' (etic) view (Polit & Hungler 1995).

Grounded theory is a research process designed to lead to generation of theory through study of a particular human context. This involves a 'search for social processes present in human interaction' (Hutchinson 1993:181).

In the course of your reading and learning about research processes in nursing you will discover that in some instances researchers mix quantitative and qualitative research processes in research design; qualitative research processes may be considered soft and less rigorous by proponents of positivist research; and that evaluative criteria for establishing the scientific validity of qualitative research are the subject of ongoing debate. As the content of this chapter is introductory, you can also expect to learn of other research traditions, paradigms and methods during your undergraduate education.

DEVELOPING RESEARCH QUESTIONS

Research ideas come from many sources. Some ideas are derived from theoretical considerations while others arise from the need to solve practical problems or to improve the quality of care. Having a good idea is often not enough – you need to translate that idea into research questions. This section discusses how to develop research questions based on the amount of knowledge and/or theory about the topic, and describes the importance of a thorough review of the literature to identify relevant theory and research.

A research question needs to be clearly stated as an 'explicit query about a problem or issue that can be challenged, examined, and analysed and that will yield useful new information' (Brink & Wood 1993:2). Although there are no specific rules and procedures for asking research questions, the way research questions are worded can have an effect on the research design and methods that follow.

Research questions can be classified into levels based on the amount of knowledge and/or theory about the topic.

Level I research studies are known as exploratory, with little or no literature on either the topic or the population to be researched. Questions at Level I are designed to explore the topic or a single population, as the area under study has not been adequately researched. Hence the question is always 'What is?' or 'What are?' The question is asked in a way that leads to an exploratory research design.

Level II research studies build on the results of studies at the first level. There is existing knowledge and theory about the topic and population. Questions at Level II examine relationships between variables. A variable is a characteristic being measured that can vary or be manipulated among the subjects under study. Level II questions ask, 'What is the relationship?' and the topic often contains two or more variables. Statistical analysis is used to determine the significance of the relationship between the variables. All Level II questions lead to correlation designs.

Questions at *Level III* require considerable knowledge of the topic. Research at this level begins at knowing the relationships between variables, therefore questions at Level III are designed to examine why this relationship exists, with a rationale and with an explanation. 'All Level III questions lead to experimental designs' (Brink & Wood 1993:16).

When formulating a research question it is important that you discuss your topic and question with your colleagues or experts in the field, as this will assist you with the development and refinement of the research question. Often the initial research question is formulated too broadly for the time frame that is available or to make the appropriate observations. Consider the following example of such a question: Do undergraduate students taught in a supportive environment increase their learning capabilities as graduates? Before this can be answered, a number of issues have to be clarified. What exactly is a supportive environment? What does it mean to increase their learning capabilities? How do we measure learning capabilities? How do we determine learning capabilities in graduates? Until you can define the terms and determine how to measure the variables they represent, you cannot answer the original question. Frequently researchers have to narrow the topic area or, in some cases, the types and number of settings or the number of participants they include in the study. This process of narrowing the topic ultimately must also be consistent with the research design and methods of the study.

Reviewing the literature

Whether you begin with a vague idea of a research study or a well-developed research plan, every research study needs to be considered an extension of previous knowledge and thereby stimulate research. There are many reasons for reviewing the literature before beginning a research endeavour. Firstly, your research question may have been addressed and answered, or a review can be the initial source of ideas for a research question. By being familiar with and understanding what has already been done with existing research and theory in an area, you can devise your research study to explore any newly identified questions (Bordens & Abbott 1996). The review will also assist you to establish a theoretical context and rationale for your study. From a practical (methodological) perspective the review can reveal research strategies, measuring instruments, experimental techniques and analysis. It allows you to learn from the strengths and limitations of other researchers' work in regard to successful outcomes and assumptions. A further advantage is that a review of the literature also keeps you up to date with current research work that has been undertaken in the area of interest.

WHERE DO WE FIND RESEARCH?

Literally hundreds of research journals, dissertations, reports and books are published each year. One of the most important steps in the research process is conducting a thorough literature review. Students are often faced with the dilemma of how extensive a review is necessary. There is no formula to determine that 60 or 120 articles will provide the necessary background for the study. The number of references will depend on how familiar you are with the area under investigation, and the scope of the review will depend on how much research is available in that area. Checking the reference list at the end of recent articles can often assist in the process. Experienced researchers know that maintaining an up-to-date review of the literature is an ongoing process throughout the research project.

To begin with, it is important to differentiate between primary and secondary sources. A primary source is a report written by the study author/s themselves. A primary source includes information on the rationale of the study, its participants, design, methods of collecting data, procedure, results, outcomes, limitations, recommendations and references. Most research articles published in professional journals are primary sources. A secondary source is one that summarises information from primary sources presented by other authors. When an author cites a previous study in the review of literature section, that is a secondary source. Both primary and secondary sources are important; however secondary sources should not be substitutes for primary sources. Avoid over-reliance on secondary sources, and make every effort to obtain the primary sources that are important to you.

Many libraries also provide reference sources in computer databases to assist students in locating references on a specific topic and to undertake their own computer searches. A computer search will generate complete bibliographic citations, often including abstracts of many articles published in a particular area of interest. A variety of indexes and databases are available, providing bibliographic listings of articles, abstracts, conference proceedings and books. The reader is recommended to consult a recent, handy research users' guide to the medical literature (Guyatt & Rennie 2002).

Indexes, abstracts and databases

Some cumulative indexes provide abstracts, while others do not publish abstracts. Abstracts are short summaries of the article. Abstracts give more information about the article, as titles can be misleading in their description of the content. All indexes provide bibliography citations, giving the authors' names, article title, journal volume and issue number, date and pages. Each academic discipline has an index to its collection of journals. Most indexes and databases in the medical field use medical subject headings. When a topic is not found in the subject headings, you need to find some related terms that have been adopted by most of the journal publishers. Many journals also publish key words with an article that refers to these headings. A valuable index and database in the health science literature for health research is the Cumulative Index to Nursing and Allied Health Literature (CINAHL) which has all nursing journals and several allied health disciplines listed. Other important indexes and databases are Indexis Medicus (MEDLINE) and Excerpta Medica (EMBASE) which provide a bibliography of medical reviews (Guyatt & Rennie 20002). MEDLINE is an attractive database for finding information because of its comprehensive coverage and its accessibility. Anyone with internet access can search MEDLINE free of charge using PubMed. However, an understanding of how to use Medical Subject Headings (MESH) is essential (Guyatt & Rennie 2002). The Cochrane Collaboration publishes the Cochrane Library, which focuses primarily on systematic reviews of controlled trials of therapeutic interventions. Updated quarterly, the Cochrane Library is available in CD-ROM format or over the internet. Other important abstract indexes that may be of relevance to your topic are: Education Resources Information Centre (ERIC), PsycINFO, Sociological Abstracts, Cancer Literature (CANCERLIT) and Dissertation Abstracts On-line.

The role of peer-reviewed journals in disseminating research

Peer-reviewed journals serve many important functions, including facilitation of expert review of manuscripts, reporting the findings of research studies or theoretical papers, dissemination of papers that have been approved for publication following peer review, and serving as a resource for scholars and researchers involved in compiling and/or developing knowledge in an area of nursing research or practice. Criteria which must be met before a paper is approved for publication in a refereed journal vary from one to another, but all editors will be concerned with a standard of excellence that must be met (particularly in regard to scientific merit), relevance of the paper in terms of its potential to contribute to incremental development of knowledge in the area, as well as the literary standard of the work. There are many peer-reviewed journals in nursing internationally. Each has its own aims and purposes and requirements which must be followed by nurses wishing to submit their work for peer review with a view to being published in the journal. Most university libraries hold extensive collections of refereed journals in hard copy across a range of disciplines, and lately some journals such as the *Journal of Advanced Nursing* are available on-line, negating the need for hard copies stored on library shelves. The Nursing Collection is a CD-ROM comprising a number of journals, which allows for downloading of full-text articles.

HOW NURSES CAN USE RESEARCH

In recent times nursing and other health professionals have been interested in the quality of patient care and establishing standards for best clinical practice, by examining the evidence base. Findings from research studies are commonly disseminated at conferences and in professional journals. Some studies are designed to inform clinical practice. For example, studies may describe a clinical practice, or compare two (or more) different ways of performing a practice. Other types of studies may shed light on patients' experiences of phenomena that are poorly understood, for example, hope or suffering.

As noted earlier, not all nurses need the ability to conduct research, but all clinical nurses need research utilisation skills in order to practise in a professional manner and in accordance with the best available evidence. Research utilisation skills involve the Four As mentioned earlier in this chapter and include abilities in *accessing* the literature, an *awareness* of important and recent studies applicable to their area of practice, an *appreciation* of the study findings, and *application* of the findings in relation to their own practice setting. These skills are important, but clearly different from the *ability* to undertake primary research. The ability to critique studies is therefore a fundamental skill for undergraduate nurses to master in preparation for professional practice as registered nurses. Current registered nurses also need these skills in terms of continuing professional development. However, the skill is not easily attained, and does not magically appear at the end of a single university research course. Rather, the ability is additive in that it is related to experience, practice and reflection over time. In fact, it is an ability that relates to 'life-long learning' as it is an area where we can always learn and improve our skills.

Evidence-based practice

The critique of an individual research paper can be extended to multiple papers on the same topic, resulting in a literature review. This is a common assessment item for university nursing students. An adaptation of this narrative literature review is a systematic review (SR), which addresses a well-defined question, provides specific information on the process undertaken to minimise bias in the review process, and uses a systematic approach to assess the quality of each study reviewed (Droogan & Cullum 1998). The question for an SR has a specific clinical focus with four components:

(1) a specific patient population and setting;
(2) a clinical condition of interest;
(3) exposure to a clinical intervention;
(4) measurement of a specific outcome.

The search strategy describes the databases (e.g. CINAHL; MEDLINE) and/or journals searched by hand. Selection of articles occurs by keywords in the article title or abstract, followed by a preliminary review prior to final selection of the papers for inclusion in the SR. Included studies are then assessed according to stated criteria. A systematic review may also include the pooling and analysis of data from the studies investigated; this process is called a meta-analysis.

A number of organisations are now developing repositories of systematic reviews to appropriately guide clinical practice (Cochrane 1972). The Cochrane Collaboration is an international network of individuals from different disciplines committed to the preparation, maintenance and dissemination of SRs of research evidence about the effects of health care (http://www.general@cochrane.co.uk). The Cochrane Library contains three main sections: the Cochrane Database of Systematic Reviews (CDSR) that includes the complete reports of all the SRs that have been produced by members of the Cochrane Collaboration and the protocols for the Cochrane SRs that are under way; the Database of Reviews of Effectiveness (DARE) that includes SRs that have been published outside the collaboration; and the Cochrane Controlled Trials Registry (CCTR) that contains the references to clinical trials that Cochrane investigators have found by searching a wide range of sources (Guyatt & Rennie 2002). A critique and examples of systematic reviews in nursing was published by Droogan and Cullum (1998).

The majority of the current systematic reviews are related to medicine. This is not surprising, given the number of studies and journals devoted to topics in the various medical subspecialties. As noted previously, the 'gold standard' for examining cause-and-effect questions in clinical practice is the randomised controlled trial (RCT). Thus, a hierarchy of study designs for studies of effectiveness have been developed (NHS Centre for Reviews and Dissemination 2001):

Level 1:   Experimental studies (e.g. RCT with concealed allocation).
Level 2:   Quasi-experimental studies (e.g. experimental study without randomisation).
Level 3:   Controlled observational studies.
Level 3.a: Cohort studies.
Level 3.b: Case control studies.
Level 4:   Observational studies without control groups.
Level 5:   Expert opinion based on pathophysiology, bench research or consensus.

It is important to remember that RCTs should rank high in the hierarchy only when they are well conducted. If there are no good RCTs, then well-conducted quasi-experimental and observational studies should be considered. Quality criteria for the assessment of all of these study designs have been produced (NHS Centre for Reviews and Dissemination 2001), though it is important to remember that quality is a construct about which there are differing views. The Centre for Evidence-Based Nursing (Droogan & Cullum 1998) is currently involved in systematic reviews of specific clinical practices that are of importance to nurses (see their websites for current projects: www.york.ac.uk/depts/hstd/centres/evidence/cebn.htm).

It should be borne in mind, however, that nursing uses a variety of research paradigms and methods to answer questions that cannot be appropriately investigated by RCTs. We therefore need to consider how to evaluate non-RCT observational studies of nursing practice so that these findings can also guide nursing care. Further, how do we incorporate findings from qualitative studies which have no generalisability to the patient group in question, but which may provide valuable insights into patient experiences in guiding quality nursing practice? The development of the necessary frameworks to address these issues is not yet formed or developed to an adequate level nationally or internationally. The aim, therefore, is to foster systematic reviews of relevant studies on clinical nursing so that quality nursing practice will be informed by the best available evidence, regardless of the research design.

CONCLUSION

An understanding of basic concepts and processes in research is central to professional nursing practice. Ideally, quality nursing care is based on the outcomes of quality research processes. It is envisaged that in time one of the hallmarks of the profession of nursing will be the utilisation of research evidence in efforts to provide the best, safest and most appropriate care. All nurses engaged in nursing practice require research utilisation skills in order to make judgements about how relevant and applicable research findings are to practice. Nursing is a complex, practice-based discipline in which a range of researchable questions will always require answers in order to extend knowledge. This in turn requires use of a range of research paradigms and methods.

REFLECTIVE QUESTIONS

(1) What processes could be followed in formulating a research problem in nursing?
(2) What advantages, if any, might qualitative research designs have over quantitative research designs in clinical nursing research?
(3) What are the critical features of a comprehensive review of the literature?

RECOMMENDED READING

Crookes, P.A. & Davies, S. (eds) (1998) *Research into Practice: Essential Skills for Reading and Applying Research in Nursing and Health Care.* Baillière Tindall, Edinburgh.
Guyatt, G. & Rennie, D. (eds) (2002) *Users' Guides to the Medical Literature: A Manual for Evidence-Based Clinical Practice.* AMA Press, Chicago.
Holloway, I. & Wheeler, S. (1996) *Qualitative Research for Nurses.* Blackwell Science, Oxford.
Martin, C.R. & Thompson, D.R. (2000) *Design and Analysis of Clinical Nursing Research Studies.* Routledge, London.
Oakley, A. (2000) *Experiments in Knowing: Gender and Method in the Social Sciences.* Polity Press, Cambridge.

REFERENCES

Bordens, K.S. & Abbott, B.B. (1996) *Research Design and Methods: A Process Approach.* Mayfield, Mountain View, California.

Briggs, A. (1972) *Report of the Committee on Nursing,* Cmnd 5115. HMSO, London.

Brink, P.J. & Wood, M.J. (1993) *Basic Steps in Planning Nursing Research.* Jones and Bartlett, Boston.

Burns, N. & Grove, S.K. (1998) *The Practice of Nursing Research: Conduct, Critique, and Utilization,* 3rd edn. Saunders, Philadelphia.

Cochrane, A.L. (1972) *Effectiveness and Efficiency: Random Reflections on Health Services.* Nuffield Provincial Hospitals Trust, London.

Crookes, P.A. & Davies, S. (eds) (1998) *Research into Practice: Essential Skills for Reading and Applying Research in Nursing and Health Care.* Baillière Tindall, Edinburgh.

D'Antonio, P. (1997) Toward a history of research in nursing. *Nursing Research,* **46**(2), 105–110.

Denzin, N.K. & Lincoln, Y.S. (1994) Introduction: Entering the field of qualitative research. In: *Handbook of Qualitative Research* (eds N.K. Denzin & Y.S. Lincoln). Sage, Thousand Oaks, California.

Department of Health (1991) *Research for Health: A Research and Development Strategy for the National Health Service.* HMSO, London.

Department of Health (1993) *Report of the Taskforce on the Strategy for Research in Nursing, Midwifery and Health Visiting.* Department of Health, Leeds.

Department of Health (1999) *Making a Difference: Strengthening the Nursing, Midwifery and Health Visiting Contribution to Health and Healthcare.* Department of Health, London.

Department of Health (2000) *Towards a Strategy for Nursing Research and Development.* Department of Health, London.

Department of Health (2001) *Research Governance Framework for Health and Social Care.* Department of Health, London.

Deyo, R.A. & Carter, W.B. (1992) Strategies for improving and expanding the application of health status measures in clinical settings: A researcher-developer viewpoint. *Medical Care,* **30**(5 suppl.), 176–186.

Droogan, J. & Cullum, N. (1998) Systematic reviews in nursing. *International Journal of Nursing Studies,* **35**, 13–22.

Germain, C.P. (1993) Ethnography: The method. In: *Nursing Research: A Qualitative Perspective* (eds P.L. Munhall & C. Oiler Boyd), 2nd edn, pp. 237–268. National League for Nursing, New York.

Greenhalgh, P. (1997) *How to Read a Paper.* BMJ Publishing, London.

Guyatt, G. & Rennie, D. (eds) (2002) *Users' Guides to the Medical Literature: A Manual for Evidence-based Clinical Practice.* AMA Press, Chicago.

Harris, M.R. & Warren, J.J. (1995) Patient outcomes: Assessment for the CNS. *Clinical Nurse Specialist,* **9**(2), 82–86.

Holloway, I. & Wheeler, S. (1996) *Qualitative Research for Nurses.* Blackwell Science, Oxford.

Hutchinson, S.A. (1993) Grounded theory: The method. In: *Nursing Research: A Qualitative Perspective* (eds P.L. Munhall & C. Oiler Boyd), 2nd edn, pp. 180–212. National League for Nursing, New York.

Martin, C.R. & Thompson, D.R. (2000) *Design and Analysis of Clinical Nursing Research Studies*. Routledge, London.

Miles, M.B. & Huberman, A.M. (1994) *Qualitative Data Analysis*, 2nd edn. Sage, Thousand Oaks.

Mulhall, A. (1995) Nursing research: What difference does it make? *Journal of Advanced Nursing*, **21**, 576–583.

Munhall, P.L. & Oiler Boyd, C. (1993) *Nursing Research: A Qualitative Perspective*. National League for Nursing Press, New York.

NHS Centre for Reviews and Dissemination (2001) *Undertaking Systematic Reviews of Research on Effectiveness*. CRD's guidance for those carrying out or commissioning reviews. CRD Report No. 4, 2nd edn. NHS Centre for Reviews and Dissemination, York.

Oakley, A. (2000) *Experiments in Knowing: Gender and Method in the Social Sciences*. Polity Press, Cambridge.

Oiler Boyd, C. (1993) Philosophical foundations of qualitative research. In: *Nursing Research: A Qualitative Perspective* (eds P.L. Munhall & C. Oiler Boyd), 2nd edn, pp. 66–93. National League for Nursing, New York.

Polit, D.F. & Hungler, B.P. (1995) *Nursing Research: Principles and Methods*, 5th edn. Lippincott, Philadelphia.

Sackett, D.L. & Wennberg, J.E. (1997) Choosing the best research design for each question: It's time to stop squabbling over the 'best' methods (editorial). *British Medical Journal*, **315**(7123), 1636.

9 A Reappraisal of Everyday Nursing Ethics
New Directions for the Twenty-First Century

Megan-Jane Johnstone

LEARNING OBJECTIVES

Upon completion of this chapter the reader will be able to:

- define nursing ethics;
- outline the development of mainstream bioethics;
- discuss the relationship between nursing ethics and mainstream bioethics;
- explore a range of 'everyday' ethical issues which nurses might face in the course of providing nursing care to clients/patients;
- discuss four areas in which a re-examination of the ethical issues faced by the nursing profession is warranted.

KEY WORDS

MORAL, ETHICS, NURSING ETHICS, BIOETHICS, SOCIAL JUSTICE.

INTRODUCTION

Nurses at all levels and in all areas of practice are confronted every day with having to make morally relevant choices and to take action on the basis of these choices during the course of their work. This 'everyday' occurrence should not be taken to mean, however, that deciding and acting morally in nursing care contexts is simply a matter of habit or 'daily routine' and therefore as something trivial requiring little knowledge, skill or attention. On the contrary. As can be readily demonstrated, dealing with everyday ethical problems requires of decision makers an exquisite moral sensibility, 'moral knowing', moral imagination, life experience, virtue (e.g. compassion, empathy, integrity, care, 'decency'), general informedness (e.g. about law, social and cultural processes, human nature, politics), and a deep personal commitment

An earlier version of this chapter was published in 1997 in the *INEN Bulletin* **5**(1), pp. 1–4 (the newsletter of the International Nursing Ethics (& Midwifery) Network, Maastricht, The Netherlands). It has been revised for inclusion in this publication.

to 'doing what is right'. In some instances 'being moral' also requires political savvy and an ability (personal and otherwise) to overcome the many obstacles that may obstruct or prevent a morally just outcome. Although it should be otherwise, there are times when deciding to act morally can require enormous courage and even 'moral heroism' on the part of those choosing to take an ethical course of action. This is especially so in the case of nurses who, despite an apparent increase in professional status in recent times, continue to lack authority in their own realm of practice, continue to be burdened with enormous responsibilities without the lawful authority to fulfil them, and continue to be forced into silence when what they have to say on important ethical issues threatens the powerful vested interests of others (Johnstone 1994, 1998).

All aspects of nursing (e.g. education, practice, management and research) have a profound ethical dimension. This dimension of nursing is distinguished from others such as the legal and clinical dimensions by the inherent moral demands to:

- promote human well-being and welfare;
- balance the needs and significant moral interests of different people;
- make reliable judgements on what constitutes morally 'right' and 'wrong' conduct, and provide sound justifications for the decisions and actions taken on the basis of these judgements.

Members of the nursing profession cannot escape these demands or the stringent responsibilities they impose. One reason for this is that no nursing decision or action (however small or trivial) occurs in a moral vacuum, or is free of moral risk or consequence – even the most 'ordinary' of nursing actions can affect significantly the well-being, welfare and moral interests of others. This is so whether in a nursing education, practice, management or research setting.

Nursing codes of ethics around the world make clear that nurses have a stringent moral responsibility to promote and safeguard the well-being, welfare and moral interests of people needing and/or receiving nursing care. These codes also variously recognise the responsibility of nurses to balance equally the needs and interests of different people in health care contexts. What is often not stated, however, is how nurses ought to fulfil their moral responsibilities to deal effectively with the many ethical issues they encounter on a day-to-day basis. 'Dealing effectively' with ethical issues in this instance includes being able to:

- identify correctly the most pertinent ethical issues facing nurses (locally and globally) at any given time;
- recognise both the short- and long-term implications of these issues for the nursing profession generally;
- develop strategies for responding effectively to these issues, once identified.

Dealing effectively with ethical issues in nursing also requires at least a rudimentary understanding of: (a) what nursing ethics are, and (b) the relationship between nursing ethics and mainstream bioethics. Let us now consider these two points.

WHAT ARE NURSING ETHICS?

In advancing this discussion, it is important first to provide a brief definition of the notion 'nursing ethics'. Nursing ethics can be defined broadly as the examination of all kinds of ethical (and bioethical) issues from the perspective of nursing theory and practice. In turn, these issues rest on the agreed core concepts of nursing: person, culture, care, health, healing, environment, and nursing itself (that is, its end and good or *telos*) (Johnstone 1999:46). In this regard, then, and contrary to popular belief, nursing ethics are not synonymous with (and indeed are much greater than) an ethic of care, although an ethic of care has an important place in the overall moral scheme of nursing and nursing ethics. Unlike other approaches to ethics, nursing ethics recognise the 'distinctive voices' that are nurses', and emphasise the importance of collecting and recording nursing narratives and 'stories from the field' (Benner 1991, 1994; Bishop & Scudder 1990; Parker 1990; Hodge 1993). Collecting and collating stories from the field are regarded as important, since issues invariably emerge from these stories that extend far beyond the 'paramount' issues otherwise espoused by mainstream bioethics (to be identified shortly).

Analyses of these stories tend to reveal not only a range of issues that are nurses' 'own', as it were, but a whole different configuration of language, concepts and metaphors for expressing them (Johnstone 1999:46). As well, these stories often reveal issues otherwise overlooked or marginalised by mainstream bioethics discourse. Given this, nursing ethics can also be described as 'methodologically and substantively, inquiry from the point of view of nurses' experiences, with nurses' experiences being taken as a more reliable starting point than other mainstream ethics discourses (texts, practices and processes) from which to advance a substantive and meaningful nursing ethics discourse' (Johnstone 1999:46–47).

NURSING ETHICS AND THEIR RELATIONSHIP WITH MAINSTREAM BIOETHICS

Contemporary nursing ethics have been profoundly influenced by the Western mainstream bioethics movement. Whether this influence has been advantageous to the development of nursing ethics, however, remains an open question and one that has yet to be fully explored by the nursing profession (see also Johnstone 1999: 45–48).

The term 'bioethics' first found its way into public usage in 1970/1971 in the USA (Reich 1994). Although originally only cautiously accepted by a few influential North American academics, the new term quickly 'symbolised and influenced the rise and shaping of the field itself' (Reich 1994:320). Significantly, within three years of its emergence the new term was accepted and used widely at a public level (Reich 1994: 328). Today, both in lay and professional circles, bioethics (and all the issues associated with it as a movement) have become the subject of major interest and debate.

Initially the term 'bioethics' was used in two different ways. The first (and later marginalised) sense had an 'environmental and evolutionary significance' (Reich 1994:320). The other, competing, sense in which the word 'bioethics' was used referred more narrowly to the ethics of medicine and biomedical research. Significantly, it was this latter sense which 'came to dominate the emerging field of bioethics in academic circles and in the mind of the public' and which remains dominant today (Reich 1994:320).

The primary focus of contemporary bioethical debate tends to be on 'exotic' issues such as: abortion, euthanasia and assisted suicide (and the associated issue of advanced directives), organ transplantation (and the associated issue of brain death criteria), reproductive technology (for example, *in vitro* fertilisation [IVF], surrogacy, genetic engineering). The debate also focuses on ethics committees, informed consent, confidentiality, the economic rationalisation of health care, and research ethics (particularly in regard to randomised clinical trials and experimental surgery). Not only have mainstream bioethics come to refer to and represent the above and other related issues but, controversially, they have given legitimacy to them – through the power of naming – as *the* most pressing (or 'paramount') bioethical concerns of contemporary health care in the Western world.

The nursing profession, like other health care professions, has responded vigorously to the modern bioethics movement. Since the late 1970s there has been a plethora of texts and journal articles published specifically on the topic of 'nursing ethics' in which a full range of the popular mainstream bioethical issues have been raised and explored; undoubtedly these works have made an important contribution to knowledge of the field, and have assisted many nurses in their quest to competently and confidently fulfil the many moral responsibilities associated with their professional practice. Nevertheless, the apparent and possibly obvious practical importance of bioethics to nurses, while recognised, is not without controversy.

One reason for this controversy is that the dominance of the more exotic ethical issues in the nursing literature has sometimes been at the expense of other areas that could be judged as being more relevant to the profession and practice of nursing. For example, while much has been written on the ethics of euthanasia and medically assisted suicide (both regarded as 'paramount' issues in the bioethics literature), comparatively little has been written on the unethical economic rationalisation (read 'decline') of expert nursing care services for people at the end stages of their lives. Similarly, while literature abounds on the subject of promoting patients' rights (abstract entitlements) in health care contexts (for example, the right to confidentiality, the right to give an informed consent to treatment, the right to die), comparatively little has been written on the promotion of patients' genuine well-being and welfare (tangible realities) which are sometimes compromised in the interests of upholding a patient's supposed 'rights' (Johnstone 1999:254–255). To further complicate the issue, there is much discussion on patients' rights to refuse medical treatment, but virtually nothing is said on patients' entitlements to request that 'everything possible to be done' including (and perhaps especially) the provision of quality nursing care from qualified and skilled nurses. And, to cite one more example, while much has been written on nurses' duties in regard to upholding patients' rights and employer interests, comparatively little has been written on nurses' rights and interests – despite the fact that, compared with other health workers, nurses are at disproportionate risk of being exploited, scapegoated, abused, injured, maimed and even killed during the course of their work (Alspach 1993; Hadfield 1991; Johnstone 1994; Kinkle 1993). On this point it is significant that, although nurses are morally entitled to be protected from these abuses, and are not obligated to 'act beyond the call of duty' in situations where their lives and genuine well-being are at risk, the issue of nurse exploitation, scapegoating, abuse and violence has rarely been addressed as an ethical issue *per se* either in the nursing ethics or mainstream bioethics literature.

IDENTIFYING AND RESPONDING EFFECTIVELY TO ETHICAL ISSUES IN NURSING

It is important to understand that ethical issues in health care contexts do not only involve the so-called 'big' or 'exotic' issues (for example when to disconnect a 'brain dead' patient from a life-support machine; whether to abort a severely disabled fetus); health care ethics also involve fundamental questions about the nature and quality of professional–client relationships. It is also about examining the more fundamental day-to-day practical ethical concerns relating to the precise impact that nurses' decisions and actions (or nonactions) have on the lives and welfare of other human beings and to 'our capacity to do harm to others while claiming scientific and professional legitimacy' (adapted from Lifton 1990:xiii).

While the so-called 'paramount' ethical issues (abortion, euthanasia, etc.) are widely discussed in the mainstream bioethics literature, health care professional literature and the lay media, it would be a mistake to conclude that these issues are the only or, indeed, the most important problems facing nurses and health care professionals. Indeed, there are many other issues that, though less 'exotic', are of equal importance and that are equally deserving of attention. However, because these matters tend to be specific to the different health care contexts in which people work, or tend to be 'too political', or both, they do not always get the attention they deserve. The ethical issues faced by nurses working in a variety of health care contexts are an example of this.

The kinds of ethical issues faced by nurses are as complex as they are varied. While until recently attention has tended to be focused on the better-known bioethical issues already identified, there has been a significant shift in the kinds of ethical issues faced by nurses and it is becoming increasingly difficult to ignore a range of other issues of relevance to the profession and practice of nursing. These issues include: (a) 'everyday' practical ethical issues faced by nurses; (b) a genuine *nursing* perspective on common mainstream bioethical issues, and (c) (the otherwise neglected) broader social justice issues associated with promoting the well-being and significant moral interests of stigmatised and marginalised groups of people.

'Everyday' ethical issues faced by nurses

As stated earlier, nurses have to deal with ethical issues every day. The nursing ethics literature does not, however, always represent or reflect the reality of these 'everyday' problems for nurses. Instead, this literature has borrowed heavily from mainstream bioethics to shape nursing ethics discourse, and that has sometimes been at the expense of nurses' own experiential wisdom.

There is considerable reason to suggest that the actual lived experiences of nurses would (and do) provide a far more reliable methodological starting point to nursing ethics inquiry than do the 'top down' theories of Western moral philosophy and the field of bioethics that derives from it (Johnstone 1999:46–47). An examination of nurses' lived experiences would yield important insights into such areas as:

- *Moral boundaries of nursing* (e.g. nurses as carers being 'in relationship' with others, as opposed to being what the North American philosopher, John Rawls (1971), describes as: 'detached observers choosing from behind a veil of ignorance').
- *Catalysts to moral action* (e.g. 'experiential triggers' such as 'the look of suffering in a patient's eyes', as opposed to abstract moral rules and principles).
- *Operating moral values* (e.g. sympathy, empathy, compassion, human understanding, and a desire 'to do the best we can', rather than an obsession to 'do one's duty').
- *Ethical decision-making processes* (which tend to be collaborative, communicative, communal and contextualised, rather than independent, private, individual, solo and decontextualised).
- *Barriers to ethical practice* (which tend to be structural rather than knowledge based – e.g. the power and authority of doctors to determine patient care, organisational norms forcing compliance with the *status quo*, and negative attitudes and a lack of support from coworkers and managers).
- *Need for cathartic moral talking* (e.g. 'talking through' moral concerns in a safe and supportive environment to help relieve the distress that so often arises as a result of trying to be moral in a world that appears to be growing increasingly amoral). For a helpful discussion on moral stress/distress and moral incident stress debriefing, see Johnstone (1998:83–88).

What talking with nurses so often reveals is that it is not the so-called paramount ('exotic') bioethical issues that trouble them, but the more fundamental issues of:

- how to help a patient in distress in the 'here and now';
- how to stop 'things going bad for a patient';
- how to best support a relative or chosen carer during times of distress and when the 'system' appears to be against them;
- how to make things 'less traumatic' for someone who is suffering;
- how to reduce the anxiety and vulnerability of the people being cared for;
- where nurses can get help for their own moral distress;
- how to make a difference in contexts where indifference to the moral interests of others is manifest.

The above and other related concerns are all issues worthy of attention and consideration within and outside the nursing profession. They are also issues that deserve to be recognised as constitutive of a substantive moral schema that might be appropriately described as nursing ethics.

A nursing perspective on mainstream bioethics

Mainstream bioethics have had as their principal concern the ethics of medicine and biomedical research, and this has been at the expense of the ethical concerns of other health care professions, including nursing (Reich 1995). One major consequence of this has been that the viewpoints of nurses on the ethics (or lack of them) of certain medical and health care practices have been either invalidated, marginalised, trivialised or ignored altogether (Johnstone 1999). In some instances, nurses have had their job security threatened and have even lost their jobs for speaking out against, or for exposing, unethical practices in health care contexts. Some examples are the 'unfortunate experiment' case in New Zealand (discussed in Johnstone 1999), the Pink case in the United Kingdom (Turner 1990, 1992) and the noted North American legal cases of *Free* v. *Holy Cross Hospital* (1987)[1] and *Warthen* v. *Toms River Community Memorial Hospital* (1985)[2] (both discussed in Johnstone 1994, 1998).

The neglect and marginalisation of nurses' concerns and experiences is seriously problematic for mainstream bioethics. Not only does such oversight render mainstream bioethics 'less than complete', but, paradoxically 'unethical', because of its discrimination against a nursing point of view in favour of the 'more legitimate' medical point of view. In failing to give due attention to the concerns and experiences of nurses, mainstream bioethics contribute to the subjugation of the moral voice of nurses and, in so doing, contribute to the subjugation of the moral interests and genuine well-being of patients. By even the most rudimentary of moral calculations, this situation is unjust, hence morally unacceptable.

Issues of social justice

Earlier it was explained that the word 'bioethics' has come to refer narrowly to the ethics of medicine and biomedical research. This has not only resulted in the marginalisation of the ethics of other professions (e.g. nursing) (Reich 1995), but in the marginalisation of other important issues which do not 'fit' with the mainstream ethical concerns of medicine and biomedical research. For example, a cursory glance of the bioethics literature will reveal a scandalous neglect of the ethical issues associated with providing health care to highly stigmatised populations – people with mental health problems, the poor, the homeless, the unemployed, the disabled, survivors of child abuse, partner abuse and elder abuse, people from different cultural backgrounds, refugees, homosexuals and transgendered persons. Significantly, the nursing ethics literature has also been relatively silent in this area. As long as nurses interact with and care for people from these stigmatised and highly vulnerable groups, they will be faced with having to make morally relevant choices associated with their care. Given this, it is morally imperative that the many special and complex ethical issues inherent in caring for people within these populations are identified and addressed as a matter of priority, and that nurses working in the field are educationally prepared to respond effectively to these special problems when they arise.

ISSUES AND RECOMMENDATIONS

It is timely to raise important questions about the nature and future directions of contemporary nursing ethics. I do not suggest that the better known issues of abortion, euthanasia, organ transplantation, reproductive technology, patients' rights to informed consent, confidentiality, etc., are not important. Clearly they are important and will

continue to be as long as people are confronted with having to make morally relevant choices related to these issues. There is room to suggest, however, that these
more 'mainstream' issues *might not have the same priority in different health care
contexts, nor necessarily be the most important ethical issues* that nurses, and indeed
other health professionals and the community at large, need to be grappling with at
this present time.

A re-examination of the kinds of ethical issues faced by nurses today is warranted,
as is the need to make visible the experiences of nurses in trying to be moral in
contexts which can be – and for the most part are – extremely demanding at both
a personal and a professional level. While it has not been possible to identify or do
justice to all the 'new' ethical issues that nurses face, perhaps the brief discussion
given here will provide a catalyst for further discussion and reflection on the nursing
profession's global task of making visible and, through this, giving legitimacy to what
might be appropriately described as the distinctive field of 'nursing ethics'.

In particular, attention needs to be given to identifying, considering and responding effectively (at local, national and global levels) to issues relevant to the following
key areas:

Nursing education: e.g. the ethics of ethics education for nurses (what to teach,
how to teach, when to teach, whether teaching ethics is possible, cross-cultural considerations); designing curricula to prepare nurses in 'preventive ethics'; devising and
teaching an 'ethics of personality' (e.g. what does it mean to be a virtuous or 'decent'
human being? Are nurses as 'decent' as they could be? Is virtue enough to fulfil the
task of ethics? Can virtue/decency be taught?); preparing nurses to take a stand (e.g.
against unscrupulous practices, conscientious objection, action lobbying on local
policy issues, broader social justice issues, professional ethical issues, law reforms
relevant to nursing ethics); global ethics (e.g. environmental, cultural and political
concerns); ethical issues in nursing education itself.

Nursing practice: e.g. the ingredients of and the processes that facilitate the ethical
practice of nursing; 'everyday' issues versus large philosophical issues; the nature and
implications of the moral boundaries of nursing and nursing relationships; catalysts
to moral action; guiding moral values; ethical decision-making processes; barriers to
ethical practice; moral distress; institutional/management support of nurses dealing
with moral quandaries; formulation of position statements by professional nursing
organisations; the unacceptable moral consequences of the economic rationalisation
of nursing care provided by qualified and skilled nurses and the increasing use by
health care agencies of lower paid, unqualified carers.

Nursing management: e.g. how best to prepare nurse managers not just to manage ethically (e.g. treat employees fairly), but to manage ethical problems effectively
in the workplace (e.g. using their positions to develop an ethical culture within
the workplace, supporting staff, providing a 'safe place' for cathartic moral talking,
institutional/unit policy development, resource mobilisation).

Nursing research: e.g. improving recognition of philosophic inquiry (of which ethics inquiry is a form) as a legitimate and important form of research within nursing;
developing an ethics research agenda (involving all research approaches); facilitation of research into ethical issues in nursing; making visible nursing's experience
of ethical issues; developing nursing ethics theory; ethical issues in nursing research
itself.

CONCLUSION

Nurses in all areas and levels of practice are confronted with ethical issues on a daily basis. In order to deal effectively with these issues, nurses must be able to identify correctly the ethical issues facing them, recognise the short- and long-term implication of these issues for the broader nursing profession, and develop strategies for ensuring moral outcomes to the ethical issues encountered in work-related contexts. Achieving these outcomes, however, requires a reappraisal of nursing ethics education, ethical nursing practice, ethical nursing management, and nursing ethics research. By undertaking such a reappraisal, members of the nursing profession will be better situated to meet the complex challenges and responsibilities of ethical nursing practice which inevitably lie ahead.

REFLECTIVE QUESTIONS

(1) Nurses are faced with ethical issues every day. In your view, what are the most pertinent and pressing ethical issues facing nurses today? What are some of the professional implications of these ethical issues for the nursing profession generally, and how might nurses best deal with these issues both locally and globally?

(2) How, if at all, might the study of nursing ethics assist nurses to practise nursing in an ethically just and responsible manner?

(3) What is the future of nursing ethics, and what influence, if any, do you envisage it will have on the broader field of health care ethics generally?

CASE REFERENCES

1 *Free* v. *Holy Cross Hospital* 505 NE 2d 118 (Ill App 1 Dist 1987).
2 *Warthen* v. *Toms River Community Memorial Hospital* 488 A 2d 229 (NJ Super AD 1985).

RECOMMENDED READING

Davis, A., Aroskar, M., Liaschenko, J. & Drought, T. (1997) *Ethical Dilemmas and Nursing Practice*, 4th edn. Appleton & Lange, Stamford, Connecticut.

Johnstone, M. (1999) *Bioethics: A Nursing Perspective*, 3rd edn. Harcourt/Saunders, Sydney.

Kerridge, I., Lowe, M. & McPhee, J. (1998) *Ethics and Law for the Health Professions*. Social Science Press, Sydney.

Tadd, G. (1998) *Ethics and Values for Care Workers*. Blackwell Science, Oxford.

Thompson, I., Melia, K. & Boyd, K. (1994) *Nursing Ethics*, 3rd edn. Churchill Livingstone, Edinburgh.

REFERENCES

Alspach, G. (1993) Editorial: Nurses as victims of violence. *Critical Care Nurse*, **13**(5), 13–14, 17.

Benner, P. (1991) The role of experience, narrative, and community in skilled ethical comportment. *Advances in Nursing Science*, **14**(2), 1–21.

Benner, P. (ed.) (1994) *Interpretive phenomenology: Embodiment, caring, and ethics in health and illness*. Sage, Thousand Oaks, California.

Bishop, A. & Scudder, J. (1990) *The practical, moral, and personal sense of nursing: A phenomenological philosophy of practice*. State University of New York Press, Albany.

Hadfield, L. (1991) Guest Editorial: Violence in the accident and emergency department: Differences across the Atlantic. *Journal of Emergency Nursing*, **15**(5), 269–270.

Hodge, B. (1993) Uncovering the ethic of care. *Nursing Praxis in New Zealand*, **8**(2), 13–22.

Johnstone, M-J. (1994) *Nursing and the Injustices of the Law*. WB Saunders/Baillière Tindall, Sydney.

Johnstone, M. (1998) *Determining and responding effectively to ethical professional misconduct: A report to the Nurses Board of Victoria*. Melbourne.

Johnstone, M. (1999) *Bioethics: A nursing perspective*, 3rd edn. Harcourt/Saunders, Sydney.

Kinkle, S. (1993) Violence in the ED: How to stop it before it starts. *American Journal of Nursing*, **93**(7), 22–24.

Lifton, R. (1990) Foreword to HM Weinstein. *Psychiatry and the CIA: Victims of mind control*. pp. ix–xiv. American Psychiatric Press, Washington DC and London UK.

Parker, R. (1990) Nurses' stories: The search for a relational ethic of care. *Advances in Nursing Science*, **13**(1), 31–40.

Rawls, J. (1971) *A Theory of Justice*. Oxford University Press, Oxford.

Reich, W. (1994) The word 'Bioethics': Its birth and the legacies of those who shaped its meaning. *Kennedy Institute of Ethics Journal*, **4**, 319–335.

Reich, W. (1995) The word 'Bioethics': The struggle over its earliest meanings. *Kennedy Institute of Ethics Journal*, **5**, 19–34.

Turner, T. (1990) Crushed by the system? *Nursing Times*, **86**(49), 19.

Turner, T. (1992) The indomitable Mr Pink. *Nursing Times*, **88**(24), 26–29.

10 Law
Issues for Nursing Practice

Helen Caulfield

LEARNING OBJECTIVES

Upon completion of this chapter the reader will have gained insights into:

- how law is made and can be influenced by nursing practice;
- why human rights are of increasing importance in nursing practice;
- the key elements of negligence;
- the key elements of consent;
- the key elements of confidentiality;
- issues surrounding euthanasia, abortion and organ donation.

KEY WORDS

NEGLIGENCE, CONSENT, HUMAN RIGHTS, LEGISLATION, CASE LAW, TRANSPLANTATION, EUTHANASIA, TERMINATION OF PREGNANCY.

INTRODUCTION

Law is an increasingly important part of nursing practice. Only 20 years ago it would have been a struggle to find even one textbook that referred to the law relating to clinical practice. Now there are many books specialising in the area, and this trend looks set to increase. The delicate balance required to maintain the professional responsibilities of clinical staff and the awareness of the rights of patients means that there is an ever-increasing reliance on the law. This chapter will set out the framework of law and provide an introduction to the main components of clinical law that affect nursing practice today. It will provide practical examples of where the law restricts or encourages nursing practice, and what nurses can do to influence its development.

WHO MAKES THE LAW: PARLIAMENT AND THE COURTS

One of the crucial issues in understanding clinical law is understanding who makes the law. This helps nurses to reflect on how any aspect of law can restrict or expand nursing practice. The law is made in two places: parliament and the courts. It is vital in any understanding of clinical law that nurses are able to identify where the law relating to that practice comes from.

Society needs a legal framework to provide a structure for the behaviour of individuals. The law is adapted according to society's demands, either through the legislative process (parliament) or through judicial decision (the courts).

The law that comes from Parliament will be contained in written documents called Acts of Parliament or Statutory Instruments. These documents contain the code of law that all citizens and public bodies have to follow. The Acts of Parliament and Statutory Instruments lay down in precise language the duties that must be carried out by various bodies, including government officials. They also lay down the penalties that can be imposed on citizens and public bodies if the rules and the codes are not followed. Even where a nurse is unaware of the law, there may be an Act of Parliament or a Statutory Instrument that sets out the parameters of practice and the penalty for not following that practice. One example of this is the Medicines Act 1968, legislation that sets out the penalties that apply in Britain where medicines are not administered according to the precise language of the Act of Parliament.

The law that comes from courts is different. Where there is no Act of Parliament or Statutory Instrument that lays down the code, it is open to the courts to decide how the gaps should be filled. There is, for example, no Act of Parliament that tells us what negligence is. The law that has been created around that has come from the courts.

Where there is an Act of Parliament or a Statutory Instrument, the courts have an important role to play in the interpretation of what the codified language means. One example of this was in the interpretation of the Human Embryology and Fertilisation Act 1990, which was intended to cover all aspects of technological fertilisation. It became apparent that this Act did not cover the use of frozen sperm where the husband had died without giving his written consent to its use. His widow went to court to ask for assistance in the interpretation of the legislation. The Court of Appeal found that the Act did not give her the right to use the sperm without this consent, and as a result, she travelled to Belgium where the law would allow its use.[1] Cases like this lead to reviews of whether the legislation should be amended to cover the gaps which later appear.

In court, the judge who hears the case is unlikely to have a clinical background or to be an expert in clinical law or nursing practice. Judges rely on the experts working with the barristers presenting the arguments to ensure that the points that affect nursing practice are covered properly in the case. It is important therefore that nurse expert witnesses ensure that they are clear about the implications of the clinical aspects of nursing practice to assist the court in its decision making.

Where there is a great deal of public disquiet about existing arrangements that are not covered by legislation, or where a gap in the existing legislation is discovered, there may be pressure on the government of the day to introduce an Act of Parliament. Media interest in any human interest story plays an increasingly important role in this regard. The arrangements for overseas adoption came under intense media scrutiny over the method used by one couple to adopt twins over the Internet. As a result, Parliament passed a Statutory Instrument that made overseas adoption more restrictive.[2]

The courts are designed to deal with disputes between two parties, and as a result, it is hard to anticipate when any particular clinical issue will be dealt with. This can be the case even where nurses identify that there is an inconsistency in a piece of legislation and want the courts to adjudicate on it one way or the other. This makes it hard for nurses to initiate case law that is decided by the courts. They need to find the parties who could make the dispute real, they need the money to employ the lawyers to bring the case, and they need the determination to see the matter through. There is an additional disadvantage for cases that are decided by the courts. There is no guarantee of which way a judge will decide the law.

WHY THE LAW IS IMPORTANT: ISSUES FOR NURSES AND ISSUES FOR PATIENTS

Why is the law so important for nurses? The reasons for this are not always straight-forward. When nurses are asked what law they know, it is generally the specific areas that apply to their practice. Mental health nurses will have a greater understanding of the relevant legislation that applies to mental health, while moving and handling nurse trainers will be very familiar with the European legislation that directs how loads, including people, can be handled manually.

Nurses are aware of the importance of accountability in their practice. This consists of the following:

- contract of employment;
- clinical law;
- regulatory guidance;
- personal ethics.

Within this framework each element is different although complementary. Clinical law is not the same as the rights and obligations contained in a nurse's personal contract of employment. It is also different from any guidance that is published by the regulatory body that sets out the limits on a nurse's practice. It is different from the personal ethics that nurses retain, whether this is around issues of transplantation, abortion, euthanasia, or keeping aspects of patient information confidential.

Clinical law is therefore an important component of nursing practice, as it can create limits that set out what nurses can and cannot do in their professional practice. The Abortion Act 1967 sets out the process that has to take place before a termination of pregnancy can be lawful. This requires that two doctors must consent to the termination taking place. A nurse cannot be part of this particular process because the Act specifies that the professional qualification for this task must be medical. A nurse who seeks to provide the authority for the termination in place of a doctor therefore commits a criminal offence. This may be the case even where the nurse is more experienced than the doctor, and has greater knowledge about the patient.

The law is important for patients. Whether the individual is taking advice from a bank manager or a solicitor, there are ways that the law can ensure that the imbalance in the power is addressed. However, health is an issue where even the most articulate assertive person can struggle to ensure that they have their health needs met in a way that they would in other areas of their life. The balance of information that nurses have over patients who may be facing a diagnosis for the first time can be very one-sided. In the event that the information or the treatment does not proceed the way that the patient wants, their first point of recourse may be to the law. This will be because patients view the law as a strong advocate for their situation. The law views the autonomy of the individual very highly and will often give greater weight to this even where it means that the patient may suffer adverse health or even death as a result. In one case in 1993, a patient at Broadmoor hospital was diagnosed with gangrene and the medical staff advised that he have an amputation of the infected leg. He refused and the court agreed that his decision should be respected even if it meant that he could die without the invasive treatment that was regarded as being in his best interests by the clinical team.[3]

HUMAN RIGHTS: ISSUES FOR NURSES AND ISSUES FOR PATIENTS

The introduction of the Human Rights Act 1998 into the legal system of the United Kingdom has been given much publicity. Citizens now can use the domestic courts to examine whether there has been a violation of human rights.

The International Council of Nurses (ICN) requires that 'individual nurses and other health care providers must play a leading role in strengthening the vital link between health and human rights and thereby contribute to prevention of disease and enhance equitable access to health care'.[4]

The Human Rights Act 1998 is intended to give all citizens of the United Kingdom a legal right to demand compliance with certain rights. These rights were originally created in 1950 in the aftermath of the Second World War when the leaders of European countries were looking for a means to prevent the types of atrocities occurring again. A series of rights was constructed to provide basic protection for the citizens of all countries who signed the Convention. The European Court of Human Rights was established in Strasbourg so that any citizen who felt that his or her rights had been violated could ask for assistance outside his or her country of origin.

The UK was one of the first signatories to the European Convention on Human Rights in 1950. However it has been one of the last countries to incorporate the Convention into its own law. This meant that in the past, if a person felt that there was an infringement of his or her rights, he or she would have to go to Strasbourg in order to make that claim. Now that the Human Rights Act 1998 is in force in UK law, it means that any citizen who claims that a right under the Convention has been infringed can ask a domestic court to decide the issue.

Reliance on the Human Rights Act does not of itself mean that treatment must be given. Resources can be taken into account, and the courts have upheld this approach in cases both before and after the Human Rights Act were enacted. In the first famous case to look at the issue of resources, a young patient in Cambridge with a particular form of cancer asked the court to compel her Health Authority to provide her with a particular type of costly treatment. The Court of Appeal said that the Health Authority was entitled to consider the balancing interests of the community, and could decide to refuse to pay for a particular type of service.[5] Even after the Human Rights Act came into force, the Court of Appeal again found that the Secretary of State was not under a legal duty to provide every health service available. The duty on the Secretary of State was to 'promote a comprehensive health service' as was his duty under the NHS Act 1977, but that he could take account of available resources.

DEVOLUTION IN THE UNITED KINGDOM: IMPLICATIONS FOR HEALTH LAW

The law that is made in different parts of the United Kingdom will have an impact on the way that Acts of Parliament and the courts decide different aspects of clinical law. As a result of devolution, the way that law is made is now slightly different in each of the four countries in the United Kingdom.

Before devolution, the law in England and Wales was identical. Following the creation of the National Assembly for Wales in the Government of Wales Act 1998, there are no powers for the Welsh to make their own Acts of Parliament or to decide court cases differently. However, the National Assembly for Wales has been given devolved powers in relation to health that allow it to decide funding and structural arrangements in the principality. It is also possible for the National Assembly for Wales to make its own Statutory Instruments. This means that there is the potential for some aspects of health law to be different in Wales from the existing arrangements for England. There is, for example, a Children's Commissioner in Wales where there is no equivalent in England under powers given to the Welsh Assembly in the Care Standards Act 2000.

The law in Scotland has always differed from the law in England and Wales, and since devolution some aspects of this in relation to health have become more apparent. The Scottish Parliament has the power to pass Acts of Parliament as well as Statutory Instruments in relation to health. In addition, the Scottish Parliament has the power to raise an additional tax on the Scottish population that could be used for a variety of purposes, including additional funding of health care. There are some striking differences in health law in Scotland from England and Wales. The Age of Capacity (Children) Act 1999 and the Adults with Incapacity (Scotland) Act 2000 only apply in Scotland. These Acts set out the age at which children are able to make their own decisions in health, and provide safeguards for the provision of health for those who suffer physical or mental incapacity. No such legislation on either matter exists in England and Wales, which means that these issues are decided by the courts in those countries.

In Northern Ireland, the impact of devolution has created the Northern Ireland Assembly by the Northern Ireland Act 1998. The Assembly has the power to make its own Acts of Parliament and Statutory Instruments. One example of this is the Family Law Act (Northern Ireland) 2001 which provides certain presumptions of parentage and for tests to determine parentage.

The impact of these differences is that they will affect the boundaries of nursing practice in each country. Where a nurse moves from one country to another in the United Kingdom, it will be important to understand where there are legal differences that affect nursing practice.

NEGLIGENCE

Nurses are responsible for performing all procedures correctly and exercising professional judgement as they carry out their work. Any nurse who does not meet accepted standards of practice or care, or who performs duties in a careless fashion, runs the risk of being negligent. Negligence is not laid down in an Act of Parliament, and is decided by the courts. Negligence may involve being reckless, such as not checking a patient's identity and administering the wrong medication. If nurses perform procedures for which they have not been trained and do it carefully but still harm the patient, a claim of negligence could be made.

In an action for negligence, these are the elements that are needed for a claim to be successful:

(1) The nurse (defendant) owed a duty of care to the patient (claimant).
(2) The nurse broke that duty by failing to act as a reasonable nurse.
(3) The patient was injured.
(4) The injury was connected to the nurse's failure to carry out the duty of care.

The duty of care is a legal concept that was established by the courts and it applies where there is a relationship of power between two people. There is a duty of care that car drivers owe to other car drivers and pedestrians. A similar duty of care applies to bank managers, lawyers and health care professionals to their clients and patients. Those who manufacture drugs or make medical equipment also owe a duty of care to those who use their products. For example, where a patient is being nursed on a specialist bed which breaks and injures the patient, there is a duty of care that exists between the patient and the bed manufacturers, even though the contract to supply and maintain the bed will be between the hospital and the manufacturers.

The duty of care is broken where the nurse fails to act in a way that is considered to be reasonable. The test of reasonableness is determined in an objective manner and is judged by the standard that is applied to a hypothetical nurse. If a nurse fails to record details of a patient's temperature, or records it inaccurately, it would appear that the duty of care has been broken. If however, the nurse can show that the reason for failing to record the temperature was that he or she was the only member of staff on duty on a busy ward, it may be found that the nurse did not break the duty of care as it would be unreasonable to expect the nurse to be able to record all details while working unaided. The legal standard of care required is that of a reasonable nurse acting in accordance with the practice expected at that time as proper by a reasonable body of nursing opinion. This test was formulated in the case of Bolam[6] and refined by the later court case in the House of Lords in the case of Bolitho.[7]

A nurse may break a duty of care and the patient may be injured, but in order to establish negligence it is necessary to show a link between the two. It may be that the nurse carries out a task in a careless manner but this has no adverse impact on the health of the patient. In such a case, there can be no claim for negligence, as the necessary link between the two has not been established.

It is possible for a patient to sue a nurse personally in an action for negligence. Generally, however, a patient will sue the hospital or employer under the principle of vicarious liability. This principle allows the employer to be sued for the negligent actions of an employee. This is based on the rule that an employer should ensure the competency of its staff and should be able to take responsibility for negligent acts or omissions of staff. It is becoming more common for the patient to add the name of the nurse as a second defendant in any action for negligence in cases where it is shown that the actions of the nurse were so reckless that the employer denies vicarious liability. In such cases, the nurse will need separate legal representation and it is advisable for all nurses to ensure adequate protection in case this occurs.

Most trades unions carry indemnity insurance as part of the services provided for the membership. This protects a nurse if a finding of negligence is made against the nurse and in order that compensation be paid to the patient. The indemnity insurance would meet the cost of compensation and the legal fees incurred.

CONSENT

The law of consent has been established in case law over a long period of time and the principles are now well established. There is no legislation that deals with the rules of consent and this has led to a debate about whether legislation would be useful in this area to protect the interests of those with a form of incapacity. The application of the principles that have been developed by the courts affects nursing practice. Consent is the legal means by which the patient gives a valid authorisation for treatment or care. The legal basis of consent is therefore identical to the professional requirement that nurses need consent before carrying out any treatment.

The case law on consent has established three requirements which must all be satisfied before any consent given by a patient can be sufficient.

(1) The consent should be given by someone with the mental ability to do so
The law assumes that anyone over the age of 16 has the mental ability to give consent. The law recognises that adults over 16 can make their own decisions about medical and nursing treatment. Adults over 16 years who do not have mental ability to make their own choices will not be able to consent to treatment or care.

Persons over the age of 18 years are allowed to make their own decisions about treatment and care. Between the ages of 16 and 18 years adolescents can consent to treatment under the provisions of the Family Law Reform Act s. 8 (1). The more problematic area concerns adolescents below the age of 16. The legal position in England, Wales and Northern Ireland is established in the famous case of *Gillick* v. *West Norfolk and Wisbech Area Health Authority*.[8]

This legal test allows adolescents under 16 years to consent to clinical treatment provided they have sufficient understanding and intelligence to enable them to understand fully what is proposed. The Age of Legal Capacity (Scotland) Act 1991 gives authority in Scotland to young persons of sufficient understanding to consent to treatment.

The court has indicated that a competent child does not have the final say in refusing treatment, and has held that any refusal of treatment by a child is not conclusive.[9] It is open to the parent or guardian to override that refusal and to consent to the treatment proposed by the health professional. Where a nurse is confronted with a strong difference of opinion between a child and a parent or guardian over proposed treatment the nurse should always seek advice to ensure the correct weight is given to the child's wishes. In some situations it may be necessary to ask the court to decide between the conflicting wishes. For example if a 14-year-old girl involved in a road accident refuses any blood transfusions because of her religious beliefs, her parents may want to override her refusal so that treatment can proceed. It may be difficult for the doctor or nurse to determine how far the child's wishes should be taken into account. In this type of situation a court would be able to hear the evidence and make a decision to be followed by all parties.

(2) Sufficient information should be given to the patient

The patient should be able to give informed consent to the proposed treatment. Many court cases concern the amount and detail of information that was given to the patient. The issue of informed consent has provoked much discussion among health professionals. Just how much information needs to be given to a patient before they have enough on which to make a decision?

The courts have held that the nurse will have fulfilled her duties in relation to informed consent by telling a patient about the material risks, alternatives to the treatment and the nature and consequences of the proposed treatment.[10] There is a duty on the nurse to assess whether the patient requires any further information. There is, however, no duty imposed by law on a health care professional to inform the patient of all the likely risks or advantages in the proposed treatment. If the patient asks questions, these should be answered truthfully.

In nursing, the standard is therefore determined by the nursing profession itself and not by reference to a particular patient. This standard of care has been criticised for failing to give sufficient weight to the patient's own circumstances, and it has been suggested that a nurse or doctor should provide the patient with all the information in their possession in order to enable the patient to make an informed decision. This has been largely rejected by the courts as being impractical and over-burdensome on the health professional.

(3) The consent must be freely given

Consent must be freely given and no threats or implied threats used. Threats such as the use of a compulsory section under the relevant Mental Health Act legislation in the United Kingdom if treatment is not accepted would nullify the consent. Whether treatment is voluntary will depend on what information is given to the patient and how this is presented. Coercion or manipulation of the patient would tend to imply that consent has not been obtained voluntarily.[11] In this situation, even where the patient signs a consent form, the consent will have been obtained in an unlawful manner and the consent will not be valid.

Once the three criteria have been established, a valid consent can be given to treatment or care.

Most hospitals require patients and clients to sign a consent form before agreeing to invasive treatment, and some health professionals have mistakenly placed too much emphasis on a signature being obtained to a form. A signed consent form does not prove that the consent is valid. It is usually good evidence that a discussion has taken place about consent. In this context, a consent form is important evidence although it should never be the only factor taken into account in establishing that full and proper consent has been obtained.

CONFIDENTIALITY

Confidentiality is a fundamental part of the nurse and patient relationship. Any information given to a nurse should remain within that relationship and should not be passed on to anyone else without the consent of the patient. The law requires that confidential information obtained in a relationship of trust should be kept private unless consent has been given for this to be disclosed. It is assumed in health law that there is an implied consent that has been given by the patient that information can be passed to other members of the health team. In this way, the GP can give information to a nurse or a consultant and vice versa without having to seek consent each time from the patient.

There are limited situations in which information can be disclosed to a third party, even where a patient has not given permission. The first situation is where the nurse is given a court order requiring specific disclosure of patient information. A court order will override the duty of confidentiality. Nurses are under a legal duty to comply with the terms of the court order, and no breach of confidentiality occurs in these circumstances.

The second situation in which information may be passed to a third party is where the nurse considers that it would be in the public interest to do so. There may be some exceptional circumstances where the nurse believes the information is so significant that she or he wants to make this known to someone else. If a patient informs the nurse that he or she has been the subject of serious crime such as child abuse or drug trafficking, it is likely that a court would find the nurse had been acting in the public interest if the nurse disclosed this information to a third party such as the police.[12]

The nurse should act sensitively in such situations. It is preferable for the patient to give permission for this information to be disclosed. The nurse will be able to communicate the seriousness of the situation to the patient if the information is withheld. In all situations, the nurse should seek to secure the patient's consent to disclosure of the information.

Where a patient believes that a nurse has broken a confidence by telling a third party of the information, the patient can sue the nurse as an individual. The principle of vicarious liability which applies in cases of negligence will not apply where a breach of confidence is alleged. As a result, in any legal action for a breach of confidence, the nurse will be sued as an individual. If the court finds that there was no justification for breaking the patient's confidence, the nurse will be obliged to pay compensation to the patient. If the public interest defence is upheld, a breach of confidence will have occurred but no compensation will be payable.

There is no duty to disclose information to a third party even where it would appear the patient is at risk and it would be in the public interest to do so. The law allows a discretion on the part of the nurse to disclose this information, but requires that there must be very serious grounds for doing so. As a result, where the police contact a nurse to ask for information about the health or identify of a patient, the only basis on which a nurse has to disclose this information is where there is a court order to do so. Where there is no court order, the nurse has to balance the powerful duty of confidentiality against the discretion of disclosure that the law allows before giving information to a third party. Where the nurse does disclose this information, he or she should be aware of the potential need to justify that action at a later date.

The seriousness of a allegation of breach of confidence means that any nurse who is considering giving information to another party without the patient's consent should consider obtaining professional or legal guidance before doing so.

SPECIFIC CLINICAL ISSUES: ABORTION, EUTHANASIA AND ORGAN DONATION

Abortion

The law in relation to the beginning and ending of life has always been emotive. The need to reconcile the current ethical and political thinking of the day with hard judgments that are binding on society has resulted in some judges reflecting their concerns that strong ethical issues are being decided by the courts in the absence of full parliamentary debate.

The complex area of termination of pregnancy has been codified to a large extent by legislation. The Abortion Act 1967 allowed terminations to be carried out with a variety of safeguards that needed to be adhered to. This Act was amended in 1990 to reflect changes in medical technology and societal attitudes to termination. It is lawful for a woman to seek a termination up to 24 weeks in her pregnancy on one of a number of grounds. The interpretation of whether a particular ground has been satisfied is a decision that is open to the two doctors who have to give their approval for the termination to take place. There have been no legal cases that have challenged these grounds. After 24 weeks, it is possible for a woman to seek a termination if she can show that the termination is needed to prevent deterioration in the physical or mental health of the pregnant woman (section 1(1) (b)) or that there is a substantial risk that the child would be seriously handicapped (section 1(1) (d)).

The law does not regard the fetus as having the same status as a person, which is why a termination is not regarded as an assault or manslaughter. In relation to fertilisation, the main Act of Parliament is the Human Embryology and Fertilisation Act 1990. This Act does not define an embryo as a person, as doing so would give a fetus more legal status than was intended. The nonlegal status allows for termination. If the fetus had been given status of a person, termination would not be allowed as there is absolute legal right to the sanctity of life for persons.

The ethical issues facing nurses in relation to termination and fertilisation were raised during the parliamentary debates at the time that each Act came onto the statute books. As a result, the legislation reflects that those who are caring for women in similar situations face professional and ethical dilemmas. In particular, the lobby from the Catholic Church in the 1960s against abortion was incorporated in a statutory right of conscientious objection. The Abortion Act 1967 and the Human Embryology and Fertilisation Act 1990 enshrine a right for any nurse to object on the grounds of conscience to any participation in a termination or selective reduction. These are the only two Acts of Parliament that give such a right to professional clinical staff. These rights of conscientious objection reflect the divergence of views that any discussions about the issues in termination or selective reduction cannot satisfy the whole population.

Any further changes in the law relating to reproductive technology will reflect the mainstream social argument of the time. This is a useful opportunity for nurses to assess whether there is a professional consensus of opinion around the use of this drug therapy, and advice given to women who find themselves in a situation of multiple pregnancy.

Euthanasia

Issues around death are no less easy for the law to decide. The legislation that sets out the parameters for this area begin from the principle that human life has sanctity and that anyone who attempts to interfere with this commits a criminal offence. The Offences Against the Person Act 1861 sets out the crimes that are committed by assaulting or ending another person's life. A deliberate intention to end another person's life will be regarded by the courts as murder.[13] Where the ending of another person's life is unintentional, it is more likely to be interpreted by the courts as manslaughter. The problems that this raises in health law relate to situations where the action of a clinician may shorten the life of another person, or where the patient requests that an omission in treatment is made so that they may die. The courts have dealt with these situations but the questions still raise many ethical issues for nurses.

The most comprehensive assessment of the law in relation to ending another person's life was discussed by the House of Lords in the case of Tony Bland, the young football fan who was a victim of the Hillsborough stadium tragedy that left him in a persistent vegetative state. The family and the health professionals were convinced that there was no prospect of recovery, but did not want to withdraw the artificial hydration and nutrition that was keeping him alive. They applied to the court for a declaration in which they asked the court to let them know that it would be lawful to take this course of action, and that this would not result in a charge of manslaughter. The House of Lords decided that it would be lawful for the doctors to withdraw the treatment where it was in the best interests of the patient.[14]

This judgment does not mean that any health professional can decide what is in the best interest of the patient and then act accordingly. There have been a number of similar situations where patients have been in persistent vegetative state since the Bland case, and it has been the court that has decided in each case whether the best interests test has been satisfied.

Where a health professional takes action that shortens a patient's life, it is a problematic area in law. The most common example of this is where pain relief is given to a patient with a terminal condition, where a secondary effect of the pain relief is that the patient dies earlier than without the treatment. There have been cases where doctors acting in what they perceive to be the best interests of their patients have been charged with murder. The most recent of these cases was heard in 1992 where a GP, Dr Cox, was charged with attempted murder because of the amount of potassium chloride that he gave to a dying patient. He was convicted, principally because the jury did not believe that his prime purpose in the administration of drugs was that of pain relief.[15]

Suicide used to be a criminal offence. The Suicide Act 1961 abolished this crime but it also introduced a criminal offence of assisting suicide in section 2. This section was challenged as to its interpretation by a dying woman who wanted the ability to decide on her own death but who does not have the physical ability to do this herself. She went to court to ask for a declaration that it would be lawful for her husband to assist her with this. The House of Lords did not agree and found that there would be a criminal activity if the husband or a member of the clinical team assisted her to kill herself.[16]

The issues around life and death will continue to be heard in the courts as new technology allows people to consider different aspects of the beginning and the ending of their lives. Nurses have a role to play in ensuring that their professional views on these matters are heard as cases come to court, so that the broadest approach to nursing practice and its development can be maintained.

Organ donation

The development of the ability to transplant tissue and organs in the latter half of the twentieth century meant that demand for organs rose. As a result, the Human Tissue Act 1961 was introduced in accordance with societal views that transplantation was both socially desirable and acceptable for health improvement. Debates around the time of the Human Tissue Act covered such issues as whether the person should retain rights over their body after they died, the value that should be placed on the views of the family at the time of transplantation, and the demand by living patients for organs. The Human Tissue Act 1961 deals with the donation of organs from those who have died.

Many of the debates around transplantation of organs from those who have died have focused on whether there should be an 'opt in' or an 'opt out' approach for the use of organs. The law in the United Kingdom follows the 'opt in' approach in which the principle of consent is maintained so that it is unlawful to remove organs from an individual without their express permission. Under this approach, it remains the decision of the individual to decide whether they want to donate their organs after death and to communicate this to their family or health professional. This approach follows the general legal principle that no touching of a patient can take place without their consent and that removal of organs after death requires this consent.

The second approach is for the 'opt out' system where it is presumed that everyone is happy to donate organs. The needs of the living are presumed to outweigh the desires of those who have died. Under this system, an individual has to make a declaration that his organs cannot be used after he or she has died and once this declaration has been made the organs cannot be used. This is not the law in the United Kingdom, although there are constant debates about whether this would be a means of ensuring that an adequate supply of organs would be made available. There are a number of countries where the 'opt out' system is being used, including Denmark, Austria, and South Africa.

In the United Kingdom, the Human Tissue Act 1961 requires that there should be a request made of the relatives that the organ can be removed, even where it is clear that the person who died had given his consent for the removal. It is this system of 'required request' that is the primary reason the current system works in a patchy manner. This can place a heavy burden on clinical staff to approach the relatives at the time of death and make the request for the organs. It requires specialist training in communication and there are a number of transplant co-ordinators who have this training.

There was no legislation that covered the donation of organs from those who were living until a few decades later. A further Act was introduced after media outrage over the way that some people from Turkey were offering organs for commercial sale. This led to the introduction of the Human Organ Transplants Act 1989 that deals with the donation of organs from those who are alive. This Act seeks to regulate the circumstances under which people may donate an organ while a person is alive. It outlaws commercial dealings in the sale of organs from both living and deceased donors. This Act therefore implies that society values a purely altruistic approach in organ donation and that adding any commercial aspect is socially unacceptable.

CONCLUSION

This chapter can give only a very broad overview of the main legal areas that affect nursing practice at the start of the twenty-first century. It is likely that there will be further need for the courts to decide on areas of dispute between those who provide health care and those who receive health care. The need for nurses to become aware of the general principles of negligence, consent and confidentiality will therefore be even more important. The impact that nurses can make on the development of health law should never be underestimated. There are countless opportunities for nurses to learn more about the general law in health care and the specific aspects of their specialist practice. At the heart of all good health care is effective communication, and this is recognised by the courts. As a result, it is therefore even more likely that nurses will be in a position of influence in the role that the courts want from health professionals. The balance that has to be made between respecting the autonomy of the patient and the desire of health staff to achieve the best health outcome for that patient will continue to challenge both the nursing profession and the courts.

REFLECTIVE QUESTIONS

(1) Have you been to a court case, either civil or criminal? If not, consider spending some of your professional updating time watching a court case in action.

(2) Are there areas in your area of practice in nursing in which you are unsure about the law? Consider looking in some of the standard legal textbooks to see where the law comes from, either parliament or the courts.

(3) Do you consider that health issues that are balanced between health professionals and patients are best decided by the courts where the judges may not be expert in this area? If not, can you think of other ways in which these issues can be debated and decided?

CASE REFERENCES

1 *R.* v. *Human Fertilisation and Embryology Authority ex parte Blood* [1997] 2 All ER 687.
2 The Adoption of Children from Overseas Regulations 2001 (SI 2001 No. 1251).
3 Re C [1994] 1 All ER 819 (Family Division).
4 ICN, *Code of Ethics for Nurses*, 2000.
5 *R.* v. *Cambridgeshire DHA ex parte B* [1995] 1 FLR 1055.
6 *Bolam* v. *Friern Hospital Management Committee* [1957] 1 WLR 583.
7 *Bolitho* v. *City and Hackney Health Authority* House of Lords 13 November 1997.
8 *Gillick* v. *West Norfolk and Wisbech Area Health Authority* [1985] 3 All ER 402.
9 Re R. [1991] 4 All ER 177.
10 *Sidaway* v. *Bethlem* RHG [1985] 1 All ER 643.
11 *Chatterton* v. *Gerson* [1981] 1 All ER 257.
12 *W* v. *Egdell* [1990] 1 All ER 835.
13 *R.* v. *Maloney* [1985] 1 All ER 1025.
14 *Airedale NHS Trust* v. *Bland* [1993] 1 All ER 821.
15 *R.* v. *Cox* 919920 12 BMLR 38.
16 *Pretty* (R. on the application of) v. *DPP*, House of Lords 29 November 2001.

RECOMMENDED READING

British Medical Association (2001) *Consent, Rights and Choices in Health Care for Children and Young People.* BMA, London.

Kennedy, I. & Grubb, A. (2000) *Medical Law: Text and Materials*, 3rd edn. Butterworth, London.

Montgomery, J. (1997) *Health Care Law.* Oxford University Press, Oxford.

Staunton, P. & Whyburn, B. (1997) *Nursing and the law*, 4th edn. WB Saunders/Baillière Tindall, Sydney.

Wikinson, R. & Caulfield, H. (2000) *The Human Rights Act: A Practical Guide for Nurses.* Whurr, London.

11 Gender Issues in Nursing

Sandra Speedy

LEARNING OBJECTIVES

On completion of this chapter, the reader will:

- have examined the role that gender plays in defining the world of nursing work;
- develop an enlarged perspective about how the health care system and health professionals are impacted on by the issue of gender;
- have briefly explored the influence that feminisms have had on the discipline of nursing;
- understand how feminist theory has influenced nursing research;
- have considered one way gender has provided an advantage to men in nursing.

KEY WORDS

GENDER, NURSING WORK, FEMINISM, PATRIARCHY, POWER, ORGANISATIONAL CULTURE.

INTRODUCTION

In order to consider a range of gender issues – which have become of increasing interest and relevance to nurses all over the world – this chapter will consider the gendered nature of nursing work. This will involve discussion about the nature of women, who provide the majority of the nursing workforce. It will also require some analysis of the nature of nursing work, as it is performed by women. Inherent in this discussion will be consideration of the role of science in determining views of the concept of woman, as well as the work they undertake. The chapter will also consider briefly the influence of feminism on nursing, and the influence of nurses and nursing on feminism. Finally, the chapter will also examine the increasing role played by men in nursing, a gender issue of utmost importance for the future of nursing.

THE GENDERED NATURE OF NURSING WORK

A consideration of the gendered nature of nursing work must examine the concept of 'woman', since the majority of nurses are women. Whatever views are held regarding women will influence perception of women's work, in this case, nursing work. Perspectives on women are influenced by 'scientific' views about the nature of women, although it might also be argued that perspectives on women influence beliefs about the nature of science.

There is a burgeoning literature that demonstrates a range of approaches and various viewpoints, on woman as object and subject. So women can be examined from sociological, psychological, biological, philosophical or political perspectives – and other viewpoints as well. Many of these viewpoints feature devaluation of women, as any examination of the concepts of essentialism, biologism, naturalism or universalism will demonstrate. Grosz (1990) suggests that all of these terms, which argue the nature of women (and men, incidentally), do fix and define the limits, because they 'are commonly used in patriarchal discourses to justify women's social subordination and their secondary positions relative to men in patriarchal society' (Grosz 1990:333).

There are problems with constructing a 'universal feminism' since allowance must be made for difference and diversity between women, just as there is between women and men. What is worthy of exploration are some of the views about women and nurses within a medical and health professions context, because these views are influenced by the concepts mentioned above. The issue of how women are constructed by science is also relevant here.

Feminist literature argues that the masculinity of science is an image that has been perpetuated for centuries. This image creation is effected by textbook representations, curriculum organisation, classroom behaviour and stereotypical beliefs and attitudes. It distorts science, yet scientific method has not been successful in filtering out patriarchal bias in the scientific construction of women. Lather (1991) is very clear about this. She says:

> The claim of positivistic researchers that their method is sufficient protection against ideological incursion is debunked by feminist critiques of the conceptual and methodological orientations that reflect and reinforce sex-based inequality. Hence the construction of women brings into question that which has passed for knowledge in the human sciences.
>
> Lather (1991:17)

The masculinity of science is only an illusion (albeit a powerful one), not an intrinsic part of its nature. Science is a social construct, and 'its development is inextricably linked with social relations, not least the relations between men and women' (Kelly 1985:76). This leads, of course, to using male as the norm and female as the referent, a strategy that has been exposed and rejected in a wide range of disciplines, including psychology, sociology, psychiatry, medicine, education and biology. As long ago as the 1970s, it was pointed out that 'male' medicine misunderstood the female body, and these debates have now extended to cover all aspects of women's health, not just those of childbirth and reproduction.

In nursing and medicine, the presence of increasing numbers of women at all levels of authority indicate a modicum of success in producing woman-friendly services and conditions. This has come about only because women have been forced to reclaim their healing role, which was given a boost by the knowledge and insights in the classic treatise written by Ehrenreich and English (1979), documenting the exclusion of women-as-healers from professionalised, modern medicine. There is now 'increasing institutional awareness of the deficiencies and sexism of specific institutional practices' (Evans 1997:42). This has had both positive and negative effects. For the latter, it has resulted in some feminists 'beating up' on nurses, earning the title of 'antinurse'. This is

> predicated on the belief that nurses willingly capitulate to male (and/or medical dominance), thereby making it difficult for 'real feminists' to achieve their goals. This … 'complicity hypothesis' … sees nurses as compliant with patriarchal demands to remain oppressed.
>
> Buchanan (1997:82)

Using this argument, nurses can be viewed as either the embodiment of the 'ideal' woman, conforming to masculine desires, or as the 'bad mother', 'thwarting women in their endeavours and assisting the medical profession in torturing women patients' (Buchanan 1997:82). In some ways this debate could be seen as unfortunate; in other ways, it suggests that there can be growth for women and nurses if we critically consider all sides of this argument.

Of course, we do not need feminists to 'beat up' on nurses – nurses do that very well to each other, whether they are feminists or not (Briles 1994; David 2000). Horizontal violence has long been recognised by a range of authors, who suggest that nurses' self-hate and dislike of other nurses is demonstrated by the lack of cohesion in nursing groups, as well as the phenomenon of 'eating our young' (Bent 1993). The systematic oppression of women can assist nurses to recognise the oppressive structures in which they practise, which includes recognising that nurses are placed in a culture that does not value their attributes, rather than 'blaming' them for ranking lower on self-esteem and higher in submissiveness in job-trait studies than do people in other occupations. Nurses must no longer assume that they are inherently inferior to the systems that surround them (Bent 1993:298).

This brings us to the work of nursing.

NURSING WORK

The role and function of nursing cannot be separated from those who undertake this activity. It is quite clear that there are particular views held about women and nursing that then create the definitions of women's work and nursing work. Cheek and Rudge (1995) point out that the low status of nursing and the way in which the work of nurses is devalued, especially when compared to other health professionals, can at least in part be explained by its gendered nature (Cheek & Rudge 1995:312).

Nursing is viewed as a natural extension of the female role, valuing nurturance, caring, support, care and concern (Bent 1993; Brykczynska 1997; Evans 1997). These characteristics have been described as encompassing a 'tyranny of niceness' (Street 1995). Nevertheless, researchers have found that these characteristics are selectively eliminated during the educational and socialisation process (Doering 1992). For example, Treacy notes that current 'nurse training' endorses 'compliance, passivity and ladylike behaviour, but it negatively sanctions other female traits such as intuition, empathy, and emotional expression' (Treacy 1989:88). The descriptors 'compliance, passivity and ladylike behaviour' are words that, it could be argued, are suggestive of 'powerlessness'. 'Intuitiveness, empathy and emotional expression' are often viewed as unscientific and hence unacceptable in the world of science. As David (2000) also points out, the gender dialectic is still so fundamental to gender politics that it permeates the traditions of nursing, such as the belief that nursing is woman's work (p. 86). Because of this, women and nurses are on shaky ground.

Evans (1997) points out that nineteenth century science and rationality perceived the 'feminine' as an abstraction, which assisted in marginalising women within institutional practices. Women, as we have seen, were constructed as hysterical and intellectually inferior, while men were expected to conform to the stereotype of masculine behaviour. Thus, 'the "soft" feminine and the "hard" masculine then received institutional recognition and confirmation in particular practices' (Evans 1997:39). Feminists have sought to demonstrate the disjunction between supposed institutional objectivity and actual institutional practice. Specifically, the institution of medicine, for example, defines its values as nongendered, while in practice they are deeply gendered (Evans 1997). This has been exposed in many areas, one example being the management of childbirth.

Because the values that dominate our health system are so pervasive and reflect the values of society at large, 'it is a struggle for nurses to remain aligned to the person rather than the institution' (Huntington 1996:170). This creates difficulties in nursing work, as the dominant discourses that shape health, illness and perceptions of what it is to be a woman (and a man, incidentally) can disadvantage the individual. As Huntington (1996) points out, 'we have been left with only male language to explain the fundamentally female practice of healing bodies' (p. 170). The only solution to this problem is to develop an alternative discourse to that constructed and dominated by orthodox scientific discourse characteristics of the medical world.

Clearly too, feminist thinking has challenged the cultural code of organisations, designed around masculinity and femininity, which suggests that 'gender is deeply embedded in the design and functioning of organisations' (Davies 1995:44). These workplaces are socially constructed, they are not gender-neutral, and operate on masculine values for their legitimation and affirmation. Nurses therefore find it difficult to function within such gendered organisations, and frequently resort to 'blaming the victim' – other nurses who also struggle with their day-to-day functioning within a hostile environment. As Davies (1995) notes, '[W]omen, in a very important sense, cannot be 'at home' in the public world – it is constructed in such a way that assumes home is somewhere else, somewhere far away and different' (Davies 1995:62).

There is a range of other scholarly work that demonstrates the further weakening of nursing's value. For example, Gamarnikow (1978) linked nursing to domesticity; Treacy (1989) suggested that the invisibility of nurses' contribution to care reflected the invisibility of much of the work contribution of women in society. Other scholars have pointed out that the sexual division of labour in the home disadvantages women in the workplace, which creates enormous stress for working women, and in this case, nurses. This taps into the work of feminist scientists who have 'identified "women's work" the "caring professions", "unpaid domestic labour", "the double shift" and other manifestations of the apparently "natural" social division of labour' (Evans 1997:59).

It has been pointed out by many scholars that caring itself is a gendered construct, since notions of professional caring are derived from traditional concepts of caring as a feminine obligation (Caffrey & Caffrey 1994; Ekstrom 1999; Falk Rafael 1996; Wuest 1997). Caring in nursing has been constructed as an inherently feminine pastime, and traditionally has received little social or economic recognition. Caring is perceived as women's work, as unintellectual, unskilled and emotional. It has long been believed that the work nurses undertake in order to provide care does not require any particular skill or knowledge; it is viewed as a quality women possess 'naturally' (Falk Rafael 1998; Henderson 2001). Nursing's detractors have long promoted the idea that nurses are 'doers' rather than 'thinkers'; that is, nurses do not need to think to do nursing, as long as they can 'do' certain tasks. This has, in no small measure, led to a significant devaluation of nursing, assisted by the unequal power relations that characterise the position of nursing *vis-à-vis* medicine. For many years this view was used to justify the low-level education provided to nurses prior to their entry into the higher education system.

That caring is assumed not to require knowledge is not without practical consequence. The replacement of registered nurses with less skilled personnel is considered less of a reflection of economic rationalism than a reflection of the idea that caring is unskilled activity intrinsic to domesticity and womanhood. To engender nurse caring as feminine, therefore positioning it as innately instinctive to women, is to deny the advanced knowledge and skills that lie within the therapeutic caring acts of nurses. Despite the fact that 'emotional labour' is a vital and necessary part of the nursing labour process, it 'tends to be marginalized as a skill that a predominantly female nursing workforce would naturally possess' (Bolton 2000:580).

Emotional labour can be conceived as a 'gift in the form of authentic caring behaviour' (p. 586), which truly reflects the state of 'being a nurse'. The fact that it is under-theorised and not appreciated is of serious concern (Henderson 2001).

It is important not to forget the value of relationships that nurses develop with their patients, with relatives and carers, all of which are part of using the self in caring mode, often critical to recovery, and which can be very demanding. Sandelowski (1997) makes the point that those who engender nursing as female inadvertently minimise or deny nursing its record of expertise and innovation within technology, the primary roles nurses have played in the deployment of technology and the power and remuneration that comes with technological knowledge and skills in a high-technology culture (Sandelowski 1997:172).

Traditional expectations that surround caring as a feminine and nursing activity involve subjugation of the self and selfless devotion to duty (Caffrey & Caffrey 1994). In some circumstances nurses may experience feelings of powerlessness and eventually burn out, as a result of suppression of their own feelings and needs (Demerouti *et al.* 2000).

For Benner (1984), caring may be experienced as an empowering, enabling process. Power and caring are gendered concepts, power as 'male' and caring as 'female', and though few studies examining gender-related differences in nurse caring have been undertaken, there is some evidence to suggest that nurse gender has an influence on how nurse caring behaviours are demonstrated (Ekstrom 1999; Greenhalgh *et al.* 1998; Jones 2001). Because of the gendered nature of power and caring, these two concepts may thus appear as oppositional. Benner (1984) associates power with caring by identifying power characteristics related to the caring dimensions of nursing practice, specifically, transformative power, integrative caring, advocacy, healing power, participative/affirmative power and problem solving.

Transformative power refers to power that patients claim for themselves in order to take control of a situation, but which is only possible because of the particular way nurses choose to care for such patients. Integrative caring refers to the care nurses provide that enables the patient to be integrated into his or her social world, despite the limitations that illness may impose. Participative/affirmative power refers to the power nurses gain from engagement and involvement with the patient by using the meanings and resources that flow from the specific situation.

Davies (1995) argues that femininity itself is what provides the threat in caring. Nursing stands for a set of qualities that are unacceptable, since they are the 'vulnerabilities and dependencies that are edited out of masculinity'. She continues:

> femininity – with its stress on dealing with dependency, acknowledging emotions and intimacy and nurturing others – comes to represent qualities that are feared and denied in masculinity, qualities that at best are seen as to be contained and allocated to a different sphere, and at worst are repressed or treated with contempt.
>
> Davies (1995:183)

On the other hand, Jones (2001) points out that claiming caring as nursing's unique essence creates serious vulnerability for nursing, particularly as caring has such widespread currency within the profession (Snellgrove & Hughes 2000; Traynor 1996).

More recently, Peacock and Nolan (2000) have expressed concern that the 'spread of outcome-oriented health services has led to care being redefined as the provision of the finest form of treatment that is financially viable' (p. 1066), or as part of a 'business model' of health care (Bolton 2000). This immediately places the concept and practice of care at risk, as it 'creates a tension at the heart of modern health care'. As Gattuso and Bevan (2000) point out, the caring relationship is hard to measure, but not to do so in the outcomes context may be dangerous for the future of nursing.

THE INFLUENCE OF FEMINISMS ON THE DISCIPLINE OF NURSING

'The feminisms' refers to the variety of theoretical approaches to the advocacy of equal rights for women, accompanied by a commitment to improve the position of women in society. It is informed by a range of theoretical propositions, and includes liberal feminism, socialist feminism, postmodern feminism and others. The argument in this chapter has been developed that women and nurses are devalued in general, although some gains have been made in recent years. Feminist nurses, and others, have provided feminist analyses of their clinical practice, their educational understandings and their research. It is most notable that the feminisms have been promoted more by nursing scholars than practitioners, which has led to some uneasiness between the two groups. This may have arisen due to the fact that the feminisms have an 'image' problem, i.e. there are stereotypical views of what constitutes a feminist, including man-hating, hairy armpits, lesbianism and antifamily activities. In reality, the feminisms are political perspectives that seek to balance societal power, to gain equalities and autonomies for women in all their diversity. These feminisms offer the opportunity for nurses to recognise and analyse the unequal power relations that have been discussed earlier in this chapter, and to develop a raised consciousness about gender issues.

While it is true that the feminisms have not been adopted wholeheartedly by nurses, they certainly have had an impact, as will be demonstrated shortly. Some feminists have been hypercritical of nursing and nurses because of the latter's inability to embrace feminist theories: they believe that nursing as a women's field needs 'rescuing', that it is a victim of patriarchy and needs help in recognising this. As previously noted, some feminists place the blame for the continuance of nursing oppression at the feet of nurses who collude with their oppressors to prevent change in the system. In this way, nurses are viewed as weak and compliant with the dominant forces that seek to retain the *status quo*.

Nursing has, however, provided fertile ground for the development of feminist theories, as they can provide useful perspectives for nurses who work with disempowered and marginalised groups in their practice. Nurses are recognising that they are also disempowered and marginalised within the health care system, and are developing understandings of these processes in order to action change. But while this is an ongoing movement, it certainly is no easy task.

One example of the way feminist theory has influenced nursing will now be explored. While feminist theories have focused on nursing and the development of nursing research, there is a significant 'halo effect' that works against the valuing of nursing research. In accepting the premise that women and nurses are devalued in general, by 'scientific' researchers in particular, nursing research itself is devalued, because it is done by women and nurses. The qualities that define a 'good nurse' are quite distinct from those defining a 'good researcher'. Hicks (1997, 1999) argues that 'research has fundamentally masculine connotations and nursing is quintessentially feminine', which in itself contributes to the relative paucity of nursing research output. Clearly, two cultures are in collision: nursing and research.

There is a long history of males who, in the past, were the academics and intellectual and political gatekeepers of Western thought. They constructed and reproduced knowledge. But with the deconstruction and reconstruction of knowledge by feminists who have challenged the 'received view', nurses can take advantage of the liberalising approach inherent in the scholarly work published since the 1970s and 1980s in academic feminism and nursing. Since this time, feminist critics of science have exposed the history and assumptions of science and identified its masculinist practices.

Evans (1997) argues that 'women then had to fight and argue their way back into science – and a scientific epistemology and community that they had had little or no part in constructing' (p. 54). Not only were they literally absent from science; there was a wider absence of the 'feminine' and an absence also from the findings and conclusions of science. This was not surprising because 'the *questions* that science identified as important were determined by the construction of the social world in which men occupied the public, and women the private, space' (Evans 1997:54). According to Huntington (1996), this created an opportunity for scientific knowledge to maintain the control of women (primarily through their bodies) as men have constructed a knowledge base that is able to be extrapolated to women. She continues: 'nurses … have not addressed the issue of the place of science in nursing nor the impact this has had on nursing generally, and the nursing of women in particular' (Huntington 1996:168). This, of course, has implications for nursing work and nursing research, as it suggests that nurses may be instrumental in maintaining a medical ideology for women patients, calculated to be negative and oppressive (Buchanan 1997).

Part of the rejection of masculinist science was fostered by scholars, intellectuals and researchers who adopted the 'emancipatory science' perspective promulgated by the Frankfurt School of Sociology and Philosophy. The inaugural address given by Habermas in 1965, entitled 'Knowledge and Interest', defined emancipatory science as 'one which reveals the relationship of knowledge and interests which the objectivist attitude conceals' (Hagell 1989:227). This included a rejection of logical positivism as the only or most appropriate approach to research; interpretive and other qualitative forms were deemed by many to be superior for the task at hand in a range of disciplines, including nursing.

In the 1960s, the nursing discipline was given opportunities for development by a nursing science that was driven by an empiricist or logical positivist philosophy. Edwards (1999) suggests that nursing was driven to claim its science base for reasons of prestige and status, as well as a need to be perceived as a 'successful' profession. Nurse researchers and scholars have long acknowledged the inappropriateness for *all* nursing research to be undertaken using the empiricist model, because many of the questions framed were not valid for nursing knowledge development (Whittemore 1999). However, if we return to the argument that has been developed, given society's attitudes to women, and hence nurses, there may be more value in conforming to the dominant culture, i.e. 'scientific research' that is acceptable to masculinist science. This is not appropriate, however, because it will not answer many of the questions nursing has.

In 1989 Hagell proposed an alternative approach for the development of nursing knowledge which was underpinned by feminist principles that could assist nurses in finding out what it is that they know, and what it is they experience. This involved reclaiming and renaming nursing's experiences and knowledge of the social world lived in and daily constructed. Doering (1992) argues for supporting other research approaches, but most particularly, feminism and poststructuralism. These she justifies as particularly relevant to nursing because they incorporate the concepts of the female experience and of power. These concepts reflect the historical, social, and political dynamics in which the discipline of nursing operates. They encompass a theme central to nursing, that of powerlessness, characterised by oppression, submission and male domination (p. 25).

It is important to note, however, that feminist research 'permits the recognition and exploration of socio-cultural factors that transcend gender' (Jackson 1997:87), which signals that, while the concept of oppression is central to feminism, it is clearly shared with other groups (Evans 1997). Thus:

> Accepting that experiences around oppression and struggle are not exclusive to women, permits recognition that institutionalised patriarchy and androcentricity are oppressive to all but those of the dominant class, race and gender.
>
> Jackson (1997:87)

This insight attempts to deal with the charge that feminist research marginalises men. Allen *et al.* (1991) raised the question of whether feminist research involving only women simply 'supports a conceptual scheme that reinforces the material subjugation of women' and thus 'perpetuates problematic social categories' (p. 50). These authors concluded, somewhat controversially, that 'a better strategy is to deconstruct the dichotomy itself and to expand awareness of the diverse contemporary and historical forms of gendered existence' (Allen *et al.* 1991:56).

It may still be reasonable to say that the value of feminist research is that it 'empowers women and addresses issues that can make a difference to the quality of life for all humankind' (Parker & McFarland 1991:66). There are those who believe that nursing research should be approached from a much broader perspective and incorporate a range of paradigms. The method used is defined by the questions being asked. Unfortunately too, the method may be driven by other motives, such as economic rationalism, and the need to obtain research funding, regardless of the ethical and moral imperatives that would normally guide research behaviour. But it is clear that the research approach must take into account the context in which it is conducted, and for nursing this has political and power implications. There is no question that gender is, once again, a critical and all-encompassing variable to be acknowledged. And it is feminist theory that has largely been responsible for raising nursing's consciousness in this domain.

MEN IN NURSING

Men have constituted less than 10% of the qualified nursing workforce in Britain, while in Australia, it is around 8%. More specifically, analyses of gender breakdown of the UK registration authority indicate that in 1990, 8.37% of registrants were male; in 2000, this figure had increased to 9.75% (http:www.ukcc.org.uk). The proportion of male nursing students in Australia has increased from 11.9% in 1987–1990, to 15.9% in 1995 (Brown 1998). Astute observers have noticed that while men are relative newcomers to nursing, they are increasingly being promoted to higher levels than women in nursing, despite their disproportionate numbers. Furthermore, they seem to have less experience and fewer qualifications (Dolan 1990). Jenkins (1989) points out that Florence Nightingale had a vision that nursing would always be under the control of women; she saw no place in nursing for men, just as there was no place for men in controlling nursing.

A study that examined senior nursing administrative positions in the UK found that, in 1987, 8.6% of registered nurses were men, but 50.3% held chief nurse/advisor posts, and 57.8% were directors of nursing education (Gaze 1987). There has been a disproportionate increase of males in senior nursing positions in the UK, which has also occurred in the USA. It should be noted however, that there was a concerted effort in the UK to 'defeminise' management within nursing, enabling men to be more easily promoted into these positions (Carpenter 1977).

Two major studies provide increasing evidence that men are being promoted to the highest levels of service in nursing, despite their numerical minority. In a national survey that examined numerical representation, seniority status and experiences of men compared to women in the university-based nursing education workforce, men were found to be over-represented at the highest levels. Fifty-two per cent of deans having control of nursing were males, 19% were professors and associate professors, and 26% were at the next level of senior lecturer (Sharman *et al.* 1996:308). The study indicated that women were supporting men in the workforce and the home, often at the expense of their own career advancement. This is a finding that has previously been highlighted in other traditionally female occupations, such as teaching, physiotherapy, occupational therapy, librarianship and social work (Williams 1992). What it demonstrates is that males are moving into powerful positions over the largest occupational group in the health workforce, nursing, an occupational group that has traditionally been 'managed, taught, disciplined and organised almost entirely by women' (MacGuire 1980:160, cited in Sharman *et al.* 1996). There is little doubt that 'the ideological climate, socialisation processes and women's family and domestic responsibilities underlie a glass ceiling for women and a glass elevator for men in non-traditional occupations' (Sharman 1998:56).

A study by Brown (1998) found that men were over-represented in senior nursing administrative positions. In this study sample, although men comprised only 8% of the registered nurse workforce, they held 22% of senior nursing positions. Brown (1998) considers a range of explanations why this is happening. One of the most compelling is that women are seen to be invading the workplace, since workplaces are constructed by men. So it is that:

> even in 'women's' occupations, such as nursing, where it may be expected that men would be perceived as not fitting in, the over-riding culture of the workplace turns this disjunction into a benefit for men (p. 21).

Thus men who enter nursing are seen to be 'lowering themselves, losing status by undertaking "women's work" ' (Brown 1998:21), yet are expected to be better workers than female nurses. They retain the benefits of their ascribed gender role: they are seen to be the 'breadwinner', to have leadership qualities, to be worth mentoring (since they are more likely to be serious about their career), and they are more likely to be assisted in accessing 'power networks' in nursing. Hicks (1999) argues that if men in these top positions behave consistently with the findings of research studies, then they are most likely to reproduce themselves at these top level positions. This will then serve to widen the gender/power divisions in nursing.

CONCLUSION

If nothing else, this last section brings into sharp focus the issue of gender in global nursing. Quite clearly there are inequities at work that can be documented with respect to control, management and leadership in nursing. Additionally, there are more subtle ways that gender impacts on nursing. This chapter has argued that nursing work in all its forms (including clinical practice, education and research), mostly undertaken by women, is affected severely by gender because of its construction and the context in which nursing is carried out. Becoming aware of such systematic oppressions is the first step in changing paternalistic structures and systems that operate to disadvantage nurses, their patients, and the overall health care system. And this is what the feminisms seek to contribute.

REFLECTIVE QUESTIONS

(1) What do you think the feminisms have to offer the discipline of nursing?

(2) Do you believe that the role and function of nursing cannot be separated from nurses who undertake it? If so, why is this? If you disagree, outline your arguments to support your position.

(3) What do you think of the fact that men in nursing, despite their numerical minority, have the majority of leadership positions? Why do you think this is? What implications does this have for nursing as a profession?

RECOMMENDED READING

Barrett, M. & Phillips, A. (eds) (1992) *Destabilizing Theory: Contemporary Feminist Debates.* Polity Press, Cambridge.

Davies, C. (1995) *Gender and the Professional Predicament in Nursing.* Open University Press, Buckingham.

Horsfall, J. (2000) Feminism in nursing. In: *Nursing Theory in Australia: Development and Application* (ed. J. Greenwood). Harper Educational Publishers, Sydney.

Lumby, J. (1997) The feminised body in illness. In: *The Body in Nursing: A Collection of Views* (ed. J. Lawler). Churchill Livingstone, Melbourne.

Speedy, S. (1991) The contribution of feminist research. In: *Towards a Discipline of Nursing* (eds G. Gray & R. Pratt). Churchill Livingstone, Melbourne.

REFERENCES

Allen, D.G., Allman, K.K.M. & Powers, P. (1991) Feminist nursing research without gender. *Advances in Nursing Science,* **13**(3), 49–58.

Benner, P. (1984) *From Novice to Expert: Excellence and Power in Clinical Nursing.* Addison Wesley Publishing Company, California.

Bent, K.N. (1993) Perspectives on critical and feminist theory in developing nursing praxis. *Journal of Professional Nursing,* **9**(5), 296–303.

Bolton, S.C. (2000) Who cares? Offering emotion work as a 'gift' in the nursing labour process. *Journal of Advanced Nursing,* **32**(3), 580–586.

Briles, J. (1994) *The Briles Report on women in healthcare. Changing conflict to collaboration in a toxic workplace.* Jossey-Bass, San Francisco.

Brown, C.R. (1998) *Gender segmentation in the paid work force: The case of nursing.* Unpublished PhD thesis, Griffith University.

Brykczynska, G. (ed.) (1997) *Caring: The Compassion and Wisdom of Nursing.* Arnold, London.

Buchanan, T. (1997) Nursing our narratives: Towards a dynamic understanding of nurses in literary texts. *Nursing Inquiry,* **4**(2), 80–87.

Caffrey, R. & Caffrey, P. (1994) Nursing: Caring or codependent? *Nursing Forum,* **29**(1), 12–17.

Carpenter, M. (1977) The new managerialism and professionalism in nursing. In: *Health and the Division of Labour* (eds M. Stacey, M. Reid, C. Heath & R. Dingwall), pp. 165–191. Croom Helm, London.

Cheek, J. & Rudge, T. (1995) Only connect … feminism and nursing. In: *Scholarship in the Discipline of Nursing* (eds G. Gray & R. Pratt). Churchill Livingstone, Melbourne.

David, B.A. (2000) Nursing's gender politics: Reformulating the footnotes. *Advances in Nursing Science,* **23**(1), 83–94.

Davies, C. (1995) *Gender and the Professional Predicament in Nursing.* Open University Press, Buckingham.

Demerouti, E., Bakker, A.B., Nachreiner, F. & Schaufeli, W.B. (2000) A model of burnout and life satisfaction amongst nurses. *Journal of Advanced Nursing,* **32**(2), 454–464.

Doering, L. (1992) Power and knowledge in nursing: A feminist poststructuralist view. *Advances in Nursing Science,* **14**(4), 24–33.

Dolan, B. (1990) Project 2000: The gender mender? *Nursing Standard,* **4**, 52–53.

Edwards, S.D. (1999) The idea of nursing science. *Journal of Advanced Nursing,* **29**(3), 563–569.

Ehrenreich, B. & English, D. (1979) *For Her Own Good: 150 years of experts' advice to women.* Pluto, London.

Ekstrom, D.N. (1999) Gender and perceived nurse caring in nurse-patient dyads. *Journal of Advanced Nursing,* **29**(6), 1393–1401.

Evans, M. (1997) *Introducing Contemporary Feminist Thought.* Blackwell Publishers, Oxford.

Falk Rafael, A. (1996) Power and caring: A dialectic in nursing. *Advances in Nursing Science,* **19**(1), 3–17.

Falk Rafael, A. (1998) Nurses who run with the wolves: The power and caring dialectic revisited. *Advances in Nursing Science,* **21**(1), 29–42.

Gamarnikow, E. (1978) Sexual division of labour: The case of nursing. In: *Feminism and Materialism* (eds A. Kuhn & A.M. Wolpe). Routledge and Kegan Paul, London.

Gattuso, S. & Bevan, C. (2000) Mother, daughter, patient, nurse: women's emotion work in aged care. *Journal of Advanced Nursing,* **31**(4), 892–899.

Gaze, H. (1987) Man appeal. *Nursing Times,* **83**(20), 24–27.

Greenhalgh, J., Vanhanen, L. & Kyngas, H. (1998) Nurse caring behaviours. *Journal of Advanced Nursing,* **27**(5), 927–932.

Grosz, E. (1990) Conclusion: A note on essentialism and difference. In: *Feminist Knowledge: Critique and construct* (ed. S. Gunew). Routledge, London.

Hagell, E.I. (1989) Nursing knowledge: Women's knowledge. A sociological perspective. *Journal of Advanced Nursing,* **14**, 226–233.

Henderson, A. (2001) Emotional labour and nursing: An under-appreciated aspect of caring work. *Nursing Inquiry,* **8**(2), 130–138.

Hicks, C. (1997) The research-practice gap: Individual responsibility or corporate culture? *Nursing Times,* **93**(39), 38–39.

Hicks, C. (1999) Incompatible skills and ideologies: The impediment of gender attributions on nursing research. *Journal of Advanced Nursing,* **30**(1), 129–139.

Huntington, A. (1996) Nursing research reframed by the inescapable reality of practice: A personal encounter. *Nursing Inquiry*, **3**(3), 167–171.

Jackson, D. (1997) Feminism: a path to clinical knowledge development. *Contemporary Nurse*, **6**(2), 85–91.

Jenkins, E. (1989) Nurses' control over nursing. In: *Issues in Australian Nursing 2* (eds G. Gray & R. Pratt). Churchill Livingstone, Melbourne.

Jones, A. (2001) Time to think: temporal considerations in nursing practice and research. *Journal of Advanced Nursing*, **33**(2), 150–158.

Kelly, A. (1985) The construction of masculine science. *British Journal of Sociology of Education*, **6**, 33–154.

Lather, P. (1991) *Feminist Research in Education: Within/Against*. Deakin University Press, Geelong.

Parker, B. & McFarland, J. (1991) Feminist theory and nursing: An empowerment model for research. *Advances in Nursing Science*, **13**(3), 59–67.

Peacock, J.W. & Nolan, P.W. (2000) Care under threat in the modern world. *Journal of Advanced Nursing*, **32**(5), 1066–1070.

Sandelowski, M. (1997) (Ir)reconcilable differences? The debate concerning nursing and technology. *Image: Journal of Nursing Scholarship*, **29**(2), 169–174.

Sharman, E. (1998) *The glass elevator: How men overtake women in the nursing higher education workforce in Australia*. Unpublished PhD thesis, University of New South Wales.

Sharman, E., Short, S. & Black, D. (1996) Why so many? The masculine mystique and men in the nursing higher education workforce in Australia. In: *Changing Society for Women's Health Conference*, Australian National University, Canberra, Australia.

Snellgrove, S. & Hughes, D. (2000) Interprofessional relations between doctors and nurses: perspectives from South Wales. *Journal of Advanced Nursing*, **31**(3), 661–667.

Street, A. (1995) *Nursing Replay: Researching Nursing Culture Together*. Churchill Livingstone, Melbourne.

Traynor, M. (1996) Looking at discourse in a literature review of nursing texts. *Journal of Advanced Nursing*, **23**(2), 1155–1161.

Treacy, M.P. (1989) Gender prescription in nurse training: Its effects on health provision. In: *Recent Advances in Nursing: Issues in Women's Health* (eds L.K. Hardy & J. Randell). Churchill Livingstone, Edinburgh.

Whittemore, R. (1999) Natural science and nursing science: Where do the horizons fuse? *Journal of Advanced Nursing*, **30**(5), 1027–1033.

Williams, C. (1992) The glass escalator: Hidden advantages for men in the 'female' professions. *Social Problems*, **39**(3), 253–267.

Wuest, J. (1997) Illuminating environmental influences on women's caring. *Journal of Advanced Nursing*, **26**(1), 49–58.

12 Becoming Part of a Multidisciplinary Health Care Team

Patrick Crookes, Rhonda Griffiths
and Angela Brown

LEARNING OBJECTIVES

Having read and understood this chapter, the reader will be able to:

- describe the characteristics of multidisciplinary health care teams;
- discuss the advantages of multidisciplinary teams as a model of providing health care;
- discuss the attributes that contribute to high levels of satisfaction and effectiveness amongst members of multidisciplinary teams;
- outline ways in which conflict may come about in multidisciplinary teams;
- describe strategies for managing conflict in multidisciplinary teams.

KEY WORDS

MODELS OF HEALTH CARE, COMMUNICATION, ROLES, SOCIALISATION, HIERARCHICAL, VALUES, CONFLICT RESOLUTION.

INTRODUCTION

The image of a health care provider engaging in a one-to-one therapeutic relationship with a patient is familiar to us all. The first point of contact for medical care is usually a general practitioner, who may refer the patient to other health service providers, e.g. to specialist personnel for diagnostic tests or treatments – interventions which, in the main, are between two people.

An alternate model of care, which has developed over the past decade and is becoming increasingly important, is the multidisciplinary team which brings cross-discipline expertise to health care consumers in a collaborative and co-ordinated way. The aims of this model are to enhance the quality of care received, support a planned and holistic approach to care, and to optimise resources.

As a student of nursing who is being prepared to work in a contemporary health care system, it is imperative that you recognise the significance and responsibilities of being an active participant in multidisciplinary health care teams. To do this requires not only an awareness of the role of nurses, but also that of others within such teams. It is also useful to be aware of factors that impact upon the nature of teams, and how they form and function. Finally it is helpful to be aware of what affects their success.

WHAT IS A MULTIDISCIPLINARY TEAM?

In its simplest form, a team is a group of people. However, Gallagher (1995:276) draws an interesting distinction between 'groups' and 'teams' in that she asserts that while both are composed of a number of individuals with some unifying relationship, the two can be differentiated by virtue of the members of a team being 'associated together in specific work or activity'. G.M. Parker (1990) furthers this point by identifying the 'high degree of interdependence ... [and being] geared toward the achievement of a goal or task' that exists within teams. The key point to be made, then, is that while people participate in all sorts of groups, a team is characterised by common goals, interdependence, co-operation, co-ordination of activities, division of effort, and shared language (Pfeffer & Schnack 1995).

A dictionary definition of a multidisciplinary team is 'a team of professionals including representatives of different disciplines who co-ordinate the contributions of each profession, which are not considered to overlap, in order to improve care' (O'Toole 1997).

The ideals encompassed by a multidisciplinary approach to care require a culture conducive to collaborative working, as well as professional ideals that are complementary to the aim of improving client/customer experiences and outcomes. Effective communication and the ability to work in groups are important characteristics of team members, if the team is to function effectively.

Lenkman and Gribbins (1994) describe the values health care organisations must demonstrate for multidisciplinary care to become reality. These include being patient-focused and service-oriented, with attention to organisational, technical and professional issues. Staff who feel empowered to 'make a difference', who are also expert in systems thinking, who feel involved, and who are dedicated to the achievement of the goals of the organisation, form the basis of effective multidisciplinary teams.

To achieve such a culture, health care facilities need to move from individualistic or parochial group activity to multidisciplinary activity. This point is raised again later in this chapter, when factors impacting upon the effectiveness of multidisciplinary health care teams are discussed. The literature provides a number of examples of multidisciplinary health care teams working in a range of settings including: acute care (Lenkman & Gribbins 1994); aged care (Wright 1993); child psychiatry (Benierakis 1995) and diabetes care (Griffiths 1996). The reader is encouraged to explore these and other readings to build knowledge and understanding of multidisciplinary teams across contexts of health care.

Why do multidisciplinary teams exist in health care?

Extending from the definition provided by O'Toole (1997) above, it could be said that the purpose of a multidisciplinary health care team is to involve professionals from various health-related disciplines, whose contributions do not overlap, in the planning and provision of ever-improving standards of health care.

This definition is simplistic and not truly reflective of clinical environments because it gives the impression that health professionals perform functions that are prescribed and confined by their discipline base. However, it does reinforce the fact that modern health care is provided by professionals from a range of disciplines, and that this multidisciplinary health care team has (or should have) as its focus, high-quality care. In practice, the demarcations that previously defined the functions and roles of each discipline are becoming blurred and increasingly complementary as collaborative models of care emerge. For example, shared care (Hoskins *et al.* 1993) and managed care (Burnell 1995) support collaborations between public and private health care providers.

Health care needs to be a team effort because no one person or any single discipline can provide the care and services required by the range of clients wishing to access health services, particularly in Western societies. This is indeed the case if one accepts the view that health care is wider than the services provided by hospitals and health centres (Hill & Becker 1995).

MEMBERSHIP OF MULTIDISCIPLINARY HEALTH CARE TEAMS

Research has demonstrated that members of a multidisciplinary team may not be well informed about the nature and scope of practice of their colleagues (McGee & Ashford 1996). An overview of the role of disciplines common to multidisciplinary health teams is presented in the following discussion.

Nurses

The role of the modern nurse is multifaceted, encompassing the promotion of wellness, the provision of curative, rehabilitative and palliative care, and the facilitation of peaceful death, all within a framework of caring practice. Such care takes place in a range of settings, both institutional and community.

In the health team situation, nurses work autonomously and collaboratively, performing functions that are independent, interdependent and dependent upon the roles and functions of colleagues. Nurses may work collaboratively when administering prescribed treatments and they independently assess their effectiveness.

Nurses are responsible for much of the care provided in both hospital and community settings, an important aspect of which involves the nurse in the role of communicator, often acting as a conduit between patients, relatives and staff from other disciplines within the team. Nurses have traditionally assumed the role of advocate for patients and their relatives, and frequently find themselves translating professional language (read 'jargon') into terms that have meaning for nonprofessionals.

The role of the nurse is challenging, intellectually demanding, and diverse. Over the past 15 years, changes in health service provision and models of care have required, and supported, increasing autonomy (and responsibility) for nurses who, in some practice settings, have assumed roles previously seen as the domain of the medical practitioner. Nursing careers are moving in new and exciting directions, as evidenced by, for example, the development of the role of nurse practitioners in a range of clinical settings.

Such a role makes nursing an interesting and rewarding profession to work within. However, it may also act as a source of irritation when colleagues fail to acknowledge or respond to nurses' input into the planning, implementation and evaluation of health care (Lenkman & Gribbins 1994). This will be discussed further shortly, with regard to the power differentials that continue to exist within multidisciplinary health care teams.

All courses leading to authority to practise as a registered nurse (RN) in the UK are now located in the higher education (i.e. university) sector, with a duration of between 3 and 4 years. You will also find enrolled nurses (ENs) working as part of the nursing team. Such clinicians have a more practical focus to their role than do RNs. This level of training was discontinued some years ago and many ENs have undergone further education to become RNs, so numbers of ENs are continually decreasing. It is also important to acknowledge that the differentiation of staff within these roles has been blurred by the introduction of 'clinical grading' in the early 1990s. Under this system individual nurses are graded according to their expertise, rather than necessarily their qualifications. The development of employment contracts between individual trusts and their nursing staff, rather than a national award system, has had a similar impact.

Medical practitioners

Medical practitioners have expertise that is, in the main, directed towards the diagnosis and treatment of disease or injury via the use of medication and/or surgery and/or other forms of therapy, e.g. psychotherapy and acupuncture. Historically, medical practitioners have been central to health service design and delivery, largely as a consequence of their rights under the law to admit patients to hospital, to prescribe diagnostic tests, medications and other treatments, and to make referrals to other health care practitioners. Medical practitioners are prepared for practice in universities and the health care sector.

Dietitians

Dietitians are a group of professionals within the wider field of nutrition who work in a number of environments and areas of specialty. Clinical dietitians work in acute care or ambulatory settings in both public and private practice, prescribing and advising individuals and groups on appropriate nutritional strategies for the dietary management of disease and for health promotion generally. Dietitians also work in the food industry, where their activities focus on nutrition promotion, informing policies and directions for food product development and acting in a consumer liaison capacity. Dietitians working in public health and health promotion positions undertake diverse roles relating to nutrition awareness, education and policy development at community and government levels. Preparation for the role is within the university sector.

Occupational therapists (OTs)

Occupational therapists focus their efforts on optimising the level of their clients' independence in undertaking everyday tasks, in both the private and public areas of their (the clients') lives. For example, after often quite detailed functional assessment they may prescribe and/or modify work-related equipment to allow an individual to continue in employment. Alternatively, they may be heavily involved in the rehabilitation process of stroke victims. Their work also involves protecting and maximising the function of joints affected by diseases such arthritis, using splints and other supportive devices. OTs should not be confused with diversional therapists, whose job is to help clients to occupy their time, not necessarily to be more independent. Currently OTs undertake a 3-year undergraduate degree in preparation for the role.

Physiotherapists

Physiotherapists are university-prepared practitioners who deal with the assessment, treatment and prevention of human movement problems. They work in a variety of settings such as hospitals, health centres, and sports centres. Their client group ranges from the very young to the aged, from the severely disabled to elite sportsmen and women. A popular misconception is that physiotherapists focus only on muscles and joints. In reality their work is much wider than this, encompassing, for example, cardiopulmonary functioning in relation to chronic respiratory disorders such as asthma and cystic fibrosis, and also cardiac rehabilitation. They can also often be seen in the postoperative phase of client recovery, aiding in the maintenance of clear airways and effective expectoration.

Social workers

In health care, social workers assist people to adjust to the changes which illness and hospitalisation can bring. They do so via the provision of psychosocial assessments, counselling, information, advocacy and referral for clients and their families. Their help can be needed in a variety of circumstances. For example, counselling could be offered following bereavement, the birth of a child, or perhaps to support the relatives of a person with a psychiatric disorder. The help may also be rather more practical; other activities include co-ordinating community support services, negotiating for hostel or nursing home placement, and linking people to relevant support agencies. Preparation for this role is currently through an undergraduate degree.

Speech and language therapists

Traditionally speech and language therapists have been involved in dealing with clients with speech difficulties such as stammering, stuttering, or problems following various forms of brain trauma. In doing so they have become focused on the functions of the mouth and throat. In more recent years the discipline has moved into other areas such as the assessment and management of clients with swallowing disorders, including poststroke patients and babies with ineffective swallowing reflexes. Speech and language therapists are prepared through an undergraduate degree.

Chaplains

Chaplains may not be an obvious inclusion in a multidisciplinary health team, however we need to recognise that clients and health professionals have spiritual needs as well as those of a physical, psychological, social and cultural nature. Clergy from a range of religions offer their services, not only in terms of 'religious' input but also as sympathetic listeners. Hospital chaplains also offer great support to staff during

times of personal and professional distress. Their importance to the team should not be overlooked.

DYNAMICS OF MULTIDISCIPLINARY TEAMS

Wright (1993) makes the point that smaller teams tend to be the most effective and productive, not least because such teams find it relatively easy to meet together – not only to communicate but also to work through to an agreement on what their 'common purpose' should be. Loveridge (1991) takes this further by asserting that committed individuals, usually working in small groups, are typically the way in which creativity (ideas) is transformed into innovation (action) within organisations. This is perhaps because collaboration between innovators has a synergistic effect (Benierakis 1995).

In practice, few multidisciplinary health care teams meet the ideals with regard to the number of members (they are usually larger) and clearly defined tasks, a point discussed later in this chapter. Nurses (and indeed other professionals within their own discipline) may therefore feel themselves to be more clearly a member of a unidisciplinary team (for example, the nurses on a ward or unit) than a multidisciplinary one, though there are of course many specialties within the profession of nursing.

The impact of tradition

Multidisciplinary health care teams are like all teams, in that each member has expected roles and functions that are influenced partly by members of the team, and partly by external factors. Health services have traditionally been organised around functional areas of professional expertise (e.g. nursing, medicine, nutrition) with a strong hierarchical structure (Fargason & Haddock 1992; Lenkman & Gribbins 1994). Individuals bring with them expectations associated with their discipline, which coalesce with the established social roles and rules (written and unwritten) associated with health care facilities. As a result multidisciplinary health care teams tend to develop along traditional hierarchical lines, partly because of the varying skill levels of members, but also 'because that's the way it's always been' (reflecting organisational norms). The result is that relationships within multidisciplinary health care teams perpetuate the hierarchical approach to decision making (Fargason & Haddock 1992) and, as such, are dominated by those with legitimated (e.g. managers) or historical/authority-based power (e.g. medical doctors). From the discussion presented thus far, it would seem obvious that this situation is at odds with the concept of multidisciplinary teams, which implies seamless care, equal recognition of skills of members, and equal recognition of members' contribution (Warelow 1996).

Health care culture

One association that has attracted attention in the literature is the nurse–doctor relationship. This association is not generally discussed within the context of multidisciplinary teams, but is rather more commonly situated within the literature on power and how it is exercised over others (Farmer 1993; Porter 1991; Roberts 1983; Stein *et al.* 1990; Warelow 1996). The origins of 'traditional' nurse–doctor interactions and the nature of their association are both relevant to a discussion about multidisciplinary teams. It has been argued that, regardless of the expected roles of team members, the most powerful team members direct the contribution of others. In that scenario the medical profession invariably dominates, and nurses (and to a lesser extent other allied health professionals) are generally submissive. This situation is maintained through an effective socialisation (societal and professional) based on gender and role differences (Bassett 1993; Coxon 1990; Warelow 1996) which are discussed at some length in Chapter 11. Meanwhile, Roberts (1983) presents a range of suggestions for nurses and nursing to free itself from domination by (particularly) the medical profession, within an excellent discussion of oppressed group behaviour and its implications for nursing.

It is unfortunate that multidisciplinary teams in health care still tend to function in ways that perpetuate the power differences. At some time in the future we may see increasing numbers of multidisciplinary teams in which the contribution of each member, regardless of professional background, will be recognised and the ideal of equality among members will be achieved. One way that this will be more readily achieved will be when nurses accept that they do play a vital role in health care, and are confident to assert that fact when working with colleagues from other health disciplines.

Senior managers in the organisation also need to recognise that, intentionally or unintentionally, they are instrumental in establishing the values and norms that set the tone of the organisation. The organisational culture is based on, and reflects, the policies, procedures and practices that are supported and reinforced at all levels. Individuals and groups then internalise the values and act out their roles accordingly. Therefore, any organisation that claims to be committed to an integrated and multidisciplinary approach to health care needs to identify clear goals for its teams, as well as putting into place the communication and organisational structures discussed earlier. If this is not the case, then the subcultures based on departments, disciplines, and charismatic individuals will continue to direct the team, the consequence of which will be that the advantages of the multidisciplinary approach will be lost to the organisation, team members and, of course, recipients of health care.

FACTORS THAT IMPACT UPON THE NATURE AND EFFECTIVENESS OF MULTIDISCIPLINARY HEALTH CARE TEAMS

A multidisciplinary team brings together individuals from diverse disciplinary and functional backgrounds. The experience and skill that members bring to the team can be a significant asset when used in problem solving, decision-making, conflict resolution and other activities that enable the team to achieve its goals. The outcomes will depend largely on how effectively the group of individuals is transformed into a team with common goals. To ensure these teams do function effectively, complex communication procedures must be established and maintained.

The literature on multidisciplinary teams indicates clearly that functional groups have elements in common. (Hein 1998; Ivancevich & Matteson 1993; Kelly-Thomas 1998). The most frequently identified attribute is the presence of effective communication. Other factors include clear roles (including leadership) and conflict resolution strategies. Inherent in these attributes is the importance of a sense of common purpose for the team, demonstrated by a mission statement and agreed goals (Lenkman & Gribbins 1994; Loveridge 1991; Pfeffer & Schnack 1995; Porter-O'Grady 1995; Wright 1993).

Effective communications

Organisations require elaborate channels of communication, both formal and informal, to ensure that everyone in the team shares a sense of common purpose, in this case the provision of high-quality health care. This may seem relatively straightforward, but in reality the various members of multidisciplinary health care teams may have very different views.

Fargason and Haddock (1992) present an interesting illustration of how poor communication can impact on the outcomes of a multidisciplinary team. In their example, a delivery-room patient record form, intended for use by obstetric and paediatric staff, was developed and approved by senior obstetric physician staff without input from other user groups. It was not surprising that the form did not fulfil its intended purpose. Fargason and Haddock conclude that in order for teams to make high-quality decisions, attention needs to be paid to group processes, including selection of team members and group decision making.

An example of a clinical specialty where one could expect to find a shared sense of purpose across the team is the hospice environment. Since the early 1970s the hospice movement, under the influence of visionaries such as Cicely Saunders, has developed to the point where there is clear agreement between the various disciplines working in this area. They concur that the focus of hospice care should be patient/family centred and holistic (not merely the relief of physical symptoms) so as to facilitate as peaceful a death as possible (Stedeford 1984; Fisher 1988). They also agree that hospice care should be provided in an environment in which staff do not see death as a failure; where staff are experts in their field yet accepting, even welcoming, the skills of others when focused towards the goal of patient comfort and well-being; all within a supportive, humanistic environment (Stedeford 1984; Fenton 1986). One outstanding feature of these teams is the sense of common purpose that is almost palpable when one comes into contact with such organisations.

Other subsets of 'effective communication' and their importance to the functioning of multidisciplinary health care can be identified within the literature. It is important, for example, that team members have a clear idea of what colleagues in other disciplines do (McGee & Ashford 1996) and the professional language they use (Wright 1993) to avoid the problems of care being fragmented through lack of a co-ordinated plan (Lenkman & Gribbins 1994). Communication between team members from different disciplines offers the opportunity to observe and acknowledge the unique contributions being made by colleagues (Benierakis 1995). Such clarity of purpose and awareness of the roles and expertise of colleagues should then enable team members to work together to achieve the (preferably) clearly stated goals of the team (Porter-O'Grady 1995). This synergy is only achieved when all members of the team are willing to co-operate (Yoder Wise 1995:280).

Benierakis (1995) and Loveridge (1991) discuss the importance of peers within teams supporting and valuing each other rather than being critically destructive of each other. If mutual appreciation occurs then trust will also tend to build up between team members, leading eventually to everyone feeling that they can put forward ideas and suggestions for improvement. Nakata and Saylor (1994) reinforce the significance of peer support, and add the view that managers should reward innovation and encourage personal accountability, perhaps through the use of a participative management style – in effect, encouraging collaboration in decision making about care, as well as actually providing that care.

Members of multidisciplinary health care teams potentially benefit greatly from the sharing of expertise and insight, not least because decisions reached and actions agreed tend to be well planned, informed by relevant experience, and 'owned' by the parties concerned, thus enhancing the chances of effecting successful change.

Clear roles

In effective teams the role each member of the team is expected to assume is generally well established and understood, albeit tacitly at times. While people fulfil these roles (norms of behaviour) then the team is likely to be functional. However, conflict can arise when a team member assumes a role that is different from that expected of her/his position in the team, or when the notion of 'equal recognition' is overlooked.

The role of nurses (who are numerically dominant in health) and doctors (who are undisputedly the dominant power group in health) has been described and analysed within the context of multidisciplinary teams (Lenkman & Gribbins 1994; McGee & Ashford 1996; Warelow 1996). In the main, the assumed roles maintain the *status quo*, with the nursing literature tending to nominate the doctor as team leader. This situation could change, albeit slowly, as new roles emerge, nurse consultant posts are increasing in number and the nurse practitioner role is established in a wider range of clinical settings.

Pfeffer and Schnack (1995) describe the 'shared governance' approach to leadership of a multidisciplinary team providing care to people with HIV/AIDS. Shared governance is a dynamic process that requires team members at every level to play key roles in the decision making that affects the team and the people it serves. As is the case in other health care environments, the nurses in that team were the only full-time primary care providers, and as a result had responsibility for clinical decisions including triaging patients, quality assurance, crisis management and conducting team meetings. If it gains momentum, shared governance will lead to changes in the structure and functioning of multidisciplinary health care teams of the future.

Leadership

The style of the leader influences significantly the performance and morale of a team (Kelly-Thomas 1998:344) although, as Barnum (1998) notes, the best leader may not always be the manager. Traditionally the leader does have responsibility for the day-to-day activities of the team. However, contemporary leadership models focus on the need for a leader to have, and to be able to articulate, a vision of what is intended and expected of the team, and to create the 'social environment' in which this can happen. According to Barnum, this shift in emphasis from manager as supervisor to

that of visionary is reflective of changing professional and community expectations. Leaders with vision are vital in health care situations where the system is changing at such a rate that health professionals require an environment that enables them to interpret, create and grow with change. The reader who is new to nursing would benefit from further reading in the area of the management of change (see, for example, Crookes & Davies 1998 or Wright 1998).

For a variety of reasons doctors are often cast in the role of leaders of health care teams. One reason for that is that when medical care is sought, the initial contact is usually with a medical practitioner (particularly GPs) and in cases where onward referral is required, it is often to other specialist doctors. Given that many people only seek to access health services when they are sick or injured, it is not unreasonable for doctors to be considered necessary and important. However, there are issues related to the conventions of this assumption of power that nurses and those in professions allied to medicine may find problematic. It is also the case that medical practitioners may not always be the best people to take the lead in multidisciplinary health care, particularly when outcomes are not 'curative' (e.g. in rehabilitation and developmental disability services). It must, however, be acknowledged that doctors occupy a key role in the care of people requiring health services, not only because the public see doctors in this light (convention again) but also because modern Western health services are orientated towards being essentially 'sick services' (Crookes 1992:228).

In the modernisation agenda for the National Health Service as outlined in *The NHS Plan* (DoH 2000), clinical leadership is seen as central to achieving the far-reaching reforms. As a result much attention is being given to developing clinical leadership skills within all members of the multidisciplinary team with the emphasis on the development of transformational leadership qualities (Bass & Avolio 1994).

The preceding discussion of roles and leadership and their impact upon the effectiveness of the multidisciplinary team leads us to the final issue related to effective teams: conflict.

THE NATURE OF CONFLICT

The traditional health care facility has been described as 'a collection of professional fiefdoms … the uniting of which requires attention to organisational, professional, and technical barriers' (Lenkman & Gribbins 1994:81). Conflict between and within groups is common, and not necessarily destructive. Functional conflict can actually enhance and benefit the organisation's performance. For example, two community health teams may agree that community-based aged care is a priority; however there may be a conflict regarding how that can best be achieved. Each team applies a different model, both of which result in improved access to services for the elderly – there is not always only one 'answer'.

However, the potential for dysfunctional conflict to interfere with the harmony and outcomes of the group is considerable, and must be addressed effectively. Umiker (1998) identifies six common causes of conflict: unclear expectations; poor communication; lack of clear jurisdiction; incompatibilities or disagreements based on difference; conflict of interest; and operational or staffing changes. Team members may be unclear about their role in the team, policies and procedures, or how outcomes will be measured. As we have discussed previously, effective communication between members of teams, and between the team and organisation, is arguably the most significant contributing factor to the team's success. Jurisdiction refers to accountability, authority and responsibility within the team. Conflict can arise when members do not comply with established expectations, either via a failure to assume expected roles, or a failure to recognise positions with legitimate authority. Conflict arising from incompatibilities, or differences of opinion, are complex situations that can spring from factors as diverse as politics, ethics, values or gender. Conflicts of interest may arise between departments, shifts and individuals, and may be precipitated by operational or staff changes.

Ivancevich and Matteson (1993) describe four factors that predispose to the development of conflict within groups: work interdependence; differences in goals; differences in perceptions; and the increased demand for specialists. Work interdependence occurs when two or more groups must depend on one another to complete their tasks; for example, conflict may arise between staff working day shift and those working night shift. Differences in goals may arise as groups become increasingly specialised, particularly when limited resources and reward structures within organisations are at stake. Differences in perceptions of reality, and disagreements over what constitutes reality, can lead to conflict, e.g. in a hospital, administrative staff may view a problem differently from the clinical staff. Increased demand for specialisation can also cause conflict between specialists and generalists.

Conflict resolution

Resolution of conflict requires clear procedures for communication (discussed earlier in this chapter) and decision making, commitment to team building, and consideration of factors such as the number of team members and their personalities. The association between the size of team and job satisfaction is significant in the discussion about health teams. Fargason and Haddock (1992) proposed that the optimum number of members in a team is five, and that a greater number predisposes to conflict manifested by increased absenteeism and reduced job satisfaction. However, multidisciplinary teams working in clinical areas usually have more than five members, some significantly more. Team size is therefore potentially a major cause of conflict within multidisciplinary health care teams.

A variety of techniques to manage conflict have been identified. Umiker (1998) described strategies such as avoidance or denial of the problem, surrender, compromise and collaboration. Ivancevich and Matteson (1993) include expansion of resources and altering the structure of the organisation as potential strategies. The model described by Tuckman and Jensen (1977) for group formation (forming, storming, norming, performing and adjourning) can be used as a framework for conflict resolution. Groups engaged in this process agree on aims, structure, leadership (forming), and then go through a stage of discussion and debate, which may include conflict (storming) to achieve co-operation, collaboration and the establishment of team norms (norming). The group is then functional (performing). Depending on the purpose of the group, it may then adjourn. A common theme in all techniques is the requirement for constructive negotiation via effective communication between the parties.

Problem solving and compromise by the parties is frequently required to resolve conflict. Fargason & Haddock (1992) are of the opinion that conflict develops in multidisciplinary teams when individuals approach problem solving in a manner that detracts from the quality of decisions made by the team. Problem solving requires meetings between the groups to debate differences and negotiate agreement. Problem solving also requires conflicting groups to display a willingness to work together to incorporate concerns into a consensus decision. Compromise can be used effectively when the goals can be divided equitably, and therefore is most useful when the conflicting parties have relatively equal power and are strongly committed to mutually exclusive goals.

Group decision making is common in organisations, with committees, working parties or teams formed to review a situation and make recommendations. However, that approach does not guarantee quality decisions (Lenkman & Gribbins 1994), or consultation with stakeholders (Fargason & Haddock 1992). The traditional, department-based, hierarchical decision-making model is not new to those who have worked in health.

While crucial and ultimately highly profitable decisions have been based on a feeling or hunch, organisations generally adopt a more scientific approach to decision making. A decision-making framework presented by Ivancevich and Matteson (1993) describes five stages that take the team through (1) the process of establishing objectives and (2) identifying alternatives; (3) evaluating the alternatives, (4) determining a course of action, and (5) the implementation of the action. Research methods frequently used to assist decision making and problem solving in nursing include the Delphi technique and the Nominal Group Technique (Jamieson *et al.* 1998). The Delphi Technique is based on structured questionnaires, with responses validated by regular feedback to participants. The Nominal Group Technique also uses structured questions, but differs from the Delphi Technique in that the results are available immediately.

Failure to attend to the 'health' of the team and/or absence of organisational commitment, impose considerable risks to outcomes. Lenkman and Gribbins (1994) refer to the 'human resource perspective' which seeks to achieve a balance between organisational and team needs. Failure to achieve that balance results in job dissatisfaction manifested in the inability to retain valued employees and attract new team members.

These authors have identified six general areas which, if addressed effectively, will significantly enhance the success of multidisciplinary teams and reduce conflict:

(1) People in the organisation must be committed to change, and opportunities and strategies for effective change must be determined.
(2) Potential barriers to success must be identified.
(3) A framework for implementation (e.g. case management, shared care) must be agreed upon.
(4) Opportunities and strategies to assist and promote change within the organisation must be identified.
(5) The organisation must provide educational opportunities for staff, and opportunities for team building.

(6) Managers within the organisation must recognise that some health professionals find working in teams more difficult than others, and provide support to those individuals.

CONCLUSION

Multidisciplinary teams are formed to achieve objectives; the most obvious (but certainly not the only) reason is to achieve measurable outcomes that are beyond the capacity of individuals or groups from the same discipline. The complexity of new therapies, increasing specialisation (and the emergence of new specialties), and the increasing diversity of services consumers expect, point to the team approach as an efficient and effective model of care. The professions represented in a multidisciplinary team will reflect local needs, priorities and resources.

Health services have traditionally been structured around functional areas of professional expertise, therefore multidisciplinary teams are unlikely to be successful until the organisation is committed to change, and group processes are in place to support communication within the group, and between the group and the organisation. The culture within the organisation will largely determine the productivity of teams and the degree of satisfaction experienced by the members.

There are potential barriers to the success of multidisciplinary teams, and these must be dealt with at both the group and organisational levels. In this chapter precipitating factors for group conflict have been discussed and strategies to prevent, or at least minimise, the effect of conflict on the team have been presented. If multidisciplinary teams are to be functional and effective, opportunities for professional development of members – which includes team-building activities – must be provided and supported by the organisation. In addition, evidence of successful problem solving, negotiation and compromise must be rewarded.

REFLECTIVE QUESTIONS

(1) What do you believe to be strengths and weaknesses of multidisciplinary teams?
(2) How could multidisciplinary teams benefit nurses and the nursing profession?
(3) Consider ways in which nurses in general, and you personally, could positively impact on the efficacy of the multidisciplinary team you may work within.

RECOMMENDED READING

Fargason, C.A. & Haddock, C.C. (1992) Cross-functional, integrative team decision-making: Essential for effective QI in health care. *Quality Review Bulletin*, **May**, 157–163.

Hein, E.C. (ed.) (1998) *Contemporary Leadership Behaviour: Selected Readings*, 5th edn. Lippincott, Philadelphia.

Kelly-Thomas, K.J. (1998) *Clinical and Nursing Staff Development: Current Competence, Future Focus*, 2nd edn. Lippincott, Philadelphia.

Roberts, S.J. (1983) Oppressed group behaviour: Implications for nursing. *Advances in Nursing Science*, **5**(4), 21–30.

Wicks, D. (1999) *Nurses and Doctors at Work: Rethinking Professional Boundaries*. Allen & Unwin, Sydney.

REFERENCES

Barnum, B.S. (1998) Leadership: can it be holistic? In: *Contemporary Leadership Behaviour: Selected Readings* (ed. E.C. Hein), 5th edn. Lippincott, New York.

Bass, B. & Avolio, J. (1994) *Improving Organisational Effectiveness through Transformational Leadership*. Sage, London.

Bassett, C. (1993) Socialisation of student nurses into the qualified nurse role. *British Journal of Nursing*, **2**(3), 179–182.

Benierakis, C.E. (1995) The function of the multidisciplinary team in child psychiatry – clinical and educational aspects. *Canadian Journal of Psychiatry*, **40**, 348–353.

Burnell, S. (1995) Case management and multidisciplinary teams. In: *Managed Care, Case Management and Nursing in Australia* (ed. P. Wilkinson). Australian Nursing Federation, Melbourne.

Coxon, T. (1990) Ritualised repression. *Nursing Times*, **86**(31), 35–36.

Crookes, P.A. (1992) The politics of health care. In: *Health: Perspectives and Practices* (eds J. Boddy & V. Rice), 2nd edn. pp. 216–232. The Dunmore Press, Palmerston North, New Zealand.

Crookes, P.A. & Davies, S. (eds) (1998) *Research into Practice: Essential Skills for Reading and Applying Research in Nursing and Health Care*. Baillière Tindall, Edinburgh.

Department of Health (2000) *The NHS Plan*. Department of Health, London.

Fargason, C.A. & Haddock, C.C. (1992) Cross-functional, integrative team decision making: Essential for QI in health care. *Quality Review Bulletin*, **May**, 157–163.

Farmer, B. (1993) The use and abuse of power in nursing. *Nursing Standard*, **7**(23), 33–36.

Fenton, M. (1986) Development of a scale of humanistic nursing behaviours. *Nursing Research*, **39**(2), 82–87.

Fisher, M. (1988) Hospice nursing. *Nursing*, **3**(32), 8–10.

Gallagher, R. (1995) Team building. In: *Leading and Managing in Nursing* (ed. P.S. Yoder Wise), pp. 275–299. Mosby, St Louis.

Griffiths, R. (1996) Australian reactions to the DCCT: Existing practices and new initiatives. *Practical Diabetes International*, **13**(2), 41–42.

Hein, E.C. (ed.) (1998) *Contemporary Leadership Behaviour: Selected Readings*, 5th edn. Lippincott, New York.

Hill, M.N. & Becker, D.M. (1995) Roles of nurses and health workers in cardiovascular health promotion. *The American Journal of the Medical Sciences*, **310**(Suppl.), S123-S126.

Hoskins, P.L., Fowler, P.M., Constantino, M., Forrest, J., Yue, D.K. & Turtle, J.R. (1993) Sharing the care of diabetic patients between hospital and general practitioners: Does it work? *Diabetic Medicine*, **10**, 81–86.

Ivancevich, J.M. & Matteson, M.T. (1993) *Organisational Behaviour and Management*, 3rd edn. Irwin, Boston.

Jamieson, M., Griffiths, R. & Jayasuriya, R. (1998) Developing outcomes for community nursing: the nominal group technique. *Australian Journal of Advanced Nursing*, **16**(1), 14–19.

Kelly-Thomas, K.J. (1998) *Clinical and Nursing Staff Development: Current Competence, Future Focus*, 2nd edn. Lippincott, New York.

Lenkman, S. & Gribbins, R. (1994) Multidisciplinary teams in the acute care setting. *Holistic Nursing Practice*, **April**, 81–87.

Loveridge, C.E. (1991) Lessons in excellence for nurse administrators. *Nursing Management*, **22**(2), 47.

McGee, P. & Ashford, R. (1996) Nurses' perceptions of roles in multidisciplinary teams. *Nursing Standard*, **10**(45), 34–36.

Nakata, J.A. & Saylor, C. (1994) Management style and staff nurse satisfaction in a changing environment. *Nurse Administration Quarterly*, **18**(3), 51–57.

O'Toole, M.T. (ed.) (1997) *Miller-Keane Encyclopedia and Dictionary of Medicine, Nursing and Allied Health*. W.B. Saunders, Philadelphia.

Parker, G.M. (1990) Team players and teamwork. In: *Leading and Managing in Nursing* (ed. P.S. Yoder Wise). Mosby, St Louis.

Pfeffer, G.N. & Schnack, J.A. (1995) Nurse practitioners as leaders in a quality health care delivery system. *Advance Practice Nurses Quarterly*, **1**(2), 30–39.

Porter, S. (1991) A participant observation study of power relations between nurses and doctors in a general hospital. *Journal of Advanced Nursing*, **16**, 728–735.

Porter-O'Grady, T. (1995) Five rules of engagement for multidisciplinary teams. *Aspens Advisor for Nurse Executives*, **September**, 8.

Roberts, S.J. (1983) Oppressed group behaviour: Implications for nursing. *Advances in Nursing Sciences*, **5**(4), 21–30.

Stedeford, A. (1984) *Facing Death: Patients, Families and Professionals*. W. Heinemann Books Ltd, London.

Stein, L.I., Watts, D.T. & Howell, T. (1990) Sounding board: The doctor-nurse game re-visited. *The Lamp*, **47**(9), 23–26.

Tuckman, B.W. & Jensen, M. (1977) Stages of small group development revisited. In: *Organisational Behaviour and Management* (eds J.M. Ivancevich & M.T. Matteson), 3rd edn. Irwin, Boston.

Umiker, W. (1998) Collaborative conflict resolution. In: *Contemporary Leadership Behaviour: Selected Readings* (ed. E.C. Hein), 5th edn. Lippincott, New York.

Warelow P.J. (1996) Nurse-doctor relationships in multidisciplinary teams: Ideal or real? *International Journal of Nursing Practice*, **2**, 33–39.

Wright, B.A. (1993) Behaviour diagnoses by a multidisciplinary team. *Geriatric Nursing*, **January/February**, 30–35.

Wright, S. (1998) *Changing Nursing Practice*, 2nd edn. Arnold, London.

Yoder Wise, P.S. (1995) *Leading and Managing in Nursing*. Mosby, St Louis.

13 Becoming Professional

The Role of Regulatory Authorities and Nursing Organisations

Judy Mannix and Irene Stein

LEARNING OBJECTIVES

After reading this chapter the reader should be able to:

- define what is meant by a 'regulatory authority' in nursing and a 'nursing organisation';
- differentiate between a regulatory authority and a nursing organisation;
- identify the major regulatory authorities and nursing organisations in Great Britain;
- understand the current role of regulatory authorities and nursing organisations in industrial, professional, regulatory and educational contexts;
- appreciate the benefits of membership of different nursing organisations;
- access relevant websites relating to regulatory authorities and nursing organisations.

KEY WORDS

ORGANISATIONS, REGULATORY, AUTHORITY, ACRONYM, REGISTRATION, INDUSTRIAL BODY, UNIONISM, POLITICS.

INTRODUCTION

Regulatory authorities and nursing organisations play a critical role in contemporary nursing. By providing structure and order these organisations aim to ensure high standards of care and safety for nursing workers and their client base. At times throughout the history of nursing it has been evident that regulatory authorities and nursing organisations do not function in isolation from one another. Rather, these organisations complement one another in many areas. In this chapter the role and place of regulatory authorities and nursing organisations are discussed in the context of contemporary nursing. Please note that a list of acronyms for the various British nursing bodies appears at the end of the chapter

KEY DATES IN BRITISH NURSING

The evolution and development of regulatory authorities and nursing organisations in any country occurs in a historical context. British nursing has a strong and a proud history. It is useful therefore to briefly review some of the key historical events that have shaped nursing in Britain.

1860 Nightingale Training School at St Thomas' Hospital, London established.
1916 College of Nursing established.
1919 Nursing Act:
       General Nursing Councils established.
1928 College of Nursing given Royal Charter.
1939 King George VI gives title Royal to College of Nursing.
1946 National Health Service Act.
1947 National Health Service (NHS) introduced based on three divisions:
       • hospital and specialist services;
       • general practitioner;
       • local authority health.
1974 Reorganisations of NHS into Regional and Area Health Authorities:
       • Department of Health and Social Security (DHSS);
       • Regional Health Authorities (RHAs);
       • Area Health Authorities (AHAs).
1978 Nurses, Midwives and Health Visitors Act.
1979 United Kingdom Central Council for Nursing, Midwifery and Health Visiting established under the Nurses, Midwives and Health Visitors Act 1979.
1981 Restructure of health with the creation of the position of chief nursing officer (CNO) in each district health authority (DHS). The role of this CNO was to provide advice to the general manager of the DHA. This position was of equal seniority to that of the other members of the district management team.
1995 Introduction of postregistration education and practice (PREP) requirements by the UKCC.
2002 Alteration of the title of the UKCC to the Nursing and Midwifery Council (NMC).

(from Applin 1991; Dean 1992; RCN 1992; UKCC 2000, 2001a,b)

REGULATORY AUTHORITIES IN BRITISH NURSING

In the United Kingdom the workforce of nurses, midwives and health visitors comprises a significant number of people. According to the United Kingdom Central Council (UKCC) over 630 000 people are registered to practise in one of these three roles (www.ukcc.org.uk). Ensuring that this large number of health workers practise within standards acceptable to both the profession and the public requires some form of control. In the United Kingdom the current regulatory body for nursing, midwifery and health visitors is the UKCC, established under an Act of Parliament in 1979. In April 2002, this regulatory body became known as the Nursing and Midwifery Council (NMC). Current registration as a nurse, midwife or health visitor with the UKCC is required before legal authority to practise is given. This registration to work as either a nurse, midwife or health visitor is issued upon initial registration and renewed every three years.

The UKCC has a number of regulatory functions that include:

- the maintenance of a register of nurses, midwives and health visitors able to practise in the UK;
- consideration of misconduct allegations;
- establishing standards for education, clinical practice and professional conduct;
- monitoring the suitability of internationally registered nurses and midwives to practise in the UK;
- carriage of the postregistration education and practice programme (PREP);
- provision of advice for practitioners. (UKCC 1996, 1999, 2001a)

Of particular significance has been the introduction of PREP by the UKCC in 1995. This mandates the level of postregistration education to be completed in a defined period in order to retain registration as a nurse, midwife or health visitor. To maintain registration in the UK it is a legal requirement that registrants meet two separate standards. These are the PREP (practice) standard and the PREP (continuing professional development) standard. The PREP (practice) standard stipulates the hours of work required for registration and the PREP (continuing professional development) standard requires that a record of continuing professional development be maintained (UKCC 1995, 1999, 2000, 2001a).

In addition to the UKCC, England, Scotland, Wales and Northern Ireland have National Boards that monitor the educational processes for nurses, midwives and health visitors in these areas. Useful websites for these National Boards are:

- www.enb.org.uk
- www.nbs.org.uk
- www.n-i.uk/NBM/
- www.wnb.org.uk

WHAT IS A NURSING ORGANISATION?

An organisation comprises a group of people functioning within a given set of aims and objectives. Within such an organisation there is usually an administrative infrastructure responsible for its day-to-day running. Whether or not these administrative functions are undertaken by elected members of the organisation or by paid employees is largely dependent on the size of the body and the way in which it is constituted. Membership of an organisation is undertaken on a voluntary basis and implies a respect for its aims and objectives, along with a desire to further these aims and objectives. Dependent on the type of organisation and the membership status of the individual, belonging to an organisation usually confers benefits on its members.

There is also a level of reciprocity with organisations and their individual members involving activities directed to benefit both the organisation and its members. These activities can range from individual members performing roles within an organisation, to an organisation acting as a voice for its members in relevant forums where representation from an interested body of people is more appropriate than that of individuals, e.g. meetings with government health authorities and organisations involved in the health care arena.

THE ROLES OF NURSING ORGANISATIONS IN THE UNITED KINGDOM

Nursing in the United Kingdom has within it a number of different nursing organisations, each of them functioning according to their specific major role. Irrespective of their primary role, nursing organisations have been and continue to be important features of the nursing landscape in the United Kingdom. In the context of nursing organisations in the United Kingdom, three primary roles or functions are evident. Nursing organisations primarily fulfil one or more of the following roles:

(1) industrial representation;
(2) professional body;
(3) specialist nursing interest organisation.

Nursing organisations with an *industrial* focus represent the interests of nurses in the industrial arena, acting on behalf of their members in pursuit of improved working conditions and wages under the relevant awards.

Professional organisations

Professional organisations play an important role in furthering the development of nursing within the health care system and the wider community. Organisations of this type represent the interests of nurses from a wide range of nursing areas. In Britain, unlike some other countries like Australia, the Royal College of Nursing (RCN) serves the dual roles of providing industrial representation and functioning as a professional body. The RCN is the largest professional organisation for nurses in the United Kingdom and offers its membership a range of professional and educational services in addition to providing trade union representation.

Granted a Royal Charter in 1928, the purposes of the RCN include the promotion of nursing education and training, raising the standing of the profession at both a national and international level, and to provide workplace support for members. Some of the services provided by RCN that meet these purposes include:

- support and advice on workplace issues and problems;
- legal representation when required;
- a variety of continuing professional development activities;
- advice on professional matters;
- counselling services;
- advice on immigration matters;
- activities to assist nursing students;
- an extensive nursing library with access to free publications on nursing, health-care and employment issues (see www.rcn.org.uk/about-rcn-workingfor-nurses.html).

Two important aspects of the work of RCN are the Association of Nursing Students (ANS) and the RCN Institute. The ANS comprises all student members of RCN and is managed by an elected committee. Policy development concerning issues affecting students is at the centre of the activities of ANS. Providing a network for students is achieved through an annual congress, regular publications, student forums and a career bulletin (see www.rcn.org.uk/student/student-anscando.html).

The RCN Institute aims to 'promote excellence through the science and art of nursing' and to enable practice development that will 'transform nursing, health and healthcare' (see www.rcn.org.uk/learning/learning_aboutthercninstitute.html). A key activity of the RCN Institute is in the area of research and practice development. Foci include competency development, evidence-based practice and advanced practice development.

As an adjunct to these services, RCN provides regular newsletters in nursing interest areas for members (for example, Link Up in the area of learning disabilities (1999)) and through corporate affiliations produces specialist materials such as the RCN Assessment Tool for nursing older people (1997). As an independent trade union, RCN negotiates working conditions for its membership, represents members in industrial forums and provides advice to members regarding workplace relations.

Specialist nursing organisations

The aims and objectives of most specialist nursing organisations generally reflect a desire to promote and represent the interests of those nurses working in the particular nursing specialty. This type of organisation has become increasingly prominent on the nursing landscape, mainly as a consequence of the growing trend towards postregistration specialisation in nursing practice. The growth in specialist nursing organisations has also occurred out of a desire by nurses, midwives and health visitors to seek greater control over their own affairs, rather than having matters such as role statements and skill standards imposed on them from outside the profession (Parkes 1994). The structure, scope and function of the different specialist interest organisations are not exactly the same, although a number of similarities do exist.

There are many nursing, midwifery and health visitor specialist organisations in the UK. These include both practitioner and education organisations. Some examples of these are:

- The Community and District Nursing Association www.cdna.tvu.ac.uk

- The Infection Control Nurses Association www.icna.co.uk
- The National Association of Theatre Nurses www.natn.org.uk
- The NHS University www.doh.gov.uk/nhsuniversity
- The Nursing and Midwifery Admissions Service (NMAS) www.nmas.ac.uk/index.html
- Student Nurse Underground www.coopshouse.freeserve.co.uk

THE SIGNIFICANCE OF REGULATORY AUTHORITIES AND NURSING ORGANISATIONS

There is little doubt that the increased professional status of nurses is directly attributable to the efforts of regulatory authorities and nursing organisations. This increased professional standing of nursing has occurred through developments such as the introduction of undergraduate tertiary education for nurses, the improvement of industrial award conditions, and the establishing of national networking and lobbying groups to influence and shape policy decisions in the health care arena.

Education

The achievements of professional nursing organisations in the area of nurse education are noteworthy. Aimed principally at postgraduate education for nurses, courses and professional development opportunities are available in many specialty nursing areas and through various education providers. Specialty clinical nursing courses available range from paediatrics through to aged care, and include nursing in acute, nonacute and community settings. Education programmes are also available for those nurses who choose to pursue a career pathway in management. Recognition of the importance of specialty nursing qualifications is evident in career pathways available for nurses, in fact, formal qualifications in a specialist area are generally an essential criterion for career advancement in nursing, irrespective of the area of practice.

Policy development

Apart from providing a forum for nurses with similar practice interests to network and develop professionally, specialist nursing interest organisations also enable nurses in a particular specialty to have a voice in matters impacting on their working lives. Many specialist nursing interest organisations provide valuable policy advice for the future development, accountability and direction of their practice areas. This advice may be sought at all levels, and may relate to nursing in particular or to the broader area of health care delivery.

Benefits of membership of nursing organisations

Nursing organisations are always seeking new members. Before joining a nursing organisation, it is advisable for an individual nurse to carefully examine its mission statement, codes of ethics and conduct, aims, objectives and spheres of both political and practical influence to ensure they are relevant to the nurse's needs. Membership of a nursing organisation can be beneficial to a nurse's professional development by providing opportunities that may be otherwise unavailable. These benefits include:

- access to up-to-date information via journals and other publications such as newsletters;
- information regarding the development of common standards and competencies for practice;
- opportunities to serve on executive and other committees of an organisation;
- providing an avenue to voice concerns to government about areas of nursing and health care;
- access to scholarships and other educational opportunities to facilitate professional development;
- providing advice concerning workplace conditions and responsibilities;
- participation in the International Council of Nursing (ICN) (www.icn.ch) activities through membership of the Royal College of Nursing.

Each of these benefits enhances an individual nurse's professional development and is available to all members of the organisation. However, the key to maximising the benefits available is to be an active member. Membership of nursing organisations is not an elitist activity, rather one that has the potential to educate and unify the profession.

CONCLUSION

It is difficult to imagine nursing in the United Kingdom without the presence of the various regulatory authorities and nursing organisations. Many distinguished British nurses have spent their political energies in the initiation, development and consolidation of these organisations. The resulting diversity of nursing organisations ensures the ongoing development of creative solutions to practice problems in nursing and health care delivery. Becoming professional is a critical focus for all nurses in the United Kingdom in order to equip nursing for the new millennium.

REFLECTIVE QUESTIONS

(1) How do industrial nursing organisations differ from specialist nursing interest groups in terms of their current roles and functions in nursing?
(2) Why do you think different nursing organisations exist in the nursing profession?
(3) For what reasons do you believe regulatory authorities are an important component of the nursing landscape in Britain?

ABBREVIATIONS

ANS   Association of Nursing Students
NMC   Nursing & Midwifery Council
PREP Postregistration Education & Practice
RCN   Royal College of Nursing
UKCC United Kingdom Central Council

RECOMMENDED READING

Applin, L. (1991) *Health and Nursing in the United Kingdom*. Royal College of Nursing, London.

Dean, D.J. (1992) *Royal College of Nursing of the United Kingdom – Working: Policy and Practice*. Royal College of Nursing, London.

United Kingdom Central Council for Nursing, Midwifery and Health Visiting (1999) *How the UKCC Works for You*. UKCC, London.

United Kingdom Central Council for Nursing, Midwifery and Health Visiting (2001) *The PREP Handbook*. UKCC, London.

United Kingdom Central Council for Nursing, Midwifery and Health Visiting (2001) *Supporting Nurses, Midwives and Health Visitors through Lifelong Learning*. UKCC, London.

REFERENCES

Applin, L. (1991) *Health and Nursing in the United Kingdom*. Royal College of Nursing, London.

Dean, D.J. (1992) *Royal College of Nursing of the United Kingdom – Working: Policy and Practice*. Royal College of Nursing, London.

Parkes, R. (1994) *Specialisation in Nursing*. ANF, Melbourne.

Royal College of Nursing (1992) *The Royal College of Nursing of the United Kingdom*. Royal College of Nursing, London.

Royal College of Nursing (1997) *RCN: Assessment Tool for Nursing Older People*. Royal College of Nursing, London.

Royal College of Nursing (1999) *Link Up*. Royal College of Nursing, London.

United Kingdom Central Council for Nursing, Midwifery and Health Visiting (1995) *PREP & You*. UKCC, London.

United Kingdom Central Council for Nursing, Midwifery and Health Visiting (1996) *Guidelines for Professional Practice*. UKCC, London.

United Kingdom Central Council for Nursing, Midwifery and Health Visiting (1999) *How the UKCC Works for You*. UKCC, London.

United Kingdom Central Council for Nursing, Midwifery and Health Visiting (2000) *The Practice Standard: Information for Registered Nurses, Midwives and Health Visitors*. UKCC, London.

United Kingdom Central Council for Nursing, Midwifery and Health Visiting (2001a) *The PREP Handbook*. UKCC, London.

United Kingdom Central Council for Nursing, Midwifery and Health Visiting (2001b) *Supporting Nurses, Midwives and Health Visitors through Lifelong Learning*. UKCC, London.

14 Meeting the Needs of Individuals

Mary FitzGerald

LEARNING OBJECTIVES

After reading this chapter the student will be able to:

- appreciate the ideal of meeting the needs of individuals;
- understand the ways that nurses can assess the needs of individuals;
- identify the systems in nursing that are conducive to individualised nursing;
- acknowledge the problems of providing an individualistic service;
- develop creative means to provide an individualistic nursing service to clients in the contemporary health care climate.

KEY WORDS

INDIVIDUALISED CARE, CONTINUUM, DEPENDENCY, NURSING ASSESSMENT, NURSING PROCESS, CARE PLANNING.

INTRODUCTION

Individualised care, or care that is specifically designed to meet the distinctive needs of each and every client nursed, is much applauded as a central and valued tenet of good nursing practice. It is supported in nursing literature, educational establishments and, to a large extent, practice. The Nursing and Midwifery Council (formerly the UKCC) code of professional conduct begins with a statement that endorses an individualised approach to nursing (N&MC 2002). It seems reasonable to assume that it is in the client's best interest to offer a nursing service that caters to each specific person, and nursing in Western countries such as Australia, the USA and the UK have certainly adopted the provision of individualised nursing as a core value. They have asserted that an understanding of the biopsychosocial needs of each person, and a service that accommodates as many of these needs as possible, is more likely to foster improvements in patients' health status, comfort and satisfaction with service than one that delivers a standard service to people according to their medical diagnosis.

In its purest form individualised nursing constitutes one end of a continuum, at the other extreme of which lies a routine service in which all people are treated the same according to their grouping (e.g. age or diagnosis) and where nurses are required to follow protocol rather than make decisions. The reality of practice probably falls somewhere between these two extremes. It is arguably one of the profession's

greatest challenges to maintain the delivery of individualised care in spite of institutional and policy pressures that militate against core nursing values such as this.
Hence the real challenge confronting nursing has less to do with the maintenance
of current practice than with the generation of creative solutions and strategies that
preserve and develop those core values that nursing has treasured.

Manthey (1980) claims that American nurses practised individualised nursing in
the 1920s:

> The nurse took care of the sick person from the time the need for care was identified
> until it no longer existed; care was personally administered by the nurse according to
> the assessment she [sic] made of the individual needs of the patient. There were no
> rules or regulations, no routine procedures, no hospital policies, time schedules, or
> supervisors. She practiced [sic] nursing with a degree of independence unheard of in
> modern hospital nursing (p. 2).

It is notable that the service described above was provided in the community, away
from the complex and medically dominated hospital system where there is a tendency for people to gain a medical diagnosis and perhaps lose some of their personal
identity. Later we will consider whether rising levels of dependency among patients
in the community might lead to the increasingly medical aspects of care detracting
from personal identity, as it has done in hospitals in the past. A strong resurgence
of interest in the individual patient returned to nursing in the 1970s against a social
backdrop of rising individualism, consumerism and the escalation of the professional
classes. The driving philosophies were existentialism and humanism. The focus of
philosophers was on the individual as an intelligent human being capable of autonomous decision making and upon the quality of individual existence. Bevis (1978), a
leading American academic, described 'humanistic existentialism' as a modern phase
in nursing, with rising value placed upon human life, uniqueness of individuals, quality of life, and freedom of human beings to choose.

The nursing theorists of the late 1970s embraced these ideals and incorporated
them, relatively uncritically, into their conceptual models of nursing (Meleis 1997;
Pearson *et al.* 1996). In turn, conceptual models of nursing and their authors have
been extremely influential in the academic and educational development of nursing
(Field & FitzGerald 1989). While they have not been used everywhere as frameworks
or guides for nursing practice they have been used to guide nursing curricula and
research. My point is that throughout their education nurses are taught in theory to
value the concept of individualised care without a great deal of theoretical consideration for the difficulties of delivering this ideal of nursing in practice. Nursing students
frequently experience a degree of disillusionment and stress in practice when they
believe that patients do not receive the kind of individual attention they are taught
and believe to be necessary.

While essentially supporting individualised nursing, I would like to present in this
chapter some perspectives that portray it as problematic. By looking at individualised
nursing in a critical way it is more likely that the forces that support or obstruct it in
practice may be understood. This should contribute to a healthily realistic approach
to its implementation and development in nursing practice. Before dealing with the
problems of individualised *nursing* there will be a section dealing with the assess-

ment of individual *needs*, for this is the starting point in any nurse/patient relationship and it is an area where a nurse's time and skill are required to reveal the patient. The systems that are conducive to the delivery of individualised care will also be discussed, along with the evidence there is for their implementation. Lastly there will be a few suggestions for improving the level of individualised care and the means of evaluating it.

ASSESSMENT OF INDIVIDUAL NEEDS

Assessment of the person who requires nursing is the crucial factor in identifying the individual needs of any client. Although assessment is usually associated with the first encounter of nurse and patient, when a history is taken on admission, the process of assessment can and should continue throughout the nurse/patient relationship. In all encounters with a patient an astute nurse is able to recognise and collect useful information that will help him or her know both the patient and the specific nursing the patient requires. Data can be collected both objectively and subjectively, but before detailing the type of data that is required some time should be spent considering the conditions that affect the collection of information.

The type of relationship that a nurse establishes with a patient affects the quality and amount of information that she or he can gather about that person. Although this may sound obvious, it is of such significance that it is worth dwelling upon. Usually relationships are built up over a period, but time to build relationships with patients is becoming scarcer for the nurse. There are some places where there is time and this should always be appreciated and capitalised upon. Consider the difference between a typical surgical ward and a nursing home that provides residential accommodation for the older person. It is far more likely in the latter institution that the nurses will know the patient and be able to cater to him or her as an individual. This is more a function of the patient's length of stay than of the amount of time available to the nurse in this setting, but it does facilitate the development of the relationship. Nurses who come into contact with people for only a short period of time require a particular skill to be able to establish a working rapport with their patients quickly. This is not necessarily a skill that can be taught, because different people will respond in their own way to particular circumstances; the astute nurse will gauge the best way to communicate with new patients in order to reassure them and encourage them to talk. New nurses should watch the skills of nurses in long- and short-stay situations and reflect upon the ways that the more experienced nurses establish, or fail to establish, relationships with patients. All nurses – new and experienced – need to reflect on the impact of the changing context of practice on the nurse/patient relationship, for it may well be that this important connection is becoming harder and harder to achieve.

In most areas of nursing, either in hospital or in the community, there are structured systems for assessing patients when they are first encountered. In selecting the form of assessment it is preferable for the team of nurses to establish a degree of consensus on the nature of nursing and what it is that they are offering patients. Without this consensus the questions may result in the collection of routine data that is unhelpful in assisting nurses who are endeavouring to offer a holistic individualised service to patients (Pearson *et al.* 1996).

In its simplest form, an assessment structure may be merely a checklist of questions required to establish the individual's bare biographical and physical benchmarks. These forms are not conducive to individualised nursing in its broadest sense, for they are not intended to extract detailed information about the person's feelings or lifestyle. However, they may be highly efficient for the service being offered (e.g. in areas where the encounter between nurse and patient is very short and the patient's main purpose is to receive treatment for a medical condition). It should also be acknowledged that not all patients require or even want a 'therapeutic relationship' with a nurse. Other frameworks for assessment are more complex and conducive to the nurse making much deeper inquiry. These assessments are commonly based on one of the theoretical nursing models, and adapted by nurses to their locale. By way of examples, I would point to the assessment frameworks given by two nursing models (Neuman 1995; Roper *et al.* 1990).

Roper *et al.* (1990) state that, at assessment, the nurse aims to establish what the patient is able or unable to do for each of the activities of living with regard to physical, sociocultural, psychological, environmental and politico-economic factors that affect the person. These well-known activities of living are:

- maintaining a safe environment;
- communicating;
- breathing;
- eating and drinking;
- eliminating;
- personal cleansing and dressing;
- controlling body temperature;
- mobilising;
- working and playing;
- expressing sexuality;
- sleeping;
- dying.

Objective information is gathered by *observation and measurement.* For example, it is possible to observe how restlessly or peacefully a person sleeps, and to measure the length of time they sleep at night. There will inevitably be an element of subjectivity in the nurse's judgment, but this should be contained in order to generate an accurate and reliable profile of the person. *Subjective information* is gathered from the person and it represents their *perception of reality.* Remember that perceptions are real in their consequences, and to that extent they are as important as objective measurement. It is this information that truly reveals the individual and enables the nurse to know how the person can be nursed most beneficially. Remember, too, that often the nurse's own subjective judgments and perceptions, coupled with all of the demands placed upon them, serve to filter and in some cases impede the reception of information from the person.

Here are some examples obtained during a phenomenological research study (Fitz-Gerald 1995) from a patient who has asthma and who consequently has extensive experience of hospital and health services:

and the senior sisters would come down on their shifts and say, 'Hello, youse back
again?' and I am in bed there – 'Oh those are lovely flowers, isn't that a pretty nightie?'
They wouldn't stop and say, 'How are you coping, do you need any help?' And I used
to think, 'Silly bloody bitches, why don't you stop and sit down and ask – just talk to
me?'

  and her job is to dismiss, err, discharge people and she comes around – it's a stupid
job she has got – and she said to me 'Ah Peggy now you're,' [as] she just rubbed my toes,
'Now you just look after yourself won't you, now you're right, aren't you, you don't need
any help when you get out?'

  When I was on the [ward] the asthma clinical sister came around – 'Ah Peggy do you
want any magazines or anything?' … [pause] … I was half dead and on a drip.

You could characterise Peggy as 'difficult' but she is a classic example of someone
who was nursed often and whose many individual needs, beyond the purely physical, were neither recognised nor met. Peggy was not just difficult. Her needs were
complex and long-standing, she had a lifetime of illness and all that goes with it, and
it is undoubtedly the case that had the nurses involved discussed these needs with her
they would quickly have found themselves out of their depth. That would have been
perfectly reasonable, and she could have been referred to the appropriate services.
However, the point is that these needs were never even identified. A thorough nursing
assessment may have afforded Peggy the opportunity to express these needs.

  In contrast to the relatively structured assessment offered by Roper *et al.* (1990),
Neuman (1995) advocates the use of just six questions to elicit information from the
patient. The questions are:

(1) What do you consider to be your major problem, difficulty or area of con-
     cern?
(2) How has this affected your usual pattern of living or lifestyle?
(3) Have you ever experienced a similar problem before? If so, what was that
     problem and how did you handle it? Was your handling of the problem suc-
     cessful?
(4) What do you anticipate for yourself in the future as a consequence of your
     present situation?
(5) What are you doing and what can you do to help yourself?
(6) What do you expect care-givers, family, friends and others to do for you?

The information, once obtained, is then inserted into a more conventional assessment format. This approach seems more likely to engage the person and thus to produce more personal profile than a checklist of questions such as Peggy was subjected
to over and again during her long hospital career. In a study to examine the practice
of individualised nursing Brown (1992) concluded that open-ended questions were
by far the most likely to elicit information that was significant to the individual.

  Individualised nursing cannot really get off the ground without an assessment,
for little is known about the characteristics of the patient. There are many ways of
obtaining information for assessment, and formal frameworks should not impede
nurses from making the most of any encounter with a patient. However, if nurses are
to work in teams that offer some reliable and consistent standard of service across

the team, assessment information needs to be written so that all nurses have information about clients readily to hand. Common sense would dictate that the nurse who initially spends time with the patient and writes the assessment is the best person to be assigned to the patient, but of course this depends upon the system of work allocation in an area. The next section of this chapter will deal with this aspect of individual nursing.

SYSTEMS FOR INDIVIDUALISING NURSING

Individualised care can mean a number of things in nursing, but it is integral to such contemporary professional developments as total patient care, the nursing process, nursing models for practice, patient-centred nursing, primary nursing, information giving and patient autonomy.

In recent years the primary vehicles used to enhance individualised nursing have been the nursing process (a written systematic process of assessment, goal setting, planning and evaluation) and total patient care (the assignment of patients to nurses for all their nursing during a shift). The nursing process was an initiative that appeared to flounder in practice, although it was hailed in theory as the most appropriate means of professional decision making geared to the individual's requirements for nursing. Total patient care has persisted, and it is now uncommon to find nursing work allocated by tasks. However, the degree to which nurses are able to meet individual needs without provision in the system for continuity of care is questionable. Primary nursing (Manthey 1980) is a system of work organisation wherein one nurse is assigned responsibility for the prescription and delivery of care to a patient, from the time they first require nursing to the time they are discharged. Primary nursing in reality incorporates both total patient care and the nursing process, because the primary nurse is responsible for the delivery of care and the written prescription of care (Ersser & Tutton 1991; Long *et al.* 1999; Pearson 1989). The primary nurse has to write an assessment and plan in order to ensure that any other nurse caring for the patient gives the same treatment and knows the person's individual needs. The most reliable way to do this is to write the nursing notes tailored to the individual's needs.

From my experience of providing individualised nursing through using the nursing process and primary nursing, I would claim associated benefits for individuals in terms of continuity of care, quality of service and accountability for nursing delivery (FitzGerald 1991, 1994). However, the amount of scientific evidence regarding the efficacy of individualised nursing is disappointing (Black 1992). Predominantly this is because the variables in clinical practice are impossible to control and it is difficult to state with certainty the cause of any improvements. While there is no conclusive empirical evidence that demonstrates the efficacy of individualised nursing, it is an integral part of the movement named by Salvage (1990) 'new nursing'. The vanguard of 'new nursing' in the UK was found in the Nursing Development Units at Burford and Oxford. On these units the primary therapy was nursing and attention was focused on the needs of individual clients. A study to compare patient outcomes and quality of care for patients who had been admitted to the nursing unit (treatment group, $n = 84$) and patients who were left to follow a normal hospital pathway (control group, $n = 74$) demonstrated the following for the treatment group:

- higher quality of care;
- higher levels of independence on discharge;
- slightly longer hospital stay;
- lower cost per day.

While the majority of studies reported higher ratings of quality after the implementation of primary nursing, it is not always apparent exactly what is the cause of the improvement. Indeed MacGuire (1991) found, in a study of the introduction of primary nursing, that both the control and the experimental wards had improved quality scores. She concluded that this was a result of increased attention to quality measures rather than primary nursing, because primary nursing was only introduced to the experimental ward.

When a team of nurses in an Australian hospital introduced and researched the effectiveness of primary nursing, they too found it difficult to prove the effectiveness of primary nursing, even though it is a system of nursing they have adopted and continue to use (Long *et al.* 1999). In Victoria, Pearson and Baker in 1992 reported consistently higher quality scores in a nursing-led ward that practised primary nursing in a 'contemporary nursing' environment, than a ward from the acute sector. The nursing-led unit nurses had a philosophy (adapted from Henderson 1964) that encouraged these nursing approaches:

- the adoption of a systematic problem-solving approach;
- the use of scientifically derived knowledge;
- the development of transforming relationships with patients;
- a holistic approach;
- active participation of the patient in his/her own care (Pearson & Baker 1992, p. 4).

This Victorian project was a small descriptive study that compared data from the nursing records by using the Phaneuf (1976) Nursing Audit to measure quality of care in the following functions:

(1) application and execution of the physician's legal orders;
(2) observations of symptoms and reactions;
(3) supervision of the patient;
(4) supervision of those participating in care (except the physician);
(5) reporting and recording;
(6) application and execution of nursing procedures and techniques;
(7) promotion of physical and emotional health by direction and teaching.

The functions where there were the biggest differences between the two wards (the nursing unit scores were consistently higher) were 2, 3, 4, and 7.

As individualised nursing is predicated on the assumption that the consumers of our services are competent and autonomous human beings, their autonomy should be respected and encouraged. Above all else, the person who knows the individual best is the individual him- or herself and nurses are technically capable of encouraging patient autonomy by a system of nursing where the patient is encouraged to identify, voice and ensure provision for his or her own needs.

In brief, the required systems for the provision of nursing that meet individuals' needs are those that provide for continuity of care, a system of record keeping that maintains a record of needs and outcomes, and one that helps to maintain and develop the patient's sense of personal autonomy within a health care setting.

THE PROBLEMS WITH INDIVIDUALISED NURSING

The first problem with individualised nursing is that on the whole it is not problematised – that is to say, individualised nursing is accepted as the ideal towards which nurses should strive. Uncritically accepting individualised nursing negates the possibility that there may be other competing ideas that have merit, and closes off any prospect of exploring those other ideas. In critiquing individualised nursing I want to traverse some of these ideas and their implications because it strikes me that there must be some middle ground that reconciles the best of individualised nursing with the needs of cost containment and the general well-being of society as a whole. For individualised nursing to survive the current reality of practice it must first be perceived as achievable in practice amid the current realities of practice, and for this the middle ground is essential.

Nurses recognise very early in their careers that the ideals they learn in their schools often bear little resemblance to the realities of practice (DHSH 1994; Kramer 1974). The disillusionment experienced by newcomers to nursing stems from a conflict between the ideals and personal expectations of individualised care on the one hand and the realities of practice on the other. The response of nurses to this discrepancy is important. Faced with a less than ideal situation, they may either see themselves as professional failures (in which case they may leave nursing or avoid promotion) or accept the *status quo* as unalterable (in which case they may steadily draw the conclusion that the ideal is unachievable and therefore not worth pursuing). Either way, individualised nursing is not advanced, and this may well be a reason why people such as Peggy (remember Peggy?) can regularly attend a hospital for more than 20 years and still perceive that they have not received individualised care from nurses. Individualised nursing should not necessarily be taught as a theoretical imperative but discussed in what Brown (1992:39) describes as its 'empirical adequacy' – that is, how it is brought about in everyday practice.

Taking a broad view, individualised nursing can be regarded as being grounded in humanism, which is a philosophy that is not universally accepted. It is firmly anchored in Western moral philosophy, but many cultures preserve an emphasis on community rather than individual needs. In these cultures – which we often, and somewhat arrogantly, like to characterise as undeveloped – nursing as we know it hardly exists. Instead, care is provided not according to need but according to the community capacity, with a far greater emphasis on public health than treatment and cure of sick individuals. When we refer to individualised nursing we are usually firmly fixed in the illness paradigm. The change of focus to public health and preventive care tends to look to the health of groups rather than individuals *per se*.

Lest we fall into the error of assuming that the influence of humanism is universally seen to be beneficial, we should look carefully at the individualism advocated by some right-wing governments as an excuse to increase individual responsibility and reduce welfare (Bowers 1989). There are social commentators (Saul 1997; Turner 1991) who are concerned about the rising individualism in Western civilisation that has resulted in an inwardly focused culture of the self to the detriment of the collective good.

At a local level an example is the patient who has absolutely no regard for the other patients in the ward, while vigorously pursuing his or her own ends. A warning has been sounded by McMahon (1996) that nurses who have responsibility for only a small group of patients are at some stage likely to make these people their priority at the expense of other patients. There is the frequently told story of the patient making a desperate request of a passing nurse being told 'I'm not your nurse'. Although that is an over-used example, these are difficulties that the ward team needs to discuss in order to arrive at a collective solution – which may well be to temper any such examples of rigid insistence upon individualised nursing.

The last problem I will mention is with regard to the operationalisation of individualised nursing. There is some resistance among nurses to the introduction of systems that change their practice and increase either their workload or responsibilities. Nurses are adept at blaming rising workloads and reduced staffing levels for most ills in the health service. They are successful in doing this because, to a large extent, it is true. However, there is an attitude amongst a proportion of nurses that resists added responsibility because it requires additional education and/or a higher commitment to work. Individualised nursing and some of the associated systems bring the patient and his or her problems closer to the nurse. As we saw from Peggy, often these problems are not easily solved and are likely to increase stress levels in a profession that is already highly stressed. I hear all sorts of explanations for resisting continuity of care, writing assessments or evaluations, or continuing education. These nurses are important because they are able to resist change, not merely by virtue of their numbers and established positions in the system, but because almost all of us are weary of change and perceive nursing development as change for the sake of change. However, the bottom line is that nurses are responsible for and accountable to patients, who enjoy an array of rights that includes the right to high-quality care. Nursing as a profession has declared that high-quality care is individual care.

MEETING THE NEEDS OF INDIVIDUALS

Rather than teach specifics, the intention of this chapter is to introduce a range of issues associated with meeting the needs of individual patients. There is an array of textbooks on the subject that will give details of how to learn skills of assessment, care planning, systems of work organisation and critical reflection. The nurse who wishes to provide an individualised nursing service to her or his patients must become skilled at establishing relationships with a broad range of people. To do this requires refining skills of personal insight, observation, measurement and listening, learning to analyse and interpret this information and, in the light of their disciplinary knowledge, using it to help the person towards health goals. This nurse also has to be able to communicate these plans to the rest of the nursing team and stand accountable for decisions.

However, it is almost impossible for a nurse with these skills to work alone to provide an individual service to patients. It must be confusing and frustrating for patients to receive care on one shift from someone who knows them, and then to meet a nurse on the next shift who not only doesn't know them, but who wants to stick to a routine of his or her own. The team needs to value individualism and work together to ensure that the patients in their area are known personally and treated in the light of this knowledge. Newcomers to an area should not, however, be too hasty in assuming – merely because the hallmarks of individualised nursing (primary nursing, etc.) are not apparent – that there is no consideration for the individual patient. Rather, they should look for alternative indicators.

One way to influence practitioners to change is to look carefully and positively at what is being done. We have already established that individualised care is a central tenet of nursing and, if this is true, forget for a while about the theory because it should be evident in nursing practice. In a very small study Brown (1992) tape-recorded the conversations between an experienced midwife and three expectant mothers. Having searched the data for examples of nursing actions that fitted the unique characteristics of the client, Brown analysed the individualised nurse/client interactions as: specific affective support, health information, decisional control, and professional/technical competencies (Brown 1992:40).

In a similar vein, nurses may look for examples of nursing that are tailored to the individual needs of patients in their practice. How is it, even though work is very busy, that some individuals' needs are catered for? The positive things need to be examined, and ways to encourage this type of care considered, reinforced and developed further. Perhaps a ward has a particularly well thought-out discharge plan that is specifically tailored to the individual and their home situation; or maybe the nursing team take particular care to deal sensitively with relatives, knowing something about their relationship with the patient and when and how to give them information. It may be that there are not many examples of individualised nursing and the team needs to consider introducing some changes. An example might be a commitment to improving written assessments, with a proviso that others in the team will read them if it is the first time they have looked after a particular patient. Another idea may be to reconsider the patient allocation system to try to reduce the number of different nurses each patient has to deal with during any treatment phase. This type of exercise brings alive the values and beliefs of the team. If they espouse a belief in individualised care they should be able to give examples from their practice that represent reality.

If a team decides that individualised care is not a priority in their area (and this could be quite legitimate) they should be able to justify this decision and articulate their priorities. It could be that the nurses on a day surgery unit believe that their main aim is to ensure the physical safety of each patient and that the number of patients treated each day is high enough to keep the waiting time for surgery down to the minimum. Their focus would be upon the identification of potential complications, information-giving and efficiency.

(British Council 2000). Information is available on the campaign website www.givi ngupsmoking.co.uk.

In primary care nursing, aggregates may be determined by the nature of the nurses' work, for example nurses who work with the learning disabled, the mentally ill or children.

The second dimension of community is the extent to which features are shared in terms of a *geographic or physical location*. This is a structural dimension, where the community may be defined by geographical or political boundaries that demarcate it as a district, region, city or neighbourhood. In the UK, determining allocation of resources to need is made through a Primary Care Trust (PCT), a defined area with a population of approximately 150 000 residents. There may be more than one PCT in any given geographical region, and within each PCT the area is broken down further into neighbourhoods. Some neighbourhoods may be rural in location, e.g Okehampton, a town in the west of the county of Devon. Or it may be a seaside loca-tion, e.g. Ilfracombe in north Devon, which has its own particular characteristics; e.g. it is an area with high teenage pregnancy rates. In addition, it has poor employment prospects, as this small seaside town is dependent on tourism for its trade and pros-perity. Tourism incurs a significant increase in demand for health service provision in summer months (http://www.northdevon.gov.uk).

Within each city neighbourhood the area is broken down further into wards in which local epidemiological and social statistics are kept. Each PCT has a duty to produce a Public Health Annual Report, highlighting pockets of deprivation and areas of 'special need' within that locality. Statistics are used to produce a Health Improvement Plan for each Health Authority. This plan compares local need with national data and identifies areas to target when planning the implementation of health service provision for the coming year.

Finally, a community may be defined by the way its residents relate to each other within a social network or social system. Members of a community may have a shared set of beliefs, values, norms, communication and helping patterns (Green & Kreuter 1991). In this type of community, individuals do not function as isolated be-ings; each person is part of a network. The network may be a family or some other group to which the individual belongs, such as a group of older people who share hostel accommodation. These networks create systems. A social system can repre-sent interrelationships of support, role fulfilment, socialisation and achievement of common goals.

An example of this may be seen as the 'travelling families' who clearly have a need for health service provision but travel widely across the country and access to health care via the primary health care teams is on an *ad hoc* basis. A further example of this would be the homeless population of Exeter, a large city in the south-west of England, a group for whom specific identified health needs have been determined and as a result now have their own health services in the form of a community nurse-led clinic.

Although the above definition of community is useful, you could explore other literature for definitions. Make a list of these definitions and decide upon a definition that could reflect your own position.

THE RHETORIC OF PRIMARY HEALTH CARE AND PUBLIC HEALTH

What drives the community health care agenda? Further to the primary health care reform initiatives in the early 1970s, the International Declaration of Primary Health Care was signed in Alma Ata in the USSR in 1978. The Declaration broadly affirms health as a state of complete physical, mental and social well-being. Although the theoretical underpinning of this health reform movement is not stated, the Alma Ata Declaration challenged health workers to address inequalities in the health status of people within the context of socio-economic order, and it established the rights of people to participate individually and collectively in the planning and implementation of their health care. Most importantly, the Alma Ata conference invited nurses, in particular, to go forward in meeting the goal of 'Health for All by the Year 2000'. In November 1986 a Canadian-sponsored international conference of the World Health Organization (WHO) took place in Ottawa. The Ottawa Charter for Health Promotion (cited in Wass 2000) provides five key health promotion action statements:

(1) build healthy public policy;
(2) create supportive environments;
(3) strengthen community action;
(4) develop personal skills;
(5) reorient health services.

Without going into too much detail, *building healthy public policy* refers to advocating a clear political commitment to health and equity in all sectors, and the *creation of supportive environments* refers to health promotion that generates living and working conditions that are safe, stimulating, satisfying and enjoyable. At the heart of the process of *strengthening community action* is the empowerment of communities through developing ownership and control over their endeavours and destinies. Health promotion supports personal and social development through the provision of information and education for health, enhancing health skills and these activities are coined as *developing personal skills*. This works to increase the options available to people for them to exercise more control over their health. *Reorienting of health services* views the role of the health sector as moving increasingly in a health promotion direction, beyond its responsibility for providing clinical and curative services. The reorienting includes expanding the health service mandate to one that is sensitive and respects diverse cultural needs.

THE NEW PUBLIC HEALTH

Since the 1970s the meaning of health promotion has shifted from an emphasis on instructing individuals to take up healthy behaviours to a recognition that people's actions are very much a part of their social environment (Baum *et al.* 1992). The Ottawa Charter illustrates this shift and goes beyond earlier individual and behavioural definitions. The social health agenda advanced by the Charter assumed that inequalities in health care could be examined and changed through the manipulation of socio-ecological or structural health determinants (gender, age, class or ethnicity). This movement constitutes the *new public health* approach to health promotion and seeks to advance the interests of groups disadvantaged by gender, age, class or ethnicity. It requires a shift in thinking about health promotion from being related to lifestyle behaviours, prevention of disease and disability to include wider social and political reform. The challenge to promote health between sectors (e.g. human services, transport and health) requires collaboration with governments, health and other economic sectors. This agenda has been particularly appealing to nurses – in fact, nurses have been expected to lead health reforms.

At a WHO International Health Promotion Conference in Jakarta in July 1997 (the third since Ottawa), Kickbush (1997a), who was the key architect of the Ottawa Charter for Health Promotion, stated:

> We know that poverty kills, that dirty water kills, that tobacco kills. We know that children thrive on love, that communities are strengthened by social cohesion and that educated and empowered women are a determining factor for the health of a society … health is definitely on the political agenda, more so than when the Ottawa Charter was adopted. Yet as the global equity gap widens, the access to a healthy life seems further removed for the citizens of some parts of the world than 10 years ago.

So it seems that the rhetoric of the new public health has not reached its target, which was Health for All by the Year 2000.

In the new public health arena, Kickbush (1997b) describes the WHO Health for All strategy as an 'open system' approach to generating health. Health was seen as a major social goal for governments; the outcome of health policy was understood to be the achievement of a socially and economically productive life for citizens. What still holds of the underlying values and the economic and epidemiological premise on which the WHO strategy was grounded? Kickbush (1997b) maintains that the 'closed system' of health is focused on service and delivery, and unable to respond adequately to the wider population needs. She claims that the contribution of health to social and economic life and, vice versa, the impact of social organisation on health, have not been adequately recognised.

In summary, primary health care can be two things: a level of service provision and an approach to health care. Although this chapter deals specifically with community nursing it is understood that, ideally, primary health care is organised within an integrated team and supported by a community network that includes as partners not only the health care workers and service providers but also the community itself. In addition, an approach to health care based on primary health care principles is valid for both acute and community care settings. The primary health care approach is to move beyond the individual and the medical and/or nursing diagnosis, clinical and curative approach, to view the larger social picture of people in the context of socio-economic, cultural and political environment, to consider the way in which the context affects health, to act upon this information, and to publish the process. It is suggested that it will become increasingly important for nursing to be more politically strategic, and develop its own professionally driven primary health care research agenda.

So what is the relationship between community nurses and the public? What are the debates around individual and population-driven primary health care?

RESPONSIVENESS OF THE PROFESSION TO THE COMMUNITY

If the primary concern of community health nurses is to improve the health of the community, can we identify the responsiveness of community nursing? Unfortunately, a professionally driven health service based on community need may be sought but not attained. Rather, responsiveness is often led by government policies and we provide the following examples from the UK.

In the United Kingdom a change in government has seen a shift in health policy. Prevalent in the 1980s and 1990s was a victim-blaming approach and this has shifted to one in which a health rather than illness focus is sought. Public health is seen as a key factor in making the UK a healthier nation (DoH 1998a, 1999a, 1999b, 2000), the goal being to reduce inequalities in health, and improve the health of the population. In 1998, the UK Labour government introduced radical changes to the NHS. *The New NHS: Modern and Dependable* (DoH 1998a) highlighted the need to produce a high quality, cost-effective and modern response to the current demands in health. This paper introduced the concept of working collaboratively with other agencies, targeting health care resources to where they are needed most and to tackle the root causes of ill health. Public health was once again leading the way in the government's health agenda.

Saving Lives: Our Healthier Nation (DoH 1999a) strategy provided a clear framework for targeting health care resources to the deprived people in society and to improve the quality of life for those who were ill. Alongside this shift from illness to health the government proposed changes in the delivery of public services, closer integrated working and 'joined-up' public services. Although the exact focus and targets for achieving these improvements differ between the four UK countries, the principles are broadly similar.

The New NHS: Modern and Dependable (DoH 1998a) abolished fund-holding and introduced the concept of Primary Care Trusts (PCTs) who have commissioning responsibility for primary as well as community and all hospital-based services. Their role is to identify those at greatest risk from serious illness. Thus health promotion and intervention will be targeted at those most in need. This fits into both the National and Local Agenda, through the process of producing local Health Improvement Plans (HIMPs) for each locality. By working in close collaboration with local authorities, primary care trusts are able to enter into agreements or to directly fund initiatives to improve the health of the population and in particular the worst off in society. The DoH introduced the notion of Health Action Zones, where deprived areas may bid for extra funding to improve the health of individuals residing in these Zones.

The clinical executive board for each primary care trust is made up of practising clinicians, with significant representation from GPs, nurses (community and health visitors), public health professionals and social services. The philosophy is that those practising clinicians in a locality are best placed to identify the health needs in a given area and decisions are made as close to the patient as possible. This has significant implications for the education of community specialist nurses who may take a role on the executive board.

Whilst primary health care service delivery is important, what has been missing until these recent reforms of the late 1990s was the incentive for reform and the approach to health as envisaged by the Ottawa Charter. Instead, prominence was given to the communities' sick care role (Baum *et al.* 1992). This view of primary health care is driven by the government and recent health care reforms reflect the UK government's desire to reflect the views of 'users' (DoH 2000). In determining service provision, the increasing costs of acute care, advances in technology, and the early discharge of patients to be nursed in their own homes are instrumental in determining the vision of future health care provision. In summary, current policy has seen a shift to concentrate more on consumers than providers; a focus upon outcomes rather than inputs; emphasis on co-ordinated care, and the particular potential of primary carers as the care managers and/or gatekeepers.

> What are the national health priorities? See if you can locate these priorities for your PCT and compare them with the national priorities. You could check with government publishers, e.g. the Health Improvement Plans for each PCT, or the Health Authority Annual Public Health Report. Ask how these priorities were decided upon.

Labonte (1997) gives a comprehensive view in *Reforming health care for health: What we know, how we know it, what we can do.* He asks: 'What is the implication for the primary health care system reform allowing consideration for socio-environmental determinants such as equity, employment, sustainable resources, respectful social relations, empowerment?' In answering these questions, he suggests that one approach would be a 'deeply' public debate with the power to raise philosophical, methodological and political challenges. So, as new practitioners, the future lies upon your understanding of the health care system and your ability to influence citizens to contribute more significantly to policy formation and debate in health care. This debate should be in partnership with the community. As Labonte (1997) argues, the 'outcome' in any primary health care system is the relationship between practitioners and the public. We need to move forward from the inadequacies of our past and certainly learn some important lessons that have relevance for the community health nurse's role. It could be argued that recent political reform is addressing this for the first time.

> Can community nurses facilitate a return to the social health agenda of new public health? There needs to be an ongoing discussion and debate about the direction primary health care and new public health should take. Can you envisage your role in this debate?

DIVERSITY AND BREADTH: THE ROLE OF NURSES IN THE COMMUNITY

Since the 1980s there has been ambiguity around the role nurses should take in district nursing, community nursing, primary health care and the larger new public health arena (Goltz & Bruni 1995; Keegan & Kent 1992; Keleher & McInerney 1998; McMurray 1993; Wass 1994). Whilst there is diversity of role experience depending upon the community in which the nurse finds him- or herself, there are also some similarities. The role descriptions below reflect what *could* be, rather than what *may* be the case. Only some role descriptions have been selected; excluded from this discussion are nurses working with indigenous communities or with immigrants, also nurses working in community health centres, e.g. practice nurses.

Community nurses are people who understand the three dimensions of the community in which they work. That is, nurses who are able to describe this community and are able to assess and articulate its needs. It is expected that such understanding works at two levels, individual and population (Baldwin *et al.* 1998). However, it is usual for the community nurse to have a specific area of expertise and he or she may focus on a service delivery level. For example, whilst aware of the needs and resources in the larger community, a district nurse works at an individual level, making a particular assessment and giving direct nursing care to clients in their home.

Assessment is the cornerstone of nursing practice, whether it be an individual or a community assessment. Further reading about researching community health, evaluation and needs assessment that makes an impact is found in the work of Baum *et al.* (1992). Nevertheless, the roles of nurses are determined by the needs of the community in which they work. Many nurses working in the community have an identifiable role that spans from the individual to a population perspective.

As discussed in the introduction to this chapter in the definition of 'community', the first dimension views the community as an aggregate of people. Accordingly, this defining characteristic is often used to describe the role of nurses working with aggregates in the community.

Health visitors work with families, groups and communities, their role is multifaceted. The focus of their work is enabling individuals, families and groups to build up their resources for health and well-being and through this, and early interventions, improve health overall. Health-needs assessment is a core tool for health-visiting practice as they seek to provide a service that is needs-led or more appropriately inequalities-led (Summers & McKeown 1996). However, in describing health-visiting practice there is a danger of trying to capture everything that might possibly be included in a health visiting remit rather than focusing on their central purpose of assessing health need and addressing this.

As an example, let us take the role of the health visitor working with aggregates of children and adolescents, and develop the role from working with individuals through to assessing population needs. The health visitor would apply knowledge of child and adolescent health needs in planning appropriate, comprehensive care at the individual level. Often the role of the nurse working with children and adolescents extends to addressing the needs of families (family as client). In addition, the role would also involve being able to identify the major indicators of child and adolescent health status and the way in which socioeconomic circumstances influence this group's health, articulating the individual and societal costs of poor health status, and being involved in public programmes targeted to children's health (e.g. immunisation).

Another example of the health visitor's role may be working with an aggregate that consists solely of gender-specific groups. We would expect that the role of the nurse working in women's health would encompass knowledge about the incidence and prevalence of gender-specific health problems. In addition, this nurse would be able to: determine the major indicators of women's health; identify the barriers to adequate health care of women; relate the impact of poverty on the health of women; articulate public policy on the health of women; discuss reproductive health in rela-tionship to the workplace, and examine significant health problems among women of all ages. Similarly, if a health visitor were to work with an aggregate of men, the role would entail being able to identify the major indicators of men's health status, discuss factors that impede men's health, and apply knowledge of men's health needs in planning gender-appropriate nursing care for men at individual, family and com-munity levels.

The aggregate for district nursing tends to be the older age group. In England, about 65% of clients seen by district nurses are aged 65 years or over. There were approximately 2.5 million first contacts in 2000/1, and of these 51% of the population were those aged 85 or over. The average duration of a district nurse episode is about two months and the majority of referrals are from the GP at 56%, with 20% from hospital staff and the remaining 24% from other sources including self-referral (DoH 2001). Wound management accounts for up to 75% of the nursing workload. In the selection of the older person as aggregate, the role of the nurse working with older persons is as varied as older people themselves. A rapidly rising ageing population raises issues significant for community health, and it is worthwhile identifying the debates around these. The focus of these debates has been the growth in the number of older people, the 'burden' of their pensions and the increased consumption of health care resources.

See if you can identify these debates in current literature.

The nurse in this role would be expected to identify the major indicators of older peo-ple's health, be able to describe the problems associated with ageing and, in an effort to counteract ageism and stereotyping of older people, consider growth and develop-ment in later life. It can be argued that the stereotyping of older persons profoundly affects the way they are perceived and consequently treated, at the societal level, as individuals in everyday interactions and, particularly, in institutions (Bernard 1998; Estes & Binney 1989; Koch & Webb 1996). Ageism manifests itself in discrimination against the old in the quality of services provided for them, exemplified by shoddy services that are inadequate and of low prestige. Ageism, it is suggested, plays a large role in care deprivation, as the process of stereotyping older people influences their health care. In addition, ageism can be viewed in the same way as sexism and racism. It can be compared with other forms of oppression in terms of stereotyping, discrimination and minority group status. However, it is deeply rooted in our social behaviour. A nurse working with older people attempts to counter these stereotypes. Here are some strategies that can be used.

If someone says that 'a woman's place is in the home', there is little hesitation in concluding that this is a sexist remark. When someone says that white people are more intelligent than black people, this will be recognised as a racist remark.

However, when someone talks about the older person as being senile or rigid in behaviour, far fewer people regard this is an ageist comment. Misconceptions about the ageing thrive and are rarely challenged, which is less likely for the corresponding notions of oppression such as sexism and racism.

 Are you prepared to take on this agenda?

Carers also occupy an important group on the community health care agenda. Research undertaken by Koch and Hofmeyer (1998) has provided evidence that emotional bankruptcy and deprivation are experienced by people who are the recipients of aged care policies. An area emphasised by the research is the existence of a sexual division of labour that leaves women with the primary responsibility for informal care. Stresses associated with caring for older partners or parents include coping with mental confusion, physical exhaustion, and lack of practical help and emotional support. What is needed now is to explore community care policies that have served to mask this enormous area of personal and financial stress borne privately, and to question why 'burdens' borne by carers are ignored by policy makers. There is a need for a reappraisal of concepts, ideas, influences and approaches that have led to recent aged and carer policies. And it is important to seek ways in which the recipients of such policies can influence the aged care agenda.

As a nurse, you may consider entering these wider debates and becoming involved in policy development.

Nurses working with the aggregates termed 'homeless' would have a role description that covers a large social health agenda. There are many meanings of the term 'homeless', not merely as 'roofless' but describing people who drift between boarding houses, shelters, squats – people who are 'roughing it'. A person's housing situation can render them homeless, regardless of whether there is 'shelter'. Being homeless could mean living where a shelter fails to meet the minimal housing conditions. It could mean that there is not a safe and secure shelter of a standard that does not damage health, threaten personal safety, or fails to provide cooking facilities or facilities that permit adequate personal hygiene. On an individual level, nurses may provide direct health care to persons with alcohol dependence, mental health problems, emotional and psychosocial health problems, acute physical disorders (respiratory disease, trauma, skin ailments, nutritional deficiencies), chronic physical disorders, infectious and communicable diseases and infestational disorders (lice and scabies). The role would also involve analysing the health problems from a social justice perspective, and lobbying effectively for housing and services for this community (Cameron & MacWilliams 1995). The typical age group of homeless people using the Personal Medical Services (PMS) pilot for the homeless in Exeter is between 20 and 40 years of age. Men form the largest group, yet homeless youth and women tend to be seen by the outreach services. The task here is to identify where homeless people are and work with them toward better health and suitable accommodation.

In the UK the shift to a primary care agenda has led to many innovative developments, including a proliferation of nurse-led clinics, telephone consultation and advice lines and nurse-led triage. Registered district nurses and health visitors are able to prescribe medications from an approved nurse prescribing formulary and work is under way to extend prescribing rights and responsibilities with the first courses to commence January 2002.

In the UK a national shortage of medical practitioners has led in part to the development of the *nurse practitioner* (DoH 2001). Following additional preparation, the accredited nurse is able to authorise diagnostic tests such as X-rays and, in some cases, manage conditions such as asthma or diabetes without reference to or approval from a doctor. The independent nurse practitioner as yet is not a recognised qualification by the regulatory bodies, however the numbers are increasing significantly.

 It would be worth considering the debates around the nurse practitioner role. You could follow these debates by exploring current literature and media coverage.

We have not yet discussed the role of nurses working in the field of community mental health. When individuals experience mental illness one could argue that the family or group with whom the client lives would also be affected, and in some cases the family may enhance or intensify the individual's experiences. If a person with an alcohol problem still resides with his or her family, it is likely that all members of the family will be affected by that person's problem.

On an individual level, one of the main roles of the nurse practitioner working in community mental health is to provide a service that reduces suffering and increases personal functioning. As an educator, the community mental health nurse instructs individuals, families or groups through community organisations about various aspects of preventive mental health, treatment of mental illness, and community management of individuals who are mentally ill (Cotroneo *et al.* 1997). On an aggregate level, the community health nurse would identify groups to target for educational activities. The assessment of a community's mental health needs is central to the role of community nurses working with these aggregates.

In summary, there is diversity and breadth in the role of nurses working in the community. In considering the position descriptions, it is quite clear that the tasks of nurses working in the community can include lobbying for housing for the homeless, working against stereotyping of older people, or as an advocate for women's or men's health. It also means recognising social health issues and being prepared to debate the issues.

MAKING NURSING PRACTICE VISIBLE

In the 1970s and 1980s nurses in the community were funded as key workers in primary health care and were geared toward embracing the new public health (Keegan & Kent 1992). Whilst nurses' work focused upon service delivery and health promotion programmes, they have not left a published record of their activities. British textbooks for health care professionals contain the rhetoric of primary health care and a shift toward the new public health (O'Connor & Parker 1995). Initially the literature was sparse; however, there is an increasing literature on community health nursing in British journals. One of the reasons could be that little research was done prior to and during the expansion of primary health care nursing. If one reviews the position descriptions of nurses in the 1970s and 1980s, it becomes obvious that nurses were not expected to base their practice upon research, nor to engage in research; this is not the case today.

Perform a CD ROM search using the terms: *research, nursing* and *community.* Can you identify the key areas of concern/topics from reading the abstracts? Is nursing practice visible?

The work of district nurses

The focus of district nursing home visits is on the individual for whom the referral is received. In addition, the nurse assesses the interaction of the individual with the family and provides education and intervention for the family as well as the client. Caring for the care-giver is central to a district nurse's practice. The primary purpose of the home health visit is to allow individuals to remain at home and receive health care services that would otherwise be offered in a health care institution. Advanced clinical practice characterises the role of the district nurse, and it has specialty positions in the areas of palliative care, intellectually disability, acquired immunodeficiency syndrome, elderly people, wound management, continence promotion and diabetes management.

The nature and characteristics of district nursing practice have not been well articulated in the professional and public domain. The definitions of expert competencies, e.g. continence promotion and wound management, are only now being developed. A clear picture of the practice of expert nurses is necessary so that those in the profession can understand and explain this expert practice and consequently direct it to the community (Bunkers *et al.* 1997). The United Kingdom has a prolific literature surrounding district nursing practice and although its district nursing services are organised along similar lines to Australia, it is surprising that not only is there no current published literature on district nursing in Australia, but that this group has escaped scholarly scrutiny, its voice has been weak in nursing matters, and it has not produced a record of its own endeavours, practice and/or research.

Nurses must take an active role in defining and establishing their practices. Maintaining a daily journal offers a strategy that can help students understand nursing and help clinicians address some troublesome practice-based issues. The phenomena of interest to students and clinicians are those identified by nurses and patients during their everyday encounters. Clinical narratives illustrate how dialogue could be, and already is, engaged by practitioners (Richardson & Maltby 1995). It makes nursing practice visible. It demonstrates that nurses are part of the setting, context and culture we seek to understand. It is also a way of understanding the political nature of work. Journal keeping can become a central activity as a student and in clinical and research practice. However, this process requires analytical skills to move it beyond mere documentation. Writing, analysing, reflecting and rewriting is a skill that does not come easily to some practitioners. Reflective skills consist 'both of the ability to think well and the ability to recognise and evaluate good thinking' (Wellard & Bethune 1996:1077). There is some literature on reflection to guide the novice (Cox *et al.* 1991; Emden 1991). The point being advanced here is that keeping a journal is an essential part of reflective practice, but the novice will need guidance.

The work of health visitors

In the UK, health visiting is unique as a profession as it is only open to registered practitioners from two other professions, i.e. registered nurses and registered midwives. It cannot be accessed directly as a profession in its own right although it is a profession under regulation. It is currently included as one of the eight community branches under the specialist practice nursing framework. Nurses in the community have tended to develop specialist roles rather than have a collective identity (Hyde 1995). This is an issue which, it could be argued, is encouraged within the current educational framework, whereby core modules are taught to primary care staff, however they are seen as eight distinct community specialisms. Specialist practice was introduced by the UKCC in 1994, and is defined as 'the exercising of higher levels of judgement, discretion and decision making' (UKCC 2001a). The incorporation of health visiting into the specialist community nursing practice framework is not without dispute. There is evidence to suggest shared learning has inhibited the flexibility of health visiting courses and has led to a focus on nursing not health visiting (Clark *et al.* 2000; Cowley *et al.* 2000; Kelsey & Hollindale 1996; Mackereth 1997; Oldman 1999). Clark *et al.* (2000) would argue this is because the differing types of community nursing may be seen to have differing philosophies and approaches.

Health visiting registration is also known as public health nursing, which clearly indicates the health visitor's role in addressing the public health agenda. As the demand for health care continued to increase, the response to this in the years of the Thatcher government during the 1980s was to 'blame' the individual. Health policy emphasised the role of the individual to take responsibility for their own health and funding for health promotion initiatives in the UK was marginalised. In spite of this, the Black Report, which was a paper commissioned by the Conservative government in 1980 (Townsend & Davidson 1992), highlighted the fact that social class, housing and poverty seriously impeded an individual's life chances.

In addition, the development of new posts of *specialist in public health* has a significant impact on the future of nurse, midwife and health visitor training and education, as the public health role grows to incorporate a wider group of professionals other than in medicine (DoH 1998b). Health visitors and community nurses working close to where people live in local communities act as advocates for vulnerable groups and people who are socially excluded, making sure that they have access to mainstream services, and are thus important in the promotion of health in the context of the broader policy agenda (DoH 1999b).

The four UK countries have clearly identified their own public health policies. The Scottish Executive (2001) proposes the development of local health care co-operatives to create the potential for public health activity through bringing together primary care, public health and other key agencies to better address the health and well-being needs of communities. In its review it recommends routine visiting, much of the current surveillance programme and some of the more routine approaches to health visiting practice should be replaced by a much greater public health focus. It will require nurses to work more openly in partnership with clients, to agree and work towards goals with families, to seek out health needs and find new and creative ways of dealing with them. Arguably this practice currently takes place, although the major focus of health visiting continues to be families with young children (Appleby & Sayer 2001). In 1999–2000, approximately 3 432 000 clients were seen by the health visiting services in England.

A survey of health visiting (CPHVA 1997) indicates health visitors encounter a vast number of issues, with dietary and housing the most common reason for consultation. Children's behaviour, mental health issues, marital breakdown and financial problems are examples of health and social conditions discussed. Other more serious social issues included child abuse, drugs and alcohol; long-term health issues include sleep problems, speech delay and family planning. Finally, one in eight health visitors surveyed helped at least one family gain access to medical services in the preceding month. This survey highlights the difficulties in monitoring health-visiting activity. A survey by its very nature suggests the majority of interventions are individualistic and related to routine surveillance, thus broader-based projects appear in isolation and are not given the recognition they deserve.

INNOVATIVE PRACTICE

Despite governments leading health care through policy direction, there are examples of innovative practice led by health visitors that are instrumental in promoting the health of disadvantaged groups in society. Farrington (1995) researched an intensive health-visiting programme targeted at families. The claim was that the incidence of juvenile crime would reduce if health visitors, who recognise the known predictors for childhood behaviour problems, delinquency and criminality, could work with these young people. In a similar vein Seeley et al. (1996) found that an increased health visitor intervention to those presenting with postnatal depression can result in a reduction in behavioural problems in children. Evaluating health-visiting intervention nonetheless is fraught with difficulties owing to the multifaceted nature of the work.

Measuring narrowly defined starting points in an intervention, e.g. routine screening, may be expressed quantitatively, even though the intervention may result in the identification of much broader social needs, which the health visitor may be able to explain qualitatively and thus inform strategies to address such needs. Measuring this intervention is much more difficult. Facilitating participation of the community in maintaining its own health was the remit for health visitors in Essex who, by utilising community mothers to use their own life experiences and understanding to provide support to parents in their locality, were successful in overcoming professional, social and cultural barriers (Suppiah 1996). The Beacon project, a health visitor led initiative in Cornwall, involved community participation in a particularly deprived area to successfully tackle its own identified health problems (Stuteley & Trenoweth 1999). Roberts and Bedford (1996) suggest that home visits have a potentially important role to play in the reduction of accidents in the home. Current innovations in health visiting practice may be elicited from the following website www.innovate.org.uk.

Health visitors have traditionally sought to influence health through education and support rather than by the use of practical skills (Robinson 1985). This is currently being challenged with the development of walk-in centres staffed by primary care nurses including health visitors. Innovations include minor injury units and minor injury clinics in GP practices, telephone consultations (DoH 2000) and nurse prescribing. Here health visitors are being asked to run nurse-led clinics or utilise a medical model and curative framework as their premise. Health visitor involvement in the Sure Start programmes in England, Wales and Northern Ireland and the Children's Services Plans and Family Centres in Scotland is aimed at ensuring that children growing up in families with few resources are offered support from an early age to give them the best start in life through promoting their development (Appleton & Clemerson 1999; Home Office 1998; Scottish Executive 1999).

RESHAPING ROLES

It could be argued there are two distinct roles developing. For example, in Scotland there is a proposal for a public health nurse and a family health nurse. Here it is suggested that some of the current health visitors and school nurses would fit into the former category and the remaining health visitors and other community nurses into the latter. It is envisaged that public health nurse interventions will be reoriented to be less individualistic, longer term and focused on high risk groups. The family health nurse will be a skilled generalist nurse with a broad range of duties, the first point of contact referring on to other specialists as appropriate. This role is very similar to the current community nurse role with its emphasis on health promotion and the prevention of ill health. Analysis of the policy documents from the four UK countries demonstrates a considerable similarity in approach albeit at different stages of evolution in each country and indicates a potentially exciting if challenging future for health visiting practice. Whatever format health visiting–public health nursing takes, it is clear there is a pivotal role for the skills of the health visitor in today's political climate and a challenge to education providers to facilitate the skills required.

> It is important to continue this dialogue, and you are in the best possible position to further this debate and seek some clarification of terms.

PREPARATION FOR COMMUNITY HEALTH PRACTICE

The principles of primary health care and an understanding of the nurse's role in creating healthy communities is essential preparation for the community health nurse. In the UK, primary care is moving at such a rapid rate it is vital that education provision keeps up with current government initiatives. The trend for community-based health care is broadening employment opportunities for nurses in community settings. As a result of decreased lengths of stay and cost-containment initiatives, fewer nurses are needed in acute care settings, indeed in some instances acute care has moved into the home. Hospital nursing is quite different from community nursing.

McMurray (1993), in an Australian study of expertise in community nursing, identified a combination of factors that influence its development. To educate for expert levels of practice, enhancement of the perceptual and analytical abilities of the learner is crucial. McMurray suggests that this can best be achieved through clinical practice opportunities, through demonstrations and case studies.

> Reading about community health nursing practice will give you some theoretical understanding and will outline some of the issues. Advancing your knowledge means that you will have located yourself in actual practice and become a reflective practitioner.

Preregistration training has recently been piloted across the UK, in which the curriculum content includes equal experience in both hospital and community settings, in addition to a 50% theory/practice split in an attempt to ensure on completion nurses are competent in both practice areas (UKCC 1999).

In the UK to undertake practice in the community as a district nurse or health visitor, it is necessary to undertake additional training in the form of a Community Health Care honours degree. This course is open to community nurses including mental health, practice nursing, child health, occupational health, school nursing and learning disability, however it is not necessary to undertake the course in these areas to work in practice. In light of current government initiatives the UKCC consultation document 'Requirements for programmes leading to registration as a health visitor' (2001b) is timely. The CPHVA response to this (Forester 2002) includes amongst other issues suggestions that the course be extended from 32 weeks to a minimum of 48, mentors in practice should be prepared to the level of a practice educator, and more resources should support education in practice. However, the introduction of benchmarking statements (QAA 2001) describing the nature and standards of programmes of study and training in healthcare, will make explicit the academic requirements. Whatever, it seems likely that provision for the education to support community practitioners will be an area of growth and change for the foreseeable future.

In the preparation of nurses who can function in local communities, clinical, professional, and interpersonal skills are important for a successful transition to community-based practice. Because community nurses cover such a large number of specialties, aggregates and terrain, specific educational role requirements are more easily acquired in the practice setting. Nursing is perceived differently from practice setting to practice setting (McIntosh 1996). For instance, people working with the community in the new public health arena require activist training (Baum *et al.* 1992). Activist training refers to learning to act upon issues with the community to promote reform and change. The ability to assess needs, either from an individual or a community perspective is one of the most important skills to foster after registration. Learning how to assess, inquire, look for evidence upon which to base practice, and striving toward a broad education are important aspects of becoming a good community nurse (Kenrick & Luker 1996). What is required is a systematic framework for role analysis, development, enactment, and evaluation. Indeed, learning to evaluate one's practice is an essential role requirement.

> Have you thought about ways in which roles can be evaluated? Why is it important to evaluate one's role?

NURSING IN THE COMMUNITY: SOME PRACTICE ISSUES

As more and more health care provision is delivered in primary care, it could be argued that confusion about the various roles, titles and differing professional certifications hinders the opportunity for an elevated status for community nursing. Services have proliferated into specialist and generalist teams, often with no clear relation to local communities (Baum *et al.* 1992). The public is often bewildered about what is available, and from where (Koch *et al.* 1998; Koch & Hofmeyer 1998). Often nurses work as *de facto* case managers of clients, families and communities, and administrative links are tenuous. Although community nursing is an integral part of the health care system, nurses and non-nurses alike express confusion about what community nursing is about (Flaherty 1995). There is also some confusion about the implications of community nursing practice for the health care delivery system as a whole (Redekopp 1997).

In the UK with the advent of personal medical services, nurse-led initiatives and telephone consultations there does appear to be a comprehensive network of nurses working in the community.

The combination of need-led service provision and consumerism in the NHS has resulted in a shift from general medical services where GPs were paid for items of service, to personal medical services whereby GPs are paid on practice outcomes. This has resulted in a sharing of skills across practices and a blurring of boundaries in terms of role, with many joint nurse/GP clinics that lead to an increased choice of service provision for the consumer. This, it could be argued, will lead to further confusion of the nurse's role in the community, particularly as the long-term vision is combined health and social care practice and education.

Data collection of community workforce practice has long been criticised for being quantitative in terms of task allocation and not truly reflecting the role of community practitioners. In a cost reduction environment where productivity (a larger number of clients visited) is valued more than the quality of care delivered, market pressures have precipitated a revisiting of the task basis of nursing. As the literature from the UK shows, many district nurses are finding themselves in unsatisfactory, often task-oriented roles (Shay *et al.* 1996). Here it is argued that nurses must be alert to health care legislation aimed at containing or reducing cost and be aware of models of delivery focused on production to contain costs (Abel 1994). There are ethical concerns regarding access to care, cost containment, and quality of health care services (Rapport & Maggs 1997). Unless nurses face these challenges, and become alert to economic and political agendas, they will lose aspects of patient and community care that they are well placed and qualified to deliver.

WHAT ARE THE ISSUES IN COMMUNITY-BASED NURSING PRACTICE?

Levels of service provision

Primary health care can be a level of service provision. Each community health nurse is responsible for making services equally available and accessible to all.

Besides access and equity issues, there is a mandate to provide a service efficiently and there is often a requirement to co-ordinate existing services. In addition to this, the community health nurse works toward decreasing client admissions to hospitals and provides continuity of care for clients discharged from hospital. Co-ordinated care, single assessment (one-stop-shop) are key concerns for nurses working in the community. With the trend to shorter hospital stays and more care in the community, continuity of patient care between hospital and community is becoming increasingly important (Armitage & Kavanagh 1996). Competition for home nursing is a reality, evidenced by the upsurge of programmes such as hospital-at-home (Clayton 1995). When nurses work only at the service provision level, there is a risk that the social health agenda of the larger population will be neglected.

CONCLUSION

Identification of the debates around community health nursing practice has been the emphasis of this chapter. Seeking your interest and involvement to work through some of the issues and debates raised are the chapter objectives. Reconsider the following:

What can nurses do? It is believed that along with political astuteness and knowledge of health care economics, research has the potential to drive practice, particularly research that will provide evidence for practice. Three domains have been identified for research within nursing: research that provides evidence for nursing practice (this is particularly pertinent to district nursing); research propelled by primary health care principles and social issues in the wider public health arena; and evaluation research, particularly in the area of alternative models of health care delivery such as nurse-led clinics (Starck *et al.* 1995).

How can nurses be responsive to the community? As McMurray (1993:204) argues, the 'first responsibility is to become well informed' and a well-prepared, well-researched, reflective practitioner. Through critically employing reflection, we must identify and explain the characteristics and essential elements of our practice, and spread this knowledge.

Do nurses have a voice? The need to have a voice in health policy development, implementation and evaluation has been well articulated by Keleher (1994), but it is time for nurses to turn rhetoric into reality. Working in the community requires a broad-based education and a sensitivity to issues of social (in)justice. Nurses with a knowledge of the economic, sociopolitical context of community issues, and a willingness to speak out on them, have the potential to drive community nursing practice forward (McDonald *et al.* 1997; Worth 1996).

What about the larger social health agenda? The language of the Ottawa Charter has mandatory currency in public health, and the concepts of reform, health promotion, empowerment, social justice, community participation and equality are assumed as desirable, but both research and practical projects in this area are devoid of theory (Rutten 1995). It is therefore important to test the assumptions underpinning the Ottawa Charter and to articulate new definitions of health that encompass a wider social view of it. Nurses should decide what role, if any, they will take in the new public health arena. If they reject the new public health agenda, they should be aware of the consequences and advantages for community health.

How can nurses participate in the debates? Following Labonte's (1997) suggestion, we must identify the issues, then facilitate and participate in debates with the community. Involving the community in action research for community health promotion is one useful strategy to engage and research with people (Kelly & Van Vlaenderen 1996; Rains & Ray 1995). Such a process allows the community to be involved in the entire process, including framing the research questions and taking action on the results.

REFLECTIVE QUESTIONS

(1) How are the following concepts defined and applied in nursing practice in the community: primary health care principle, the new public health, community health?
(2) What is health promotion?
(3) What constitutes advanced nursing practice in a community setting? How would you know it is advanced practice?

RECOMMENDED READING

Appelton, J.V. & Cowley, S. (2000) *The Search for Health Needs: Research for Health Visiting Practice.* Macmillan Press, London.

Blackie, C. (1998) *Community Health Care Nursing.* Churchill Livingstone, London.

Lawton, S., Cantrell, J. & Harris, J. (eds) (2000) *District Nursing: Providing Care in a Supportive Context.* Churchill Livingstone, Edinburgh.

Littlewood, J. (1999) *Current Issues in Community Nursing 2: Specialist Practice in Primary Health Care.* Churchill Livingstone, Edinburgh.

Sines, D., Appleby, F. & Raymond, E. (eds) (2001) *Community Healthcare Nursing.* Blackwell Science, Oxford.

REFERENCES

Abel, E. (1994) Productivity versus quality of care: Ethical implications for clinical practice during health care reform. *Nurse Practitioner Forum,* **5**(4), 238–242.

Armitage, S. & Kavanagh, K. (1996) Hospital nurses' perceptions of discharge planning for medical patients. *Australian Journal of Advanced Nursing,* **14**(2), 16–23.

Appleby, F. & Sayer, L. (2001) Public health nursing–health visiting. In: *Community Healthcare Nursing* (eds D. Sines, F. Appleby & E. Raymond). Blackwell Science, Oxford.

Appleton, J. & Clemerson, J. (1999) Family based interventions with children in need. *Community Practitioner,* **72**(5), 134–136.

Baldwin, J.H., Conger, C., Abegglen, J. & Hill, E. (1998) Population-focused and community-based nursing – moving toward clarification of concepts. *Public Health Nursing,* **15**(1), 12–18.

Baum, F., Fry, D. & Lennie, I. (eds) (1992) *Community Health Policy and Practice in Australia.* Pluto Press, Sydney.

Bernard, M. (1998) Back to the future? Reflections on women, ageing and nursing. *Journal of Advanced Nursing,* **27**(3), 633–640.

British Council (2000) *Health Insight,* March 2000- http://www.britishcouncil.org/health

Bunkers, S., Michaels, C. & Ethridge, P. (1997) Advanced practice nursing in community: Nursing's opportunity. *Advanced Practice Nursing Quarterly,* **2**(4), 79–84.

Cameron, J. & MacWilliams, J. (1995) Health care needs of homeless people. In: *Issues in Australian Nursing: The Nurse as Clinician* (eds G. Gray & R. Pratt). Churchill Livingstone, Melbourne.

Clark, J., Buttigieg, M., Eaton, N. *et al.* (2000) *Recognising the Potential: A Review of Health Visiting and School Health Services in Wales.* University of Wales, Swansea, unpublished.

Clayton, L. (1995) Hospital at home: Offering customer choice for post acute care. In: *Issues in Australian Nursing: The Nurse as Clinician* (eds G. Gray & R. Pratt). Churchill Livingstone, Melbourne.

Community Practitioner and Health Visitor Association (1997) A month in the life of a health visitor. *CPHVA Omnibus, 1997.* CPHVA, London.

Cotroneo, M., Outlaw, F., King, J. & Brince, J. (1997) Integrated primary health care: Opportunities for psychiatric-mental health nurses in a reforming health care system. *Journal of Psychosocial Nursing and Mental Health Services,* **35**(10), 21–27, 41–42.

Cowley, S., Buttigieg, M. & Houston, A. (2000) *A first steps project to scope the current and future regulatory issues for health visiting.* Report prepared for the UKCC. UKCC, London.

Cox, H., Hickson, P. & Taylor, B. (1991) Exploring reflection: Knowing and constructing practice. In: *Issues in Australian Nursing: The Nurse as Clinician* (eds G. Gray & R. Pratt). Churchill Livingstone, Melbourne.

Department of Health (1990) *The NHS and Community Care Act.* HMSO, London.

Department of Health (1998a) *The New NHS: Modern and Dependable: A National Framework for Assessing Performance.* The Stationery Office, London.

Department of Health (1998b) *Chief Medical Officers project to strengthen the public health function in England: A report of emerging findings.* HMSO, London.

Department of Health (1999a) *Saving Lives: Our Healthier Nation.* HMSO, London.

Department of Health (1999b) *Making a Difference: Strengthening the Nursing, Midwifery and Health Visiting Contribution to Health and Health Care.* HMSO, London.

Department of Health (2000) *The NHS Plan: A Plan for Investment, a Plan for Reform.* HMSO, London.

Department of Health (2001) *National Statistics Summary Information for 2000–01, England* – http://www.doh.gov.uk/public/kc560001/index.htm

Emden, C. (1991) Becoming a reflective practitioner. In: *Issues in Australian Nursing: The Nurse as Clinician* (eds G. Gray & R. Pratt). Churchill Livingstone, Melbourne.

Estes, C. & Binney, E. (1989) The biomedicalisation of ageing: Dangers and dilemmas. *The Gerontologist,* **29**(5), 587–596.

Farrington, D. (1995) Intensive health visiting and the prevention of juvenile crime. *Health Visitor,* **68**(3), 100–102.

Flaherty, B. (1995) Advanced practice nursing: What's all the fuss? *Journal of Nursing Law,* **2**(3), 7–25.

Forester, S. (2002) UKCC Consultation on standards for health visitor education. *Community Practitioner and Health Visitors Association,* **75**(1), 14–15.

Goltz, K. & Bruni, N. (1995) Health promotion discourse: Language of change? In: *The Politics of Health. The Australian experience* (ed. H. Gardner), 2nd edn, pp. 510–546. Churchill Livingstone, Melbourne.

Green, L. & Kreuter, M. (1991) *Health Promotion Planning. An Educational and Environmental Approach*, 2nd edn. Mayfield Publishing, Mountain View, California.

Home Office (1998) Supporting Families: A consultation Document. HMSO, London. http://www.northdevon.gov.uk/dris/main-mnu.html

Hyde, V. (1995) Community nursing: A unified discipline? In: *Community Nursing: Dimensions and Dilemmas* (eds P. Cain, V. Hyde & E. Howkins), pp. 1–26. Arnold, London.

Keegan, F. & Kent, D. (1992) Community health nursing. In: *Community Health Nursing Policy and Practice in Australia* (eds F. Baum, D. Fry & I. Lennie), pp. 156–169. Pluto Press, Sydney.

Keleher, H. (1994) Public health challenges for nursing and allied health. In: *Just Health: Inequalities in Illness, Care and Prevention* (eds C. Waddell & A. Peterson). Churchill Livingstone, London.

Keleher, H. & McInerney, F. (1998) *Nursing Matters: Critical Sociological Perspectives*. Churchill Livingstone, Sydney.

Kelly, K. & Van Vlaenderen, H. (1996) Dynamics of participation in a community health project. *Social Science & Medicine*, **42**, 1235–1246.

Kelsey, A. & Hollindale, P. (1996) Equal but different: Health visiting and the new curriculum. *Health Visitor*, **69**(11), 457–458.

Kenrick, M. & Luker, K.A. (1996) An exploration of the influence of managerial factors on research utilisation in district nursing practice. *Journal of Advanced Nursing*, **23**(4), 697–704.

Kickbush, I. (1997a) Think health – what makes a difference? Address given at *WHO 4th International Health Promotion Conference*, Jakarta July 1997.

Kickbush, I. (1997b) Designing the future: Strategic directions for primary health care in economically advanced countries. Paper given at *Centre for Primary Health Care National Conference*, Queensland, Australia, 12–14 March 1997.

Koch, T. & Hofmeyer, A. (1998) *Exploring the experience of caring for a person with Alzheimer's Dementia living at home: listening to the voices of caregivers*. Unpublished report, Royal District Nursing Service of SA Inc, Glenside SA.

Koch, T. & Webb, C. (1996) The biomedical construction of ageing: Implications for nursing care of older people. *Journal of Advanced Nursing*, **23**(5), 954–959.

Koch, T., Tooke, E. & Marks, J. (1998) *Evaluation Report: RDNS Disabilities Service*. Unpublished report, Royal District Nursing Service of SA Inc, Glenside, SA.

Labonte, R. (1997) Designing the future: Strategic directions for primary health care in economically advanced countries. Paper given at *Centre for Primary Health Care, National Conference*, Queensland, Australia, 12–14 March 1997.

Mackereth, C. (1997) Health visiting: Is it a nursing matter? *Health Visitor*, **70**(4), 155–157.

McDonald, A., Langford, I. & Boldero, N. (1997) The future of community nursing in the United Kingdom: District nursing, health visiting and school nursing. *Journal of Advanced Nursing*, **26**(2), 257–265.

McIntosh, J. (1996) The question of knowledge in district nursing. *International Journal of Nursing Studies*, **33**(3), 316–324.

McMurray, A. (1993) The political and economic context, Chap. 5. In: *Community Health Nursing: Primary Health Care in Practice*, 2nd edn. Churchill Livingstone, Melbourne.

National Health Service Executive (1999) *Primary Care Trusts: Establishing Better Services.* HMSO, London.

O'Connor, M. & Parker, E. (1995) *Health Promotion Principles and Practice in the Australian Context.* Allen and Unwin, Sydney.

Oldman, C. (1999) An evaluation of health visitor education in England. *Community Practitioner and Health Visitor,* **72**(12), 392–395.

Quality Assurance Agency for Higher Education (2001) *Subject Benchmark Statements: Healthcare Programmes.* Quality Assurance Agency for Higher Education, Gloucester.

Rains, J. & Ray, D. (1995) Participatory action research for community health promotion. *Public Health Nursing,* **12**, 256–261.

Rapport, F. & Maggs, C. (1997) Measuring care: The case of district nursing. *Journal of Advanced Nursing,* **25**(4), 673–680.

Redekopp, M. (1997) Clinical nurse specialist role confusion: The need for identity. *Clinical Nurse Specialist,* **11**(2), 87–91.

Richardson, G. & Maltby, H. (1995) Reflection-on-practice: Enhancing student learning. *Journal of Advanced Nursing,* **22**(2), 235–242.

Roberts, I. & Bedford, H. (1996) Does home visiting reduce the risk of childhood accidents? *Health Visitor,* **69**(7), 268–269.

Robinson, J (1985) Health visiting and health. In: *Political Issues in Nursing: Past, Present and Future* (ed. R. White). John Wiley, London.

Rutten, A. (1995) The implementation of health promotion: A new structural perspective. *Social Science & Medicine,* **41**(12), 1627–1637.

Scottish Executive (1999) *Towards a Healthier Scotland: A white paper on health, (CM4269)* The Stationery Office, Edinburgh.

Scottish Executive (2001) *Nursing for Health: A Review of the contribution of nurses, midwives and health visitors to improving the public health in Scotland.* Scottish Executive, Edinburgh.

Seeley, S., Murray, L. & Cooper, P. (1996) The outcome for mothers and babies of health visitor intervention. *Health Visitor,* **69**(4), 135–138.

Shay, L., Goldstein, J., Matthews, D., Trail, L. & Edmunds, M. (1996) Guidelines for developing a nurse practitioner practice. *Nurse Practitioner: American Journal of Primary Health Care,* **21**(1), 72, 75–76, 78 passim.

Starck, L., Mackey, T.A. & Adams, J. (1995) Nurse managed clinics: A blueprint for success using the Covey framework. *Journal of Professional Nursing,* **11**(2), 71–77.

Stuteley, H. & Trenoweth, P. (1999) The Beacon Project – Falmouth, Cornwall. Cornwall Health Care Trust. Unpublished.

Summers, A. & McKeown, K. (1996) Health needs assessment in primary care: A role for health visitors. *Health Visitor,* **69**(8), 323–324.

Suppiah, C. (1996) Working in partnership with community mothers. *Health Visitor,* **67**(2), 51–53.

Swanson, J. & Nies, M. (1997) *Community Health Nursing Promoting the Health of Aggregates,* 2nd edn. WB Saunders, Philadelphia.

Townsend, P. & Davidson, N. (1992) *Inequalities in Health: The Black Report and the Health Divide.* Penguin, London.

United Kingdom Central Council for Nursing, Midwifery and Health Visiting (1999) *Fitness for Practice: The UKCC Commission for Nursing and Midwifery Education.* UKCC, London.

United Kingdom Central Council for Nursing, Midwifery and Health Visiting (2001a) *Registrar's Letter Relating to Standards for Specialist Practice and Education*, 11/2001.UKCC, London.

United Kingdom Central Council for Nursing, Midwifery and Health Visiting (2001b) *Requirements For Registration as a Health Visitor–Consultation Document*. UKCC, London.

Wass, A. (1994) Health promotion in context: Primary health care and the new public health movement. In: *Promoting Health: The Primary Health Care Approach* (ed. A. Wass), pp. 5–31, Harcourt Brace, Sydney.

Wass, A. (2000) The Ottawa Charter for Health Promotion Appendix 2. In: *Promoting Health: The Primary Care Approach*, 2nd edn. pp. 267, 272, Harcourt Brace, Sydney.

Wellard, S. & Bethune, E. (1996) Reflective journal writing in nurse education: Whose interests does it serve? *Journal of Advanced Nursing*, **24**(5), 1077–1082.

Worth, A. (1996) Focus. Identifying need for district nursing: towards a more proactive approach by practitioners. *NT Research*, **1**(4), 260–269.

16 Meeting Health Care Needs in Culturally Diverse Societies

(I)Rena Papadopoulos

LEARNING OBJECTIVES

Upon completion of this chapter the student should be able to:

- understand the various reasons that have contributed to the formation of culturally diverse societies;
- become familiar with the main concepts associated with the study of culture and health;
- discuss some of the challenges of living in culturally diverse societies;
- identify and discuss the differences between assimilation, multiculturalism, antiracism, and the elimination of health inequalities;
- critically examine some of the current challenges to health care and relate these to nursing;
- appreciate the relevance of culturally competent care, and become familiar with at least one model that aims to promote cultural competence amongst nurses.

KEY WORDS

CULTURE, CULTURAL DIVERSITY, MIGRATION, REFUGEES, MULTICULTURALISM, ANTIRACISM, SOCIAL EXCLUSION, INEQUALITIES, CULTURAL COMPETENCE.

INTRODUCTION

This chapter will begin by examining when and why culturally diverse societies have come to exist. It will then briefly raise some of the existing challenges that are the result of misconceptions and propaganda. Some of the main approaches that have been tried to promote harmony in the culturally diverse UK are then discussed. Recent challenges to and relevant policies for health care provision are then examined. All these form important background information that will help you to understand some of the nursing issues related to meeting health care needs in culturally diverse societies.

Although the chapter is written from a UK perspective, I believe that its content is relevant to nurses working in other European countries. It is also important to state that I have used the terms 'cultural/culturally' and 'ethnic/ethnically' as though they are synonymous; they are of course closely related, and some may argue that we can use them interchangeably without causing any confusion, but strictly speaking they are not the same. There are a number of good articles and books that deal with the analysis of these complex and politically charged concepts, which you can refer to (Fernando 1991; O'Hagan 2001). I have also used these terms in general ways, which may be perceived to imply that the majority or dominant cultural group in a country, or that its minority cultural groups, are homogeneous. This is not so, as I am sure you will already be aware of many differences in values and practices among members of your own cultural/ethnic group. Finally, I have used the terms 'culturally competent' and 'transculturally competent' synonymously as they are used in this way in the literature, and because nobody as yet has proposed any conceptual differences between the two, if these indeed exist.

THE FORMATION OF CULTURALLY DIVERSE SOCIETIES

In 1992 the World Health Organization declared that among the possible trends in a future Europe is increased migration both from within and outside Europe.

Population movements of a size and complexity unprecedented since World War II have resulted in the displacement – mostly involuntary – of large numbers of people from many countries of the world. Ethnic conflicts, wars, oppressive political regimes, the on-going effects of colonialism, and natural disasters continue to inflict poverty and illness to millions of people around the globe. Such unfortunate disasters are largely responsible for this epidemic of mass migration that has affected almost every region of the world, including Europe. At the beginning of the year 2001 the number of people needing protection and assistance from the United Nations High Commission for Refugees (UNHCR) was almost 22 million. Of them, 12 million were refugees, six million were internally displaced people, almost one million were asylum seekers, almost another million were returned refugees, and another two million came under various other categories.

The current politicisation of refugeedom and asylum seeking as well as the negative sensationalism surrounding the plight of refugees, asylum seekers and economic migrants by the popular news media, create the impression that migration is a recent phenomenon. This of course is not true. Even though the scale of migration in the twentieth century (and the twenty-first century) is reported to be much larger than that of past centuries, people have been migrating almost since the beginning of time for a variety of reasons. We only have to take a quick look at our own country's history to discover when and why people migrated from it or when and why people migrated to it. For example, Cyprus, my birthplace, has a 9000-year history, during which we can trace the migration to it of the Achaean Greeks, and later, of a number of post-Trojan war heroes. No doubt, a few Phoenicians, Assyrians, Egyptians, Persians, Romans, French and English people as well as many Turks migrated to Cyprus as a result of having control over the island at different times of its history. At the same time small numbers of Cypriots were migrating to other countries. More substantial migration occurred in the twentieth century when, for example, there were three major migration waves of Greek Cypriots to the UK. The first major group of Greek Cypriots (just over 1000) arrived in the UK in the 1930s. As Cyprus was a British colony, young men seeking employment made their way to the UK. The second wave of migration occurred in 1960–61 when 25000 Cypriots left for the UK at the time Cyprus became a republic. The last wave of emigration occurred in 1974 following the conflict between the two major ethnic communities (the Greek Cypriots and the Turkish Cypriots) when almost 50% of its people became displaced, many of whom subsequently sought refuge in other countries.

 Take a few moments to reflect on the migration patterns of your country of birth and (if different) your adopted country. How culturally and ethnically diverse is the country you are living in?

I can report that members of my family have migrated from Cyprus to the UK, America, Canada and South Africa. For example, poverty and a search for a better life were the reasons behind some of my relatives' decision to migrate to America in the 1930s, 1940s and 1950s. Stories about opportunities and riches motivated some to migrate to South Africa in the 1950s and 1960s. On the other hand, my older brother arrived in the UK in 1950 to further his education, since tertiary education was not existent in Cyprus at the time. He subsequently settled in the UK and was the main reason for my choosing to migrate to the UK after becoming a refugee in 1974.

Try to plot the geographical whereabouts of your family starting from your grandparents (or earlier if you can). What made your family members migrate to another country?

Over many centuries the UK received immigrants from many different countries and cultural backgrounds. For example, during the nineteenth century a large number of people migrated from Ireland to escape famine. During the twentieth century many thousands of Jews from Germany and Eastern Europe fled to the UK to escape persecution by the Nazis. After World War II, labour shortages led to active recruitment of people from the former colonies of the Commonwealth. Asians and African-Caribbeans responded to the promise of a better life in the UK but, as history reveals, many faced tremendous hardship and discrimination. Although the number of migrants having these ethnic origins was relatively small compared to the Irish and Jews, and despite the fact that they contributed greatly to the rebuilding of the UK by taking on the least popular but nonetheless vital jobs, the hostility they experienced was primarily due to their skin colour (Solomos 1993).

Each European country has its own historical, political, economic and other reasons for being a country whose people have migrated either from it, or to it. The creation of the European Union (EU) is enabling nationals of the 15 member states to move without any difficulty between the EU countries. The forthcoming enlargement of the EU will result in greater cultural diversity within each member state. As a result, many of us end up living hundreds or even thousands of miles away from our motherlands or birthplaces, with people who may not share our beliefs, values, and culture in general.

THE CHALLENGES OF LIVING IN CULTURALLY DIVERSE SOCIETIES

Although multicultural societies are becoming the norm, this does not mean that all individuals within them enjoy equal and fair treatment, and have their human rights respected and protected. Many migrants continue to view themselves as guests in their adopted country even though they may have lived there many more years than they did in their own country of birth. In the case of black and Asian people Robinson (2001) reports that, despite the fact that they have been settling in the UK for more than 300 years they have yet to overcome the stigma of being labelled as 'outsiders' or 'others', and they continue to be labelled as 'problems' by many British people. This may be the same for other less visible UK migrant communities, and there is no reason to believe that this is very different in other European countries. In 1999 the UK Audit Commission found that a large section of the British news media was clearly xenophobic. In a survey of 161 newspaper articles collated by the Refugee Council, the Commission found that only 6% of the stories had cited any positive contribution made by refugees and asylum-seekers. On the other hand 28% of the stories focused on housing or employment difficulties, allegedly being exacerbated because of asylum-seekers, and 15% concerned crimes and offences committed by asylum-seekers.

However, UK Home Office research into migration (Glover *et al.* 2001) found that there is little evidence that migration damages the employment prospect of the existing resident workers. On the contrary the report suggested that managed migration could help to fill labour market shortages, improve public finances and contribute to the development of new industries and jobs. This view was echoed by Robinson (2001) who proposed that the UK will have to encourage more immigration in the twenty-first century to help pay for the pensions and health care of the ageing population. Thus both the Home Office and the Robinson reports state that migrants have made significant cultural, social and economic contributions in UK society.

- Think of six examples of positive contribution made by the migrant population of your country.
- List six 'good things' about living in a culturally diverse society.
- List six 'challenges' or 'negative aspects' about living in a culturally diverse society highlighted in the newspapers where you live.

In your reflections you may have decided that one of the positive contributions made by some migrants in your country is their diet. One of the 'good things' about living in a culturally diverse society often mentioned by many English people, is the availability of a larger range of food products, a direct result of the migrants' different dietary habits. However, whilst the notion of being different could be viewed as positive and enriching by many, it can also be viewed as a problem by some. Those who wish to promote xenophobia exaggerate the differences between what they view as 'us' (the indigenous majority population) and 'them' (members of minority cultural/ethnic groups).

PROMOTING UNDERSTANDING
OF EACH OTHER'S CULTURE

In culturally diverse societies, fear of the unknown is one of the causes which sustains the existence of first class citizens – those who believe that they are the true members of a particular society and should enjoy all the rights afforded by it – and second class citizens – those whom the first class citizens view as inferior and alien. There is mounting evidence which confirms the view that cultural minorities suffer inequalities and discrimination sometimes due to government policies and legislation but most frequently due to people's negative attitudes and ignorance.

To enhance harmony in a culturally diverse UK, a number of approaches have been tried over the years (Papadopoulos 2001). In the 1950s and 1960s the focus was on assimilation, which meant that members of minority cultural groups were encouraged to take on the values and lifestyles of the larger society, thus losing their distinctiveness. Migrants were encouraged to believe that holding onto their cultural identities would be detrimental to them. Since each one of us is a product of the culture into which we have been born and brought up, it soon became evident that although migrant communities wished to adapt and become a part of the host society, they were not prepared to abandon the central tenets of their cultural values, beliefs and practices.

The next approach to be tried in the UK in the 1970s and early 1980s, was that of multiculturalism. This was based on the theory that the promotion of understanding of each other's culture would reduce the unfounded fears of the majority cultural group whilst at the same time helping minority cultural groups to adapt to their adopted country. We therefore see the gradual acceptance of diversity and the acknowledgement that through better understanding and prolonged contact between cultural groups, the migrant groups will incorporate values and behaviours from the host culture (a process called acculturation), whilst the host culture would learn to accept cultural differences. What happened in reality was that the dominant cultural group used the culture of minority groups to assign blame or explanation to any health problems faced by their members (a process known as essentialism) (Ahmad 1996).

During the 1980s and early 1990s, the antiracist movement occupied centre stage. Many leading academics and political activists from minority cultural groups put forward the position that the inequalities experienced by a large number of people from minority ethnic groups were due to racist policies and structures within society, as well as racist attitudes of the majority group. These attitudes have their roots in the domination by British colonialists of many of the countries from which migrant communities come. Thus, according to the antiracists, unless British people acknowledge the injustices they committed in the past, they will not be able to eradicate contemporary racism and the resultant inequalities experienced by migrants in the UK (Ahmad 1993). Although this approach had strong supporters, it was also criticised by many, including members of minority groups, as too aggressive and counterproductive.

From the mid-1990s onwards a new combined approach is being used. This has elements of both multiculturalism and antiracism, with an emphasis on the promotion of equality and good citizenship.

In England and Wales, there are an estimated 3 million people of minority ethnic origins, constituting 6% of the total population. In some areas of inner cities, such as Brent in London, this rate is as high as 45% (OPCS 1992).

 Do you know the demographic ethnic breakdown of the city/town where you live? Do you know which are the three largest minority ethnic groups in the city/town where you live? How much do you know about the culture of these groups?

CHALLENGES FOR HEALTH CARE

It is now widely recognised that a person's health depends not only on their biological make-up but also on sociocultural, psychological, environmental and other factors. Dahlgren and Whitehead (1991) illustrated this by using a four-layered model of health determinants that surround the individual's core (or fixed) components, which are age, sex and hereditary factors. The first layer consists of the individual's lifestyle factors such as smoking, diet and physical activity; the second consists of their social and community networks; the third is made up of the person's living and working conditions, education, transport and access to health services, whilst the fourth layer describes the general economic, cultural and environmental conditions present in society as a whole.

This understanding of health is akin to that espoused by the World Health Organization's (WHO) 'Health for All' strategy (1992) which emphasises the need to eradicate poverty, as one of the main causes of ill health, and the importance of providing the basic prerequisites for health such as good nutrition, appropriate housing and education, reduction of crime, and access to effective health care.

There are two important messages that can be drawn from the above explanations. Firstly, that poverty, which is often the cause of, and the result of both exclusion and inequality, has now been strongly linked to poor health, and secondly that our cultural background has an important influence on most of the components of health.

The UK government has accepted this definition of health, and particularly in the past 10 years, it has steadily worked towards addressing these health components. At the same time, the UK government has recognised that minority cultural groups often suffer more inequalities and disadvantage compared with the majority cultural (indigenous) group. Many studies (Amin & Oppenheim 1992; Jones 1993; Modood *et al.* 1997) have established the following:

- Unemployment rates for most minority ethnic groups are considerably higher than those of the majority indigenous group.
- Low-paid occupations such as catering employ a disproportionate number of people from minority ethnic groups.
- Poor working conditions such as shift work, night work and home-working are experienced by a greater proportion of people from minority ethnic groups.
- Poverty, defined in various ways, is also experienced by a greater proportion of people from minority ethnic groups.

- Housing tenure exhibits marked ethnic patterns with poorer quality housing being experienced by minority ethnic groups.

In 1998 the report of the *Independent Inquiry into Inequalities in Health* (Acheson 1998) was published. It emphasised, as others did before it, that the roots of ill-health lie in such determinants as income, education, employment, environment and lifestyle. The report included a section on ethnicity that began with the problems surrounding the issues and difficulties of defining the various terms associated with minority ethnic/cultural health, but chose a definition that focused on cultural identity, place of origin and skin colour, which means that both white and nonwhite minority groups were included. It went on to highlight the problem of not having accurate ethnic data and the total absence of such data for some groups. The report dealt with issues around mortality, morbidity and socioeconomic status; it stated that people from minority ethnic groups have higher than average rates of unemployment and that there is a clear association between material disadvantage and poor health.

The quality of services as well as access to services was also criticised by the report, which catalogued a number of problems encountered by people from minority ethnic groups such as:

- People from minority ethnic groups have longer waiting times in the doctor's surgery.
- They feel that the time spent with the doctor is inadequate.
- They are less satisfied with the outcome of the consultation.
- They are less likely to be referred to secondary and tertiary care.

However, the report failed to acknowledge in any clear way that health inequalities may result from some racist organisational structures and the racist attitudes of some health care professionals. It stated that part of the problems the inquiry had identified may be related to communication barriers, and some may be due to cultural differences between the doctor and the patient. It recommended that health workers are trained in cultural competency but failed to define what the inquiry meant by it. It went on to recommend that further development of services that are sensitive to the needs of minority ethnic people, and which promote greater awareness of their health risks, are needed. In addition, the report recommended that the needs of minority ethnic groups are specifically considered in needs assessment, resource allocation, health care planning and provision.

The most recent UK government health policies such as *Saving Lives: Our Healthier Nation* (1999a), *The NHS Plan* (2000), and *Reducing Health Inequalities: an action report* (1999b) all focus on modernising the National Health Service (NHS), and reducing health inequalities. Other initiatives such as Health Action Zones, Employment Action Zones, Education Action Zones, Healthy Living Centres, and The National Strategy for Neighbourhood Renewal – to name but a few – have been implemented in order to address the causes of deprivation, material disadvantage and inequalities whilst at the same time promoting social networks amongst people and collaborative partnerships amongst the various agencies.

What are the advantages and disadvantages of the current health policy that subsumes the management of culturally diverse health needs into the 'inequalities' agenda?

CHALLENGES FOR NURSES

If we acknowledge that most of us live in culturally diverse societies, if we agree that our cultural backgrounds play an important role in the construction of our health beliefs and practices, and if we accept the evidence about health inequalities suffered by people from minority ethnic cultures, then we must try to:

- learn more about the cultural backgrounds of the people we care for;
- understand the causes of inequalities suffered by these people;
- gain the skills which will enable us to deliver culturally competent care.

Madeleine Leininger, the founder of transcultural nursing, made the following statement:

> Our world continues to change and is bringing people close together in one world with many diverse cultural values, beliefs, and lifeways. With these global cultural changes, have come new expectations and challenges in nursing to prepare nurses through transcultural nursing education to become competent, sensitive, and responsible to care for people of diverse cultures in the world (1995:3).

She defined transcultural nursing as:

> a humanistic and scientific area of formal study and practice in nursing which is focused upon the comparative study of cultures with regard to differences and similarities in care, health, and illness patterns, based upon cultural values, beliefs, and practices of different cultures in the world, and the use of this knowledge to provide culturally-specific and/or universal nursing care to people (1984:42).

I would add that transcultural nursing requires a commitment for the promotion of anti-oppressive, anti-discriminatory practices. Since transcultural nursing emphasises the importance of empowering clients to participate in health care decisions, health care professionals must recognise how society constructs disadvantage. In my view no other nursing philosophy and framework places so much emphasis in such an explicit way towards the promotion of equality and the value of individuals as this does.

A number of transcultural theories and models have been developed to help nurses deliver culturally competent care (or transculturally competent care – the two terms will be used synonymously). These include Leininger's Sunrise Model (1988), Campinha-Bacote's model of culturally competent care (1991), Papadopoulos *et al.*'s model for developing cultural competence (1998), and Purnell's model for cultural competence (1998).

The Papadopoulos *et al.* model emphasises the preparation of the nurse rather than the use of the model in the assessment of patients. My colleagues and I believe that once nurses are prepared in transcultural ways using our model then they can deliver transcultural nursing within any nursing framework that is used in their working environment. We define cultural/transcultural competence as the capacity to provide effective healthcare taking into consideration people's cultural beliefs, behaviours and needs.

MODEL FOR DEVELOPING CULTURAL COMPETENCE

Our model consists of four stages as seen in Fig. 16.1. A conceptual map is provided for each stage as a guideline only. Educators who are well versed in this area of learning may add other concepts or modify the proposed ones to suit the type and level of students.

The first stage in the model is cultural awareness, which begins with an examination of our personal value base and beliefs. The nature of construction of cultural identity as well as its influence on people's health beliefs and practices are viewed as necessary planks of a learning platform.

Cultural knowledge (the second stage) can be gained in a number of ways. Meaningful contact with people from different ethnic groups can enhance our knowledge around their health beliefs and behaviours as well as raise understanding around the problems they face. Learning from our clients/patients will undoubtedly contribute towards avoiding making ethnocentric judgements. Sociology informs debates around power, ideology and the way in which the state constructs images of normal-

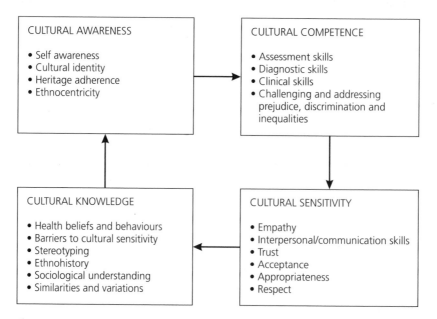

Fig. 16.1 The four-stage model for developing cultural competence (Papadopoulos *et al.* 1998:179).

ity. It particularly considers the power of the professions and the role of medicine in social control.

An important element in achieving cultural sensitivity (the third stage), is how professionals view people in their care. Dalrymple and Burke (1995) have stated that, unless clients are considered as true partners, culturally sensitive care is not being achieved; to do otherwise means that professionals are using their power only in an oppressive way. Equal partnerships involve trust, acceptance and respect as well as facilitation and negotiation.

The achievement of the fourth stage (cultural competence) requires the synthesis and application of previously gained awareness, knowledge and sensitivity. Further focus is given to practical skills such as assessment of need, clinical diagnosis and other caring skills. A most important component of this stage of development is the ability to recognise and challenge racism and other forms of discrimination and oppressive practice.

The model promotes the view that cultural competencies can be both generic and specific. Gerrish and Papadopoulos (1999) argued that in order to be transculturally competent, nurses need to develop both culture-specific and culture-generic competence. Culture-specific competence refers to the knowledge and skills that relate to a particular cultural group that enable the nurse to understand the values and health practices of the client. Culture-generic competence is defined as the acquisition of knowledge and skills that are applicable across cultural groups.

Think of a client/patient you nursed recently who comes from a different cultural background from your own. What culture-specific information did you need in order to provide culturally competent care?

If I were nursing a dying elderly Pakistani woman I would want to know what her religion was. If she were a Muslim, then I would want to know what specific religious and cultural practices Pakistani Muslims adhere to. For example, she might wish to lie facing towards Mecca or she might wish her relatives to recite prayers around the bed.

 Can you think of any culture-generic competencies that may apply to the above scenario?

My culture-generic competence includes my awareness that not all Muslims are the same. Thus I am aware that I should not stereotype this woman. I should consult her, or her immediate family, as to her wishes and their wishes regarding their religious and cultural practices, and should communicate this in a sensitive way without causing any offence.

CONCLUSION

Purnell and Paulanska (1998) state that all clients and staff have the right to be understood, respected, and treated as individuals despite their differences. Nursing people involves ethical responsibility. Service to society also requires assurances that practitioners are competent. Culturally incompetent nursing is not only unethical but it is also unsafe. This chapter has demonstrated the imperative of transcultural nursing by highlighting some of the challenges facing culturally diverse societies and their health care systems. It is evident that cultural and structural factors influence the quality of health and nursing care. If nursing fails to consider these factors, then it is failing to provide individualised care to all its clients. Valuing diversity in health care enhances the delivery and effectiveness of health care for all people, whether they are members of a minority or a majority cultural group.

REFLECTIVE QUESTIONS

(1) Consider the health care policies that guide the health care practice of your work area. Which one of the four approaches discussed in this chapter mainly describes the approach taken by management? Is this different from that which underpins the ethos and practice of the nurses you work with? Give examples to justify your views.

(2) It could be argued that nursing is a powerful profession because of its size and the centrality of its role in terms of health care delivery. Do you think that the nursing profession is using this power to reduce health inequalities? Give examples to justify your views.

(3) List the advantages of utilising a model for the development of culturally competent nurses.

USEFUL WEBSITES

www.unhcr.ch
The website of the United Nations High Commission for Refugees.

www.refugeecouncil.org.uk
The UK's largest provider of direct help to people seeking asylum.

www.cre.org.uk
The Commission for Racial Equality (UK) is the government body for monitoring and advising on race issues in the UK. The website covers areas such as law, publications and facts about racism together with a comprehensive list of contacts.

www.doh.gov.uk
This is the UK's Department of Health website. Contains the latest policy documents, is searchable and has links to almost all government websites.

www.homeoffice.gov.uk
This is the UK's Home Office website. Contains downloadable policies and statistics about migrants and refugees.

www.mdx.ac.uk/www/rctsh/homepage.htm
This is the website of the Research Centre for Transcultural Studies in Health, Middlesex University, UK. It contains information about the work of the Centre and

its publications. It has many links to sites dealing with culture, ethnicity, refugees, migrants, transcultural health care and so on.

www.health.qld.gov.au/hssb/cultdiv/cultdiv/home.htm
Queensland Health (Queensland Government, Australia) has sponsored the development of this site, which is a guide for health professionals to support the provision of culturally-sensitive health care in hospitals and community health services.

www.tcns.org
The site aims to promote the field of transcultural nursing, provide information about this field to those who are interested in the topic, encourage nurses who want to further their education in transcultural nursing and promote the interactions of those who are interested in transcultural nursing.

www.culturediversity.org/index.html
This is an interactive site containing case reports and anecdotes of actual problems that occur as a result of cultural differences. It also has a discussion forum, case studies and a useful reading list.

RECOMMENDED READING

Leininger, M.M. (1995) *Transcultural Nursing: Concepts, Theories, Research and Practices*, 2nd edn. McGraw-Hill, New York.
O'Hagan, K. (2001) *Cultural Competence in the Caring Professions*. Jessica Kingsley, London.
Papadopoulos, I., Tilki, M. & Taylor, G. (1998) *Transcultural Care: A Guide for Health Care Professionals*. Quay Books, Wilts.
Purnell, L.D. & Paulanska, B.J. (1998) *Transcultural Health Care: A Culturally Competent Approach*. F.A. Davies Co., Philadelphia.
Smaje, C. (1995) *Health, Race and Ethnicity: Making Sense of the Evidence*. King's Fund Institute, London.

REFERENCES

Acheson, Sir Donald (Chair) (1998) *Independent Inquiry into Inequalities in Health*. The Stationery Office, London.
Ahmad, W.I.U. (1993) Making black people sick: race, ideology and health research. In: *'Race' and Health in Contemporary Britain* (ed. W.I.U. Ahmad). Open University Press, Buckingham.
Ahmad, W.I.U. (1996) The trouble with culture. In: *Researching Cultural Differences in Health* (eds D. Kelleher & S. Hillier). Routledge, London.
Amin, K. & Oppenheim, C. (1992) *Poverty in Black and White Deprivation and Ethnic Minorities*. Child Poverty Action Group, London.
Campinha-Bacote, J. (ed.) (1991) *The Process of Cultural Competence: A Culturally Competent Model of Care*, 2nd edn. Transcultural C.A.R.E. Associates, Ohio, USA.

Dahlgren, G. & Whitehead, M. (1991) *Policies and Strategies to Promote Equity in Health.* Institute for Future Studies, Stockholm.

Dalrymple, J. & Burke, B. (1995) *Anti-oppressive Practice: Social Care and the Law.* Open University Press, Buckingham.

Department of Health (1999a) *Saving Lives: Our Healthier Nation.* Department of Health, London.

Department of Health (1999b) *Reducing Health Inequalities: An Action Report.* Department of Health, London.

Department of Health (2000) *The NHS Plan.* Department of Health, London.

Fernando, S. (1991) *Mental Health, Race and Culture.* Macmillan and Mind Publications, London.

Gerrish, K. & Papadopoulos, I. (1999) Transcultural competence: The challenge for nurse education. *British Journal of Nursing,* **8**(21), 1453–1457.

Glover, S., Gott, C., Loizillon, A. *et al.* (2001) *Migration: An economic and social analysis.* RDS Occasional Paper No 67. Home Office, London.

Jones, T. (1993) *Britain's ethnic minorities.* Policy Studies Institute, London.

Leininger, M.M. (1984) Transcultural nursing: An essential knowledge and practice field for today. *Canadian Nurse.* **Dec**, 41–57.

Leininger, M.M. (1988) Leininger's theory of nursing: Culture care diversity and universality. *Nursing Science Quarterly,* **1**(4), 152–160.

Leininger, M.M. (1995) *Transcultural Nursing: Concepts, Theories, Research and Practices,* 2nd edn. McGraw-Hill, New York.

Moodood, T., Berthoud, R., Lakey, J. *et al.* (1997) *Ethnic Minorities in Britain.* Policy Studies Institute, London.

O'Hagan, K. (2001) *Cultural Competence in the Caring Professions.* Jessica Kingsley, London.

Office of Population Censuses & Surveys (1992) *1991 Census.* HMSO, London.

Papadopoulos. I, Tilki, M. & Taylor, G. (1998) *Transcultural Care: A Guide for Health Care Professionals.* Quay Books, Wilts.

Papadopoulos, I. (2001) Antiracism, multiculturalism and the third way. In: *Managing Diversity and Inequality in Health Care* (ed. C. Baxter). Baillière Tindall, Edinburgh and Royal College of Nursing.

Purnel, L.D. & Paulanska, B.J. (1998) *Transcultural Health Care: A Culturally Competent Approach.* F.A. Davies Co, Philadelphia.

Robinson, V. (2001) *Jewels in the Crown: the Contribution of Ethnic Minorities to Life in Post-War Britain.* Moneygram International, London.

Solomos, J. (1993) *Race and Racism in Britain.* Macmillan Press, Basingstoke.

World Health Organization (1992) *Targets for Health for All: The Health Policy for Europe.* (Summary of the updated edition September, 1991) WHO Regional Office for Europe, Copenhagen.

17 Becoming a Critical Thinker

Steve Parker and Judith Clare

LEARNING OBJECTIVES

At the completion of this chapter, the student will be able to:

- describe the essential nature of critical thinking;
- describe the main characteristics of a critical thinker;
- explain the basic structure of an argument;
- apply the basic structure of an argument to various areas of nursing practice;
- identify resources for further reading and study of critical thinking.

KEY WORDS

THINKING, REFLECTION, ACTION, EVALUATION, ARGUMENT, INDUCTION, PREMISE, NURSING PROCESS, DECISION MAKING.

INTRODUCTION

There is a variety of definitions of critical thinking and, as Richard Paul (1993) suggests, we need to be careful about relying on any one definition. In essence, however, critical thinking refers to the activity of *questioning what is usually taken for granted*.

Whether one is aware of it or not, all behaviour is based on certain values, assumptions and beliefs. These form the basis for a person's decisions to act in certain ways. In a professional context such as nursing practice, everything that is thought, said and done is the result of a complex web of beliefs, values and assumptions that have formed throughout one's life experiences. As people grow up in their family, attend school, participate in religious communities, associate with friends, watch television, read newspapers, work for various employers, they develop a 'pair of spectacles' through which they understand and interpret the world and all that happens in it. Just as people who wear glasses eventually becomes unaware that they are even wearing them, so too do individuals adjust to their world view 'spectacles' until, often, they are completely unaware what values, beliefs, and assumptions are influencing them in a specific situation.

Critical thinking means stopping and reflecting on the reasons for doing things the way they are done or for experiencing things the way they are; focusing on what is frequently taken for granted and evaluating the values, beliefs and assumptions that are held, and asking whether or not what is done and thought is justifiable or not. These characteristics of critical thinking imply a self-consciousness of what, how, and why we are thinking, with the intention of improving thinking. In short, 'critical thinking is thinking about your thinking while you're thinking in order to make your thinking better' (Paul 1993). Improving thinking is essential because it is intimately related to the many decisions that need to be made each day. The quality of our lives is determined by the quality of our decisions, and the quality of our decisions is determined by the quality of our reasoning (Schick & Vaughn 1995).

An important aspect of critical thinking is healthy scepticism. This scepticism is necessary because there are many attempts to persuade people to accept various claims. These attempts to persuade also occur in professional contexts. For example, research reports suggest changes to practice; peers argue that their way of acting is the right one; therapists promote various interventions; administrators argue that certain changes need to be made to the workplace, and so on. Often these claims are contradictory, so they cannot all be acceptable.

Practitioners need to sort through all these, often competing, claims. To accept them all without question will, at best, be highly confusing and, at worst, may endanger the lives of others if actions are based on wrong information or conclusions. To adopt an attitude of healthy scepticism means cautiously to listen to or read the claims that others make, carefully evaluating their legitimacy, and not rushing to accept a conclusion without careful thought.

It is possible, of course, to become too pedantic, resulting in inaction because one is not prepared to accept anything that is not 100% proven. This is why the scepticism needs to be healthy. There is a limit to what can be known for certain. And part of critical thinking is knowing these limits and making the best evaluation under the circumstances.

THE RELATIONSHIP BETWEEN CRITICAL AND CREATIVE THINKING

A brief comment needs to be made about creative thinking. Critical thinking is not the same as creative thinking. According to Miller and Babcock (1996) creative thinking is, among other things, more divergent, messy, unpredictable, provocative, spontaneous and playful than critical thinking. They describe critical thinking as selective, orderly, predictable, analytical, judgemental and evaluative.

Creative thinking, although different from critical thinking, is an essential, complementary process to critical thinking. As a practitioner, there are many situations that arise that do not fit with the ideal or that are not predictable. No individual person for whom nurses care ever fits the 'average', because each person and situation is unique. In order to solve problems for these unique situations and individuals the practitioner needs to be able to develop new approaches and solutions, so that all parties have their needs met. Miller and Babcock (1996) suggest that:

> Creative thinking is very useful when what we know and what we know how to do are not working, including the rules of reason, common sense, gravity, and routine. The

creative thinker is willing to think wildly, without having any idea where her or his path of thinking may lead. Deliberative cognition is temporarily held in abeyance (p. 120).

Because creative thinking is so 'chaotic' it means that it needs to be evaluated to ensure that any conclusions that are reached are appropriate. In this regard, Ruggiero (1998) understands the mind to have two phases:

> It both produces ideas and judges them. These phases are intertwined; that is, we move back and forth between them many times in the course of dealing with a problem, sometimes several times in the span of a few seconds (p. 81).

In the past, critical thinking has often been presented apart from creative thinking. However, in practice, creative and critical thinking go hand-in-hand. Without creative thinking, critical thinking would be dry and mechanical. Without critical thinking, creative thinking would be chaotic and inefficient. As Ruggiero (1998:81) asserts, '[t]o study the art of thinking in its most dynamic form [where creative and critical thinking are intertwined] would be difficult at best.' Consequently, in practice, we need to consider them separately. However, although critical thinking and creative thinking are distinct from each other, they should never be separated.

THE CHARACTERISTICS OF CRITICAL THINKING

So what are the characteristics that a critical thinker will demonstrate? Jacobs *et al.* (1997) have developed a set of observable skills that indicate the presence of critical thinking. These are grouped into four categories.

Firstly, a critical thinker needs the ability to integrate information from all relevant sources by being able to distinguish between relevant and irrelevant data; validate data that is obtained; recognise when data is missing; predict multiple outcomes; and recognise the consequences of actions.

Secondly, to think critically means to be able to: examine assumptions by recognising them when they are present; detect bias; identify assumptions that are not stated; recognise the relationships of action or inaction; and transfer thoughts and concepts to diverse contexts or develop alternative courses of action.

Thirdly, it is important for the critical thinker to be able to identify relationships and patterns. This includes recognising inconsistencies or fallacies of logic; working out generalisations; developing a plan of action consistent with a model, and where appropriate, seeking out alternative models.

Jacobs *et al.* (1997) offer a definition of critical thinking that incorporates all these characteristics:

> Critical thinking is the repeated examination of problems, questions, issues, and situations by comparing, simplifying, synthesizing information in an analytical, deliberative, evaluative, decisive way (p. 20).

Many more examples of ways of describing the characteristics of critical thinking could be offered. One way of summarising these is to focus on critical thinking as reasoning. The heart of reasoning is the argument. In what follows, the nature of argument will be described, followed by a survey of the ways in which arguments 'appear' in nursing. Suggestions will then be offered regarding the way in which the principles of critical thinking might be applied in these areas. By doing so, the way in which this approach synthesises the skills of critical thinking will become obvious.

WHAT IS AN ARGUMENT?

In colloquial language the word 'argument' is often used for a shouting match between two people who are having a disagreement where the participants are very angry, abusive, or physically aggressive. There may be shouting, pointing of fingers, threats, crying, name-calling, and so on.

However, in critical thinking, the term 'argument' does not apply to these situations. In fact, these situations are the very opposite of critical thinking. In critical thinking an argument consists of a conclusion and one or more reasons that are intended to support the conclusion. Figure 17.1 shows the relationship between these parts of an argument. Each reason may or may not have evidence that is intended to support the reason or reasons.

Here is an example of an argument:

> Every person has the right to choose how they live their lives. Therefore, every person has the right to choose to practise life-threatening behaviours if they wish.

This is an argument because it has a conclusion ('A person has the right to choose to practise life-threatening behaviours if he or she wishes') and a reason intended to support that conclusion ('Every person has the right to choose how they live their lives').

At this stage, it is of no concern whether this is a good argument or not, only with what makes something an argument. If it were desirable, a person presenting this argument could provide some evidence for the first statement by drawing attention, for example, to various statements of human rights, the constitutions of countries, or discussions about ethics.

So an argument needs to have the following:

- a conclusion;
- one or more reasons intended to support the conclusion.

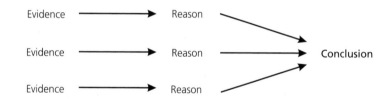

Fig. 17.1 The components of an argument.

What makes a sound argument?

For an argument to be sound, three criteria need to be met. Firstly, the reasons need to be acceptable to the person evaluating the argument. Secondly, the reasons need to be relevant. And thirdly, the reasons need to provide adequate grounds for accepting the conclusion.

Govier (1992) offers a useful way to remember these three criteria, which she calls the conditions of argument. If the first three letters of the word argument (ARG) are taken on their own, each letter stands for one of the conditions of argument, thus:

A Acceptability
R Relevance
G Grounds

Govier's definitions of each of these conditions is also useful:

Acceptability: 'The premises are acceptable when it is reasonable for those to whom the argument is addressed to believe these premises. There is good reason to accept the premises – even if they are not known for certain to be true. And there is no good evidence known to those to whom the argument is addressed that would indicate either that the premises are false or that they are doubtful' (p. 68).

Relevance: 'Premises are relevant to the conclusion when they give at least some evidence in favor of the conclusion's being true. They specify factors, evidence, or reasons that do count toward establishing the conclusion. They do not merely describe distracting aspects that lead you away from the real topic with which the argument is supposed to be dealing or that do not tend to support the conclusion' (p. 68).

Grounds: 'The premises provide sufficient or good grounds for the conclusion. In other words, considered together, the premises give sufficient reason to make it rational to accept the conclusion. This statement means more than that the premises are relevant. Not only do they count as evidence for the conclusion, they provide enough evidence, or enough reasons, taken together, to make it reasonable to accept the conclusion' (p. 69).

The following example illustrates these criteria:

(1) Nurses must have a practising certificate to be employed as a nurse.
(2) Sue does not have a practising certificate.
(3) Therefore, Sue is not permitted to be employed as a nurse.

Statements 1 and 2 are both reasons that are intended to support the conclusion in Statement 3. If this is a sound argument, then the reasons must be relevant and acceptable and they must provide adequate grounds for accepting the conclusion.

Statement 1 is certainly acceptable. Most countries have a requirement that nurses need to be licensed to practise. Statement 2 is hypothetical, so we will assume that it is true for the sake of the discussion. All the reasons, then, are acceptable. The two reasons are also relevant to the issue under consideration.

The next question is whether these reasons provide adequate grounds for accepting the conclusion. We can test this out by asking: is it possible to reject the conclusion and still believe the reasons to be true? In other words, could one believe that Sue could practise and still believe that the two reasons offered are true? In this case, the answer is No. If it is true that a nurse must have a practising certificate to practise, and Sue does not have one, one is 'compelled' to accept the conclusion that Sue cannot practise. This argument, then, is a sound one.

Another example will illustrate a poor argument:

(1) Everyone's hair falls out when undergoing chemotherapy.
(2) Jo is undergoing chemotherapy.
(3) Therefore, Jo's hair will fall out.

First, are the reasons acceptable? Does people's hair fall out when they are undergoing chemotherapy? Some people's does, but not necessarily everyone's. So this reason is not acceptable because, although some people's hair falls out, not everyone's does. For the sake of this discussion, the second reason can be accepted (that Jo is undergoing chemotherapy).

Both of the reasons are relevant and so the final question is whether the reasons offered provide adequate grounds for accepting that Jo's hair will fall out. The answer is No because the first reason was false. Although it might be true that Jo's hair will fall out, it is not possible to predict it because not everyone's hair does when they are on chemotherapy.

To summarise:

(1) An argument consists of a conclusion with one or more relevant reasons that are intended to support the conclusion.
(2) Evidence may or may not be offered to support each reason.
(3) A sound argument is one in which the reason(s) are acceptable and provide adequate grounds for accepting the conclusion.

There are a few technical terms that need to be remembered in regard to what has been covered so far.

(1) A *reason* can also be called a *premise*.
(2) The question of whether reasons provide grounds for the conclusion is a question of *validity*. In everyday conversation, the word validity often has a broader meaning. In critical thinking, it is used to refer to the logical relationship between the reasons and the conclusion.
(3) When an argument has reasons that are acceptable and is valid (i.e. the reasons provide adequate grounds for accepting the conclusion) then the argument is said to be *sound*.

It is important to note that an argument can be valid but unsound. For example, the following argument is valid but unsound:

(1) All nurses are female.
(2) Alex is a nurse.
(3) Therefore, Alex is female.

Statement 1 is not true, of course. Some nurses are male. Statement 2 can be assumed to be true. Because Statement 1 is false, we already know that this argument is unsound. But is it valid? Yes it is. If Statement 1 were true, the acceptance of Statement 3 would be unavoidable. This means that the argument is logically valid, but it is not sound – that is, it is not a sound argument.

THINKING CRITICALLY

Critical thinking, in essence, means being able to identify the presence of an argument in any form and evaluate it. Once what makes a sound argument, and the questions needed to be asked to evaluate it are known, it is possible to assess any argument that is encountered. Critical thinking means applying to this task thinking which has the characteristics discussed above.

Critical thinking in nursing

The basic approach outlined above can be applied to many areas within nursing. In the following sections some examples of these areas will be surveyed, how the basic framework introduced above applies to that area will be discussed, and some guidelines for thinking critically about issues in the respective area will be offered. The overlaying of the structure of argument onto the various areas in nursing builds on the work of Mayer and Goodchild (1995) in their discussion of critical thinking in psychology.

Clinical practice
In clinical practice, decisions are constantly being made to act in certain ways for the benefit of clients. These actions can be beneficial or have serious consequences for the health and well-being of the people a nurse is working for or with. It is essential that these interventions be considered critically. Figure 17.2 illustrates the application of the basic argument framework to clinical practice.

As can be seen, very little alteration is necessary. The equivalent of the conclusion is the particular action that has been, or will be, performed. It should be possible to justify each of a nurse's actions by appealing to an appropriate set of reasons. These reasons, in turn, must be based on high-quality evidence.

In the past, many of the actions and interventions of nurses have been based on tradition, folklore, or no evidence at all. In recent years, however, the developing

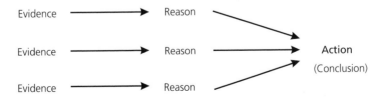

Fig. 17.2 The basic argument framework applied to clinical practice: the conclusion will be manifest as *action*.

professional status of nursing has resulted in more concern about the basis for nursing action. There is a growing and strengthening movement called evidence-based practice that promotes an attitude of thinking critically about what is done by nurses and asking on what basis what is done can be justified.

The increasing interest of consumers in their own health care has also had an effect. People are no longer willing to allow health professionals to make all the decisions for them and are demanding higher quality care. The increasing incidence of litigation has also motivated a concern for basing nursing action on high quality evidence.

On an individual level, a nurse should be able to justify any action performed on behalf of a client. The reasons need to be based on solid evidence. The source of this evidence may take many forms including personal experience, traditions handed down between 'generations' of nurses, and what is taught during nurse education. However, on their own, these sources of knowledge are not adequate. A formal process for exploring nursing knowledge is needed that allows the testing of ideas and the validation of actions and interventions.

The activity of formal research provides this opportunity. Nursing research will be examined below from a critical thinking perspective. First, however, there are a number of questions that can be asked about practice, which will help nurses think critically about it. When reflecting on an action or intervention, ask the following questions:

(1) What are the reasons for acting or intervening in the way that is planned?
(2) What evidence is available which supports the reasons for acting in this way?
(3) Are the reasons relevant to the issue that is being considered?
(4) Are there other reasons that need to be considered?
(5) Is there any evidence that raises questions about the manner of acting or intervening?
(6) Do the reasons provide adequate grounds for acting in the planned way?
(7) Are there alternative actions or interventions that could be chosen and the reasons still be acceptable in these situations?

THE NURSING PROCESS

The nursing process is a common framework for making practice decisions in nursing, therefore it will be briefly explored in relation to critical thinking. The steps of the nursing process are:

(1) collection of subjective and objective data;
(2) arrival at a diagnosis of the client's problem(s);
(3) planning of appropriate nursing interventions in response to the problem(s);
(4) implementation of the planned intervention(s);
(5) ongoing evaluation of the effectiveness of the intervention(s) in relation to the client's problem(s).

The nursing process can be summarised in three 'phases':

(1) diagnosis;
(2) intervention;
(3) evaluation.

Each of these three phases can be understood as an argument (remember the technical meaning of the term argument). Figure 17.3 illustrates this.

The diagnosis is the equivalent of the conclusion in an argument. The data that is collected comes from observations of the patient as well as information provided by the client, relatives, friends, past history, and so on. This raw data needs to be interpreted and takes on meaning in the context of developing a diagnosis. Finally, on the basis of the meaning of the data, a conclusion is arrived at in the form of a diagnosis.

Of course, the description here is somewhat simplistic. The actual process is much richer and more complex than this. However, understanding the process of diagnosis as an argument leads us to ask questions like the following:

- Is the data collected accurate? If not, how reliable is it?
- Has the data been understood and interpreted correctly?
- Is the data and its interpretation relevant to the diagnosis that has been chosen?
- Does the interpretation of the data provide adequate grounds for arriving at the diagnosis?
- Are there any other diagnoses which could possibly fit the data that has been collected? Are any of these more consistent with the data?

A similar process applies to the intervention and evaluation phases. Intervention and evaluation criteria must be justified to support claims of improvement, deterioration, or preservation of the status quo. Figures 17.4 and 17.5 illustrate the structure of argument related to these two phases.

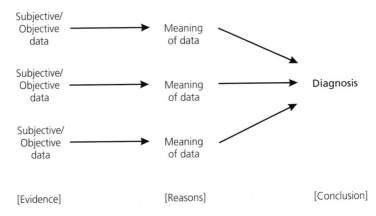

Fig. 17.3 The three phases of the nursing process represented as an argument.

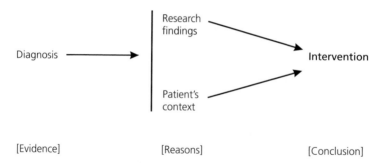

Fig. 17.4 The intervention phase represented as an argument.

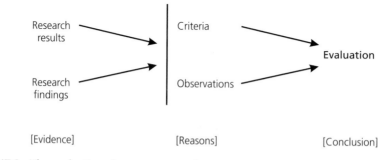

Fig. 17.5 The evaluation phase represented as an argument.

THINKING ABOUT RESEARCH

The need for nursing research and the current focus on evidence-based practice has been described above. Nursing research provides the evidence nurses need to evaluate the appropriateness of nursing practice, helps to raise new questions for nurses to explore, and provokes new ways of looking at what nurses do.

Nurses may relate to research in three ways. A nurse may be a 'consumer' of research, a researcher, or both. In this discussion, we will be focusing particularly on the role of research consumer.

It has already been argued that nurses must base their practice on high-quality evidence. The results of nursing research form the most significant source of this evidence for nurse practitioners. Nurses must avail themselves of the latest research in their area of practice and this means that some understanding of the process is important.

Every research project suffers from limitations and flaws of some sort or another. So nurses cannot take a research report and automatically assume that it provides them with the best guidance for practice. The nurse needs to think critically about research reports. Understanding a research report to be an argument assists in thinking critically about the conclusions it draws (Mayer & Goodchild 1995). Mayer and Goodchild (1995) discuss the way in which any research can be understood as an argument. Figure 17.6 illustrates this approach.

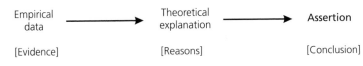

Fig. 17.6   Research represented as an argument.

Thinking critically about research

Given this understanding, it is possible to formulate a number of questions to help think critically about research:

(1) What is the assertion that is being made in the research report? What type of assertion is it? What type of evidence would be needed to be convinced of the truth of the assertion?

(2) What sort of evidence is offered to support the assertion being made? Is the evidence relevant to the assertion being made? Is adequate information provided to convince the reader that the evidence has been collected rigorously?

(3) Does the evidence offered provide adequate grounds for accepting the assertion that is being made? Is it possible to think of any other conclusions that could be drawn from the evidence offered? Are these alternative solutions more reasonable than the assertion made in the report?

(4) Does the theoretical explanation make sense? Are there alternative explanations that make more sense? Does the application of Occam's Razor (the principle that the simplest explanation is most likely to be the right one) make any difference to the likelihood of the explanation being correct?

Asking these questions in relation to any research report heightens one's awareness that the conclusions of research are not always correct, nor is the process in arriving at that conclusion automatically sound. This promotes a careful assessment of new nursing practice proposals and consequent higher levels of safety in practice.

THINKING ABOUT ETHICS

Another essential area of which nurses need to be aware is ethics. Thinking ethically means being able to justify what is done in terms of ethical principles. All behaviour needs to be ethical. Although there are high-profile issues such as euthanasia, abortion, and organ transplantation that demand a great deal of attention, they are, perhaps, not the most important issues for nurses.

Issues such as the style of communicating with a patient; the facilitation of the signing of a consent form; communication with other professional colleagues and patients; the management of work rosters; the provision of child care for employees; the influencing of clients in choosing treatment options – all need to be considered in ethical terms if the individual nurse is to practise with integrity and fulfil his or her obligations to clients.

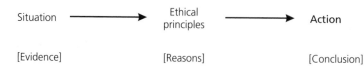

Fig. 17.7 Ethical thinking represented as an argument.

Most professional bodies have documented codes of ethics and the nursing profession is no different. For example, the *Code of Ethics for Nurses in Australia* (Australian Nursing Council Inc 1993) contains six value statements for nurses to 'use as a guide in reflecting on the degree to which their practice demonstrates the stated value.' As the Code points out, however:

> A Code of ethics is not intended to provide direction for the resolution of specific ethical dilemmas, nor can this document [the Code] adequately address the definitions and exploration of terms and concepts which are part of the study of ethics. Nurses are encouraged to undertake discussion and educational opportunities in order to clarify for themselves issues related to the fulfilment of their moral obligations.

Because of this, nurses need to develop skills to be able to think through these issues and evaluate various options for practice. Understanding ethical thinking as an argument can help in this task. Figure 17.7 illustrates the components of an ethical argument. Each of these components will now be examined in relation to critical thinking.

The situation

Ethical thinking is often taught using highly controversial case studies that involve an often unresolvable dilemma between competing principles. However, a number of false impressions may be gained from this. One possible false impression is that 'the continued use of controversial examples serves to exaggerate the extent to which morality, as distinct from moral theory, is controversial' (Coope 1996).

In reality, ethical thinking should pervade all activities, and ethical questions about practice should be continually asked. Ethical thinking should be an everyday activity, which may not always be about problems.

Usually, we find ourselves in situations where a decision needs to be made about how to act towards another person. These situations continually occur for nurses. For example, a patient might require a sponge in bed. This may not appear to be a situation where ethical thinking needs to take place. However, as this example is explored below, it will be seen that ethical thinking is fundamental to ensuring that the best care is provided.

The first thing to do when thinking ethically is to be aware of as much about the situation as is possible. Too often assumptions are made on the basis of past experience, but every person is different and has unique needs.

The principles

Everyone has a system of principles (values) that guide their lives and how they act. Some of these will be conscious; others may be unconscious. In health care, four principles have been identified as an essential starting point for ethical thinking. They are:

- Autonomy: the right a person has to direct their own life and make their own decisions.
- Beneficence: the responsibility of doing good.
- Non-maleficence: the responsibility to avoid doing harm.
- Justice: the responsibility to be fair in the way we treat others.

After gaining a knowledge of the situation, the next step is to ask which of the principles (values) are relevant to consider in the particular situation in which the nurse finds him- or herself. In the example of the person who needs to be washed in bed, the issue of autonomy is clearly relevant. How is autonomy to be ensured in this particular situation? How will patients be empowered to make their own decisions about their hygiene and the way they wish to maintain it?

The principle of beneficence is also relevant. The whole reason for instituting the patient-washing in bed is because it is believed it is good to promote hygiene. It is possible, however, that beneficence may spill over into a denial of the person's autonomy. When this happens, nurses are acting paternalistically – doing what they think is best for the patient – even if the patient does not agree with the nurse. Paternalism needs to be rigorously justified because it over-rides a person's fundamental right to autonomy.

Many examples can be found of situations where paternalism occurs: imposing medication on a psychotic individual; legally enforcing a blood transfusion for a child of a Jehovah's Witness parent. Unfortunately, on many occasions paternalistic attitudes prevail without adequate ethical justification.

Action

Once the situation is understood and the implications of the relevant ethical principles have been thought through, it is necessary to make a decision about how to act. Often this will not be easy. Sometimes ethical principles conflict with each other (such as when beneficence and autonomy conflict). Nurses do not live and practise in an ideal world, and so it is necessary to be satisfied with the best decision that can be made under the circumstances. The point is not that perfect decisions have to be made; that is never possible. It is rather that, whatever decisions are made and whatever actions are performed, they have been carefully thought through and can be justified by appeal to accepted ethical principles.

THE ETHICS OF CRITICAL THINKING

Often, when people learn the tools of critical thinking they become highly critical of others. It is important that critical thinking be viewed primarily as a set of tools applied to one's own thinking. When evaluating the ideas of others, critical thinking skills are used to decide whether an idea is acceptable or should be rejected. The identity of the other person is usually irrelevant. Furthermore, when critical thinking skills undermine or attack other people, then the purpose of critical thinking is lost. One of the most important distinctions to remember is that between an idea and the person who presents the idea.

The critical thinker always needs to think critically within the framework of well-developed interpersonal relationship skills. Critical thinking skills are not weapons to be wielded to cut another person down to size. They are tools of personal growth that allow one to travel through an often confusing landscape and keep one's bearings while providing the best possible quality care for those to whom one is responsible and accountable.

DEVELOPING CRITICAL THINKING SKILLS

There is no magical solution to actually developing critical thinking skills. An awareness of what critical thinking is and where it can be applied is an appropriate start. Like anything, it requires continual practice. Ultimately, it is about developing a conscious attitude of reflection during daily and professional life. Halpern (1998) suggests a number of attitudes and dispositions that support the development of critical thinking. They are: willingness to plan, flexibility, persistence, willingness to self-correct, being mindful ('the habit of self-conscious concern for and evaluation of the thinking process'), and consensus-seeking. As Halpern says:

> No one can become a better thinker just by reading a book. An essential component of critical thinking is developing the attitude and disposition of a critical thinker. Good thinkers are motivated and willing to exert the conscious effort needed to work in a planful manner, to check for accuracy, to gather information, and to persist when the solution is not obvious or requires several steps (pp. 10–11).

Although it is hard work to develop new skills in critical thinking, the time and energy are well worth the rewards that come with the ability to think clearly.

CONCLUSION

Critical thinking is a vital skill to have as a nurse. Nurses are engaged in providing care to people who have a right to high-quality professional conduct and health services. Nurses have a responsibility to make sure that their actions are based on rigorous evidence and can be justified with acceptable reasons. Although developing the skills to think critically may at times be difficult and demanding, thinking critically provides a greater level of confidence and satisfaction as nurses interact with colleagues, and it promotes high-quality, safe practice.

REFLECTIVE QUESTIONS

(1) How has your understanding of thinking changed as a result of reading this chapter?
(2) What areas of your professional life would benefit from applying the principles of critical thinking to them?
(3) What will you do now to further develop your skill in critical thinking?

RECOMMENDED READING

Bandman, E.L. & Bandman, B. (1998) *Critical Thinking in Nursing*, 2nd edn. Appleton & Lange, Norwalk, Connecticut.
Browne, M.N. & Keeley, S.M. (1998) *Asking the Right Questions*, 5th edn. Prentice Hall, Upper Saddle River, New Jersey.
Miller, A. & Babcock, D.E. (1996) *Critical Thinking Applied to Nursing*. Mosby, St Louis.
Paul, R.G. & Elder, L. (2001) *Critical Thinking: Tools for Taking Charge of your Learning and your Life*. Prentice Hall, Upper Saddle River, New Jersey.
Rubenfeld, M.G. (1995) *Critical Thinking in Nursing: an Interactive Approach*. J.B. Lippincott, Philadelphia.

REFERENCES

Australian Nursing Council Inc (1993) *Code of Ethics for Nurses in Australia*. ANCI, Canberra.
Coope, C.M. (1996) Does teaching by cases mislead us about morality? *Journal of Medical Ethics*, **22**(1), 46ff.
Govier, T. (1992) *A Practical Study of Argument*, 3rd edn. Wadsworth Publishing Company, Belmont, California.
Halpern, D.F. (1998) *Critical Thinking Across the Curriculum: A Brief Edition of Thought and Knowledge*. Lawrence Erlbaum Associates, Mahweh, New Jersey.
Jacobs, P.M., Ott, B., Sullivan, B., Ulrich, Y. & Short, L. (1997) An approach to defining and operationalizing critical thinking. *Journal of Nursing Education*, **36**(1), 19–22.
Mayer, R. & Goodchild, F. (1995) *The Critical Thinker*, 2nd edn. Brown & Benchmark Publishers, Madison.
Miller, M.A., & Babcock, D.E. (1996) *Critical Thinking Applied to Nursing*. Mosby, St Louis.
Paul, R. (1993) *Critical Thinking: How to prepare students for a rapidly changing world*. Foundation for Critical Thinking, Santa Rosa, California.
Ruggiero, V.R. (1998) *The Art of Thinking: A Guide to Critical and Creative Thought*, 5th edn. Longman, New York.
Schick, T.J., & Vaughn, L. (1995) *How to Think about Weird Things: Critical thinking for a new age*. Mayfield Publishing Company, Mountain View, California.

18 Writing Nursing, Writing Ourselves

Jennifer Greenwood

LEARNING OBJECTIVES

Upon completing this chapter the reader will be able to:

- distinguish 'thoughtful' from 'reflective' practice;
- describe the constituent elements of reflective practice and how they interrelate;
- discuss the three levels of reflectivity through which nurses can explore their practice;
- discuss the important benefits of systematic reflection;
- compare the benefits of written and verbal reflections.

KEY WORDS

REFLECTIVE PRACTICE, CLINICAL KNOWLEDGE, ANALYTICAL THINKING, JOURNALLING, ACTION, ACQUISITION OF SKILLS.

INTRODUCTION

Although it may not be obvious from the title, this chapter focuses on reflection and reflective practice. What should be obvious from the title, however, is that reflection, if it is to realise the considerable benefits that both I and a range of other scholars believe it should, hinges critically on *written* reflections. Why this is the case is discussed fully below. I hope to demonstrate clearly that it is through written reflections that we explore nursing and ourselves and identify ways to improve, reconstruct or reinvent nursing and ourselves.

The decision to omit the terms 'reflection' and 'reflective practice' from the title was a strategic one. Reflection has become 'commonplace' in nursing and nursing education (Cox *et al.* 1991; Hagland 1998; Hulatt 1995; Pierson 1998) and what might be construed as just another chapter to add to the already substantial literature on reflection and reflective practice might not engage the interest of readers to the degree I would like. Be assured, therefore, that although this chapter is, in a sense, just another piece on reflection, it is not *just* another piece. I sincerely hope readers will find it sufficiently stimulating to commence (or continue, for those who are already doing it) serious, systematic and disciplined reflective practice.

This chapter was first published in *Transitions in Nursing: Preparing for Professional Practice* (eds E. Chang & J. Daly), MacLennan & Petty Publishers, Sydney, Australia, 2001.

Overkill, therefore, is one reason why 'reflection' and 'reflective practice' are received unenthusiastically by nurses; there are, however, two other reasons. The first is that, generally speaking, these practices are poorly taught and supported (Foster & Greenwood 1998). The second is that nurses genuinely believe they are already reflective practitioners (Reid 1993). This chapter attempts to address both these issues. I argue that nurses are not reflective practitioners (at least, not as reflective practice is defined in this chapter) and I also provide some guidelines on how to go about learning to become seriously reflective. The chapter, therefore, includes some definitions of reflection, a comparison of thoughtful and reflective practice, some discussion on the benefits and risks associated with reflection and how to go about reflective journalling. Having read the chapter, I do hope readers will be enthusiastic advocates of reflection rather than cautious critics of it (Foster & Greenwood 1998).

WHAT IS REFLECTION?

John Dewey (1993) was the first philosopher to recognise the centrality of reflection in human thinking; he defined 'reflection' thus:

> Active, persistent, and careful consideration of any belief or supposed form of knowledge in the light of the grounds that support it and further conclusions to which it leads.
>
> Dewey (1993:9)

Boyd and Fales (1983) defined it slightly differently:

> The process of creating and clarifying the meaning of experience (present or past) in terms of self (self in relation to self and self in relation to the world). The outcome of the process is *changed conceptual perspective.*
>
> Boyd & Fales (1983:101)

By 'changed conceptual perspective' Boyd and Fales simply mean coming to see things differently. They make explicit what Dewey leaves implicit – that is, that serious reflection results in seeing things differently and it is this that differentiates *reflective* from *thoughtful* practice. Thoughtful practice is what every nurse inevitably engages in; all nurses think about or recall aspects of their practice. This 'thinking about' or recalling is spontaneous and goes on automatically. It does not necessarily lead to any changes in behaviour. Reflective practice, in contrast, requires that nurses learn from their reflections, revise their conceptual perspectives appropriately and act differently in future, as a result (Andrews 1996; Jarvis 1992).

Opinions differ with respect to the number of constituent elements of reflective practice. Schon (1983, 1987) considers there are two elements to it, namely, reflection-in-action and reflection-on-action.

Reflection-in-action means to think about what we are doing while we are doing it and it is usually stimulated by surprise, by something that puzzles the practitioner concerned. As practitioners try to make sense of the situation they confront, they ask themselves questions, such as: 'What features do I notice when I recognise … ?'

'What procedure am I enacting when I use this skill?' Thus they reflect on the under-standings that have been implicit in their actions, the feelings that led to the adoption of this particular course of action and the way they structured the problems initially; they bring all these to the surface, criticise them, restructure and embody them in further action. Reflection-in-action, therefore, serves to reshape what we are doing as we are doing it.

In contrast, reflection-on-action involves a cognitive postmortem (Greenwood 1993); practitioners look back on their experiences to explore again the understand-ings they brought to them in the light of their outcomes.

Van Manen (1990), Greenwood (1993) and Boud *et al.* (1985) disagree with Schon; they all consider that there are three constituents to reflective practice and they agree as to the nature of the third constituent. They all identify anticipatory reflection (Van Manen 1990), or reflection-before-action (Greenwood 1993), as a critically important component. This is because, in unfamiliar or problematic situations, intelligent pro-fessionals should think carefully (reflect) about what they intend to do and why they intend to do it before actually doing it. Reflection-before-action, therefore, should reduce human error.

What is it about the practice of nursing, discerning readers may ask, that requires reflective rather than merely thoughtful practitioners? Donald Schon (1983) provides the answer; he characterised all professional practices (which include nursing) as consisting of:

> a high hard ground overlooking a swamp. On the high ground, manageable problems lend themselves to solutions through the application of research-based theory and tech-nique. In the swampy lowland, messy, confusing problems defy technical solution.
>
> Schon (1983:3)

What Schon (1983) is referring to here are the two kinds of knowledge that inform professional practice. He argues that practice requires knowledge, which is derived from both sciences and from experience. (Prior to Schon, the scientific community recognised only scientifically derived knowledge as legitimate bases for practice. This 'technical rationality' view, as it was called, saw practice as merely the 'appli-ance of science'.)

To recognise that knowledge gained through experience is important in profes-sional practice is one thing; to render that knowledge explicit – that is, to articulate or express it – is, however, clearly another (Greenwood 1993). Knowledge gained simply through practical experience is notoriously difficult to articulate because it is constructed largely unconsciously as nurses go about their everyday nursing activities (Berry & Dienes 1993; Garnham & Oakhill 1994).

This knowledge is constructed by working with or alongside other nurses who already possess it; we generally term the gradual acquisition of this knowledge 'pro-fessional socialisation'. It includes, therefore, all the implicit beliefs, norms and values that characterise nursing. Thus, largely unconsciously, simply through engaging in repetitious everyday activities, nurses learn what to do, to whom, when, where, how, with what resources and with what end in view. Such knowledge is, as we say, *embed-ded* in their practice and becomes manifest, typically, only in practice. It is learned in practice and expressed in practice.

There is a very serious limitation to experiential knowledge, however, and it is this. Since nurses are not aware that they possess it, they are generally not aware when they are expressing it in their actions, nor are they aware of its relative appropriateness, in either technical or ethical terms, to the clinical situation in which it is being used. This is critically important in terms of therapeutic nursing practice because this everyday practical knowledge is, as its name implies, used in everyday practice – not infrequently, occasionally or sometimes – it is used *every day*. In terms of quality care, therefore, it is enormously important. For this reason alone, nurses should ensure that their everyday practical knowledge is therapeutic – that is, appropriate both technically and ethically. Reflective practice is a means of assisting them to do this.

Reflective practice enables nurses to explore their practice at three levels (Van Manen 1977). At the very least, it enables them to improve what they do, the technical aspects of their work – for instance, improving their aseptic dressing technique. It should also enable them to appreciate the theoretical or scientific bases of practice; for example, understanding the microbiological basis of aseptic technique. This is particularly important in a practice discipline where much of what is done is done because it has always been done that way or because senior colleagues prefer it that way (Waterman *et al.* 1995).

Lastly, and probably most importantly, it enables nurses to identify the sociopolitical and economic influences that govern the choices they make in clinical situations and the ways they behave in them. These influences include cultural norms, beliefs, values and the systems and structures in which they are institutionalised in health care. Kemmis and McTaggart (1988) suggest that these cultural norms, sociopolitical and economic influences find expression in the language we use, the activities we engage in and the social relationships we establish and maintain.

You may find it salutary to reflect on the different language used by different health professionals to describe their work with patients and clients. Physiotherapists, occupational therapists and social workers work *with* patients and clients. Nurses work *on* or *do* patients and clients ... 'I'm doing (beds) 11 to 16 today.' Equally salutary would be reflections on the activities undertaken as legitimate aspects of the role of different health care professionals. Allied health therapists and social workers will undertake serious patient/client assessment and care planning prior to initiating care. Consider how this differs from the typical activities of nurses. As to relationships, how often, for example, do nurses interrupt doctors on clinical rounds or in case conferences? Is the reverse true?

THE BENEFITS OF REFLECTION

Because reflection can proceed at these three progressively more sophisticated levels it results in some important benefits for nursing and for nurses themselves. Reflection helps nurses to:

- improve analytic thinking skills (Durgahee 1996; Kobert 1995);
- facilitate integration of theory and practice (Landeen *et al.* 1995; McCougherty 1991; Wong *et al.* 1995);

- develop individual theories of nursing, to influence practice and generate nursing knowledge (Emden 1991; Parker *et al.* 1995; Reid 1993);
- advance theory at a conceptual level to lead to changes at professional, social and political levels (Emden 1991; Smyth 1992, 1993);
- heighten the visibility of the therapeutic working of nurses (Johns 1994a, 1995);
- enable the monitoring of increasing effectiveness over time (Johns 1995; Landeen *et al.* 1995);
- explore and come to understand the nature and boundaries of their own role and that of other health professionals (Johns 1994a; Kobert 1995);
- come to an understanding of the conditions under which practitioners practise and, in particular, the barriers that limit practitioners' therapeutic potential (Emden 1991; Johns 1994a,b, 1995);
- accept professional responsibility (Johns 1994a, 1995);
- allow the generation of a knowledge base that is more comprehensive because it is directly tuned into what practitioners know about practice (Parker *et al.* 1995; Smyth 1992, 1993).

As well as construing reflection in terms of three levels, it can be construed as single- and double-loop; this is because it can result in single- and double-loop learning (Argyris *et al.* 1985). Single-loop reflection focuses on the effectiveness of the nursing action or intervention in light of its goal – that is, on how and why a nurse did what she or he did. Double-loop reflection focuses not only on the outcome(s) in light of goal(s) and plan(s) but also on the beliefs, norms, values and sociopolitical and economic influences that 'informed' the selection of the goals in the first place (Greenwood 1998a). The quotation marks surrounding 'informed' here are important. They imply that, although all selections/choices must necessarily be informed, much of this information is implicit; that is, the actor (nurse) is not aware of it.

HOW TO REFLECT

By now it should be obvious to readers that reflection, or the ability to reflect, is a sophisticated intellectual skill and is learned, like all such skills, through feedback-governed practice (Greenwood 1990). Aspirant reflective practitioners, therefore, require someone with whom they can share and explore their reflections and who can provide them with thoughtful and constructive feedback (Cox *et al.* 1991). Ideally, such a person will facilitate a progressively more double-loop orientation to reflection (see above) by focusing whenever possible on structural rather than individual influences on behaviour (Cox *et al.* 1991).

Similarly, the acquisition of the skills of reflection will be facilitated and expedited through the use of a reflective framework, typically constructed as a series of questions, to structure reflection. Again, and ideally, such a framework will be double-loop oriented. There are a number of such frameworks available in the literature – for example, Smyth (1989), Smith and Russell (1991), Burrows (1995) and Johns (1995). Figure 18.1 is a framework I have constructed; clearly, it has been informed by the work of these other scholars.

Level 1

What *exactly* did I do?
i.e. how, where, to whom, with what or whom?

To prepare the patient, carer, equipment, students, clinical environment (including communication with/involvement of other nurses/health professionals)
To implement the procedure, intervention
To monitor my ongoing performance
To complete the procedure, intervention (patient, carers, equipment, etc.)
To evaluate the effectiveness of the procedure, intervention, on its completion

Why did I do what I did?
Have I done this before?
When? Where? To whom, etc.?
Did I or did they behave or react the same?
— How do I feel about this?

What did I learn from this procedure, intervention?

What will I do differently next time?

Level 2

Why exactly did I do what I did?
What assumptions, beliefs, values, and attitudes do my actions express?
Are these consistent with those of therapeutic nursing?
— How do I feel about this?

What nursing and nursing-related theories and/or rituals and traditions informed my choices?
What have I learned from examining the rationale of my actions?
— How do I feel about this?
Why will I do things differently next time?

To prepare, implement, monitor, complete and evaluate the procedure, intervention

Level 3

What values, beliefs, cultural norms, sociopolitical and economic factors were influential in determining my choices?
Whose interests are served by these norms and influences?
— How do I feel about this?
— How might I minimise/obviate their influence in the future?
Who will be affected by these strategies?
What negative consequences are possible or problematic for me, for patients, for other nurses, other health professionals, etc. if I try to implement these minimising strategies?
— How can I minimise/obviate these?
— Whose assistance can I solicit?

Fig.   18.1 A framework for reflection.

Readers will note that Level 1 is exclusively single-loop in orientation, Level 2 is both single- and double-loop and Level 3 is exclusively double-loop. Importantly, however, all three levels include a consideration of how actions (and the possible consequences of actions in Level 3) might be adapted and improved in future. Such adaptations, therefore, are a result of reflection-on-action and it is these that should be included in a nurse's reflection-before-action when he or she confronts similar clinical situations in future.

REFLECTIVE JOURNALLING

I said in the introduction that I hoped to demonstrate clearly in this chapter that it is through written reflections that we explore nursing and ourselves and identify ways to improve nursing and ourselves; it is now appropriate to do this. I begin by outlining the benefits of journalling. It is important that readers consider these carefully since nurses are notoriously reluctant to journal. The reasons for this reluctance include nursing's oral culture (Corbett 1997), lack of time (Corbett 1997; Cox *et al.* 1991; Holly 1984; Wellard & Bethune 1996), and a passive resistance to exploring practice (Wellard & Bethune 1996). Some reflection on such passive resistance would be an extremely valuable exercise. We express our values and beliefs as much in the activities we do not undertake as in those we do.

The benefits of journalling:

- the imposition of order on what are often chaotic experiences (Cooper 1991; Kobert 1995);
- the bringing to light of connections and meanings that would otherwise remain hidden (Welty 1984);
- the clarification of ideas, perceptions and attitudes through writing them down (Cooper 1991);
- an appreciation of one's own role and influence in clinical situations (Kobert 1995);
- the exploration of culture, customs, history, values and beliefs, and their influence on self and others (Witherell 1991);
- the encouragement of an analytic approach to practice (Hagland 1998).

What this means, essentially, is that writing improves nurses' thinking skills. It is through writing that a nurse clarifies and elaborates her thoughts and ideas and notices patterns, regularities, gaps and inconsistencies (Greenwood 1998b; Lubinski 1990; Sorrell 1994). Nurses become more analytical (able to identify components and elements in relationships), more synthetical (able to reconfigure them in unfamiliar and innovative ways) and, thereby, more creative by writing (Van Manen 1990). In a beautifully written paper, Rolfe (1997) observes that we create ourselves through writing. This is because our thoughts, ideas and attitudes are, in an important sense, part of us. I would go further: through writing we create and recreate (reconstruct, reinvent) ourselves and nursing because the practice of nursing is merely the expression of the beliefs, values and attitudes that we as nurses possess. Journalling also provides the opportunity for catharsis and for dealing with difficult issues that we would prefer to avoid (Hodges 1996). Furthermore, of course, journalling, if it is done as systematically and carefully as it should be, assists nurses to express themselves more clearly and improve their writing skills.

A caution: there is a downside to journalling, too, which readers should be aware of. It can be emotionally painful to journal events that are largely self-critical (Conway 1994; Gray & Forsstrum 1991). This is why reflective practitioners should always search for structural or systematic influences on their work rather than concentrate on their own individual actions.

JOURNALLING

Serious journalling should always be undertaken in a quiet, undisturbed place and it should be done as soon as practicable after an interesting clinical event. By 'interesting', I mean an event that caused the nurse to reflect-in-action. Reflection-on-action very frequently focuses on nurses' prior reflections-in-action.

Only two rules govern journalling. The first relates to Spradley's (1980) verbatim principle and the second to his concrete principle. The *verbatim principle* enjoins nurses to record verbatim what people in the clinical (or other) situation said. (Recall, above, that Kemmis and McTaggart (1988) suggest that we express our beliefs and values, implicit as well as explicit, in our language as well as our practices.) Nurses do call their patients names like 'Smellie' and they do talk of 'doing' (rather than 'working with') patients … . Unless their language is recorded precisely as spoken, the implicit beliefs and values it expresses will not be identified (and, if they are not identified, they cannot be revised).

The *concrete principle,* similarly, enjoins nurses to use concrete language to describe situations and to provide as much precise detail as possible on what was seen, heard, smelled, felt, tasted, etc. This level of concrete detail adds depth and substance to an account and this is required if real insights about cultural meanings and norms are to be realised.

What Spradley's (1980) two principles indicate, rather obviously, is that what a nurse can get out of (i.e. learn from) journalling is directly proportional to what she puts into it by way of effort.

The size of a nurse's journal is merely a matter of individual preference. Some prefer small, pocket-sized notebooks that can be carried into clinical areas and important words or phrases (e.g. 'I'm going to <u>do</u> old <u>Smellie</u> now') jotted down for further elaboration later. Some prefer larger notebooks that are kept away from clinical areas (and away from the risk of loss and discovery by others).

Irrespective of the size of the journal, it is recommended all entries are dated (for repeated, subsequent analysis) and that only one page of a double-page spread is used for entries; the opposite page can then be used for comment, memos and analysis (Heath 1998; Holly 1984). Memos and repeated analyses are important learning tools; they help a nurse to see patterns and inconsistencies and to trace his or her own double-loop development.

Writing to reflect involves a cyclical pattern of reflection: first, reflecting on experiences before or as you write; and, then, reflecting on the journal entries themselves at some later stage, which may provide material for further reflection and writing, and so on (Holly 1984).

The insights a nurse can gain from reflection, in terms both of self-knowledge and knowledge about nursing, are gained primarily from *analysis* of reflections. Analysis may sound difficult, but it need not be. A relaxed mind will automatically notice regularities and patterns emerging in regular, detailed reflections. The same people may be involved, the same type of unit, the same language, the actions undertaken and their results might be the same. Importantly, too, the mere anticipation or expectation of actions and/or events, including your own, may serve to pre-empt situations.

'Unpacking' – that is, analysing antecedent and concurrent influences on these sorts of similarities – will allow you to see how they occur. You will then be in a position to prevent their recurrence by planning strategies to avoid them.

Analysis is assisted through writing memos; do write memos to yourself. If you generate a hunch about an event or a person, memo this: ('Is she uncomfortable dealing with people from non-English-speaking backgrounds?'). If you think certain values and beliefs could underpin certain utterances or behaviours, memo ... ('Why do I want to get all my patients showered by 10 AM, even when I know this is unnecessary?'). If you think you are beginning to discern connections between organisational structures and individual actions, memo this, too: ('Could qualitative research be getting "bashed" because most of the research experts on the research ethics committee are medical (quantitative) scientists?').

Analysis is also assisted through drawing diagrams. This allows you to represent situations and events pictorially; it is particularly helpful for analysing the causes (antecedents) and results (consequences) of actions and events. Figure 18.2 illustrates this; it would appear on the page opposite the detailed narrative of the event in your journal.

You will notice immediately that the consequences of cancelling the operations of three patients and, indeed, the cancelling of their operations, could easily have been avoided. You will also notice the amount of blaming that resulted; as yet, no one has asked what antecedents were contributory. Yet, clearly, rostering three new graduates on a late shift on an operation afternoon was excessive. In addition, allowing the nurse educator to attend an emergency meeting when senior RNs were off sick and leaving the unit to be staffed largely by inexperienced nurses, who would have required the nurse educator's advice and support, seems mistaken.

You will be surprised how much you will learn both about yourself and your clinical worlds through reflective analysis.

There is only one further aspect of journalling to deal with. It relates to what, in terms of both amount and nature, nurses should share from their journal with their reflective partner. There are no hard and fast rules here; it is entirely up to the journalling nurse. Decisions on how much and what to share will depend critically on the degree of trust that exists between them and their partner. Typically, however, they will start with relatively innocuous situations, where appraisal of their own performance is not overly negative; they will progress to more emotionally charged situations as trust develops.

There are three very useful strategies to facilitate the development of trust. The first is for both nurses to agree to be reflective partners for each other. This establishes the relationship as a reciprocal one where both share the benefits and risks equally.

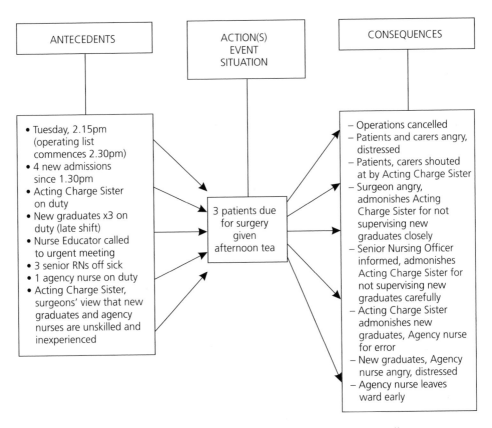

Fig.   **18.2** A 'diagram' of an event represents situations and events pictorially.

The second is to spend enough time together to allow the growth of trust. Regular reflective dialogues (e.g. at least once a month for an hour) should be arranged. The third is to contract formally on what will be reflected on, to what end and the degree of confidentiality of the information shared (Bond & Holland 1998).

CONCLUSION

All human language, actions and institutions implicitly express the beliefs, values and norms of cultures and subcultures. Such implicit beliefs and values are learned and exercised by cultural indigents (in our case, nurses) merely by engaging in repetitive, everyday activities; the acquisition of these beliefs and norms constitutes a person's socialisation.

Systematic and disciplined reflection enables nurses to examine the language, activities and social institutions that typify contemporary health care for evidence of these implicit beliefs and values. Through systematic reflection, they identify them and critically appraise their suitedness to therapeutic nursing. Where appropriate, they replace them with those more consistent with therapeutic nursing and plans to ensure their future expression in nursing care.

Written reflection is more valuable than verbal reflection. Through writing, nurses improve their thinking skills. Through writing they clarify and refine their beliefs and values and notice patterns and inconsistencies in language and activities (and, therefore, the beliefs and values that underpin them).

Reflective journalling should observe Spradley's (1980) verbatim and concrete principles and analysis is assisted through a set of reflective questions. Such questions, ideally, will promote double-loop as well as single-loop analysis and learning.

Single- and double-loop analysis is also assisted through the use of memos and diagrams. Both strategies encourage the development of nurses' analytic and synthetic thinking skills.

Through reflective writing, nurses 'discover' themselves and nursing (by 'discovering' their own beliefs and values and those that underpin nursing). Equally importantly, through writing they also recreate or reinvent themselves and nursing (by rejecting the inappropriate beliefs and values they 'discover' and replacing them with those more fitting to therapeutic nursing).

REFLECTIVE QUESTIONS

(1) When you are next having coffee or lunch with colleagues, ask them if they think they are reflective practitioners, and why. If necessary, explain to them the difference between thoughtful and reflective practice. Check that they understand.

(2) Think of an event or situation in your clinical practice that recently engaged your attention. Using the journalling guidelines and the framework for reflection provided in this chapter, record the event or situation and then analyse it through reflection levels 1, 2 and 3. (Allow yourself about an hour to do this.)

(3) Listen to the language your nursing colleagues typically use to describe patients/clients and the nursing care they routinely undertake. What sort of values does such language use reflect?

RECOMMENDED READING

Cox, H., Hickson, P. & Taylor, B. (1991) Exploring reflection: knowing and constructing practice. In: *Towards a Discipline of Nursing* (eds G. Gray & R. Pratt), pp. 373–390. Churchill Livingstone, Melbourne. (A beautifully written chapter on reflection from a critical social theory perspective.)

Foster, J. & Greenwood, J. (1998) Reflection: a challenging innovation for nurses. *Contemporary Nurse*, **7**, 165–172. (Elaborates on some of the challenges of introducing reflective practice into clinical areas.)

Greenwood, J. (1998) The roles of reflection in single- and double-loop learning. *Journal of Advanced Nursing*, **27**, 1048–1053. (This paper includes a description and a critique of Burrows, Johns and Smyth's reflective frameworks.)

Holly, M. (1984) *Keeping a Personal–Professional Journal*. Deakin University Press, Victoria. (See especially Parts 2 and 3 for some very practical guidelines on journalling.)

Wellard, S.J. & Bethune, E. (1996) Reflective journal writing in nurse education: whose interests does it serve? *Journal of Advanced Nursing*, **24**, 1077–1082. (A really interesting, alternative view on reflective practice.)

REFERENCES

Andrews, M. (1996) Using reflection to develop clinical expertise. *British Journal of Nursing*, **5**(8), 508–513.

Argyris, C., Putman, R. & Smith, D.M. (1985) *Action Science*. Jossey Bass, San Francisco.

Berry, D.C. & Dienes, Z. (1993) *Implicit Learning: Theoretical and Empirical Issues*. Lawrence Erlbaum Associates Ltd, Hove, Sussex.

Bond, M. & Holland, S. (1998) *Skills of Clinical Supervision for Nurses: A Practical Guide for Supervisees, Clinical Supervisors and Managers*. Open University Press, Buckingham.

Boud, D., Keogh, R. & Walker, D. (1985) Promoting reflection in learning: a model. In: *Reflection: Turning Experience into Learning* (eds D. Boud, R. Keogh & D. Walker), pp. 18–40. Kogan Page, London.

Boyd, E.M. & Fales, A.W. (1983) Reflective learning: a key to learning from experience. *Journal of Humanistic Psychology*, **23**(2), 99–117.

Burrows, D.E. (1995) The nurse teacher's role in the promotion of reflective practice. *Nurse Education Today*, **15**(5), 346–350.

Conway, J. (1994) Reflection, the art and science of nursing and the theory-practice gap. *British Journal of Nursing*, **3**(3), 114–118.

Cooper, J.E. (1991) Telling our own stories: the reading and writing of journals or diaries. In: *Stories Lives Tell* (eds C. Witherell & N. Noddings), pp. 96–112. Teachers College Press, New York.

Corbett, N.A. (1997) *Writing a Journal: A Strategy for Lifelong Learning as a Reflective Practitioner*. Proceedings of the 1st International Conference on Correcting Conversations: Nursing Scholarship and Practice, Reykjavik, Iceland, 20–22 June 1995.

Cox, H., Hickson, P. & Taylor, B. (1991) Exploring reflection: knowing and constructing practice. In: *Towards a Discipline of Nursing* (eds G. Gray & R. Pratt), pp. 373–390. Churchill Livingstone, Melbourne.

Dewey, J. (1993) *How we Think*. Regnery, Chicago.

Durgahee, T. (1996) Reflective practice: linking theory and practice in palliative care nursing. *International Journal of Palliative Nursing*, **2**(1), 22–25.

Emden, C. (1991) Becoming a reflective practitioner. In: *Towards a Discipline of Nursing* (eds G. Gray & R. Pratt), pp. 335–354. Churchill Livingstone, Melbourne.

Foster, J. & Greenwood, J. (1998) A challenging innovation for nurses. *Contemporary Nurse*, **7,** 165–172.

Garnham, A. & Oakhill, J. (1994) *Thinking and Reasoning*. Blackwell Publishers, Oxford.

Gray, J, & Forsstrum, S. (1991) Generating theory from practice: the reflective technique. In: *Towards a Discipline of Nursing* (eds G. Gray & R. Pratt), pp. 355–372. Churchill Livingstone, Melbourne.

Greenwood, J. (1990) *Learning to care: thought and action in the education of nurses*. Unpublished PhD thesis. Leeds University.

Greenwood, J. (1993) Reflective practice: A critique of the work of Argyris and Schon. *Journal of Advanced Nursing*, **19**, 1183–1187.

Greenwood, J. (1998a) The role of reflection in single- and double-loop learning. *Journal of Advanced Nursing*, **27**, 1048–1053.

Greenwood, J. (1998b) The write advice, or how to get a journal article published. *Contemporary Nurse*, **7**(2), 81–90.

Hagland, M.R. (1998) Reflection: a reflex action. *Intensive and Critical Care Nursing*, **3**, 96–100.

Heath, H. (1998) Keeping a reflective practice diary: a practice guide. *Nurse Education Today*, **18**, 592–598.

Hodges, F. (1996) Journal writing as a mode of thinking for RN-BSN students: a leveled approach to learning to listen to self and others. *Journal of Nursing Education*, **35**(3), 137–141.

Holly, M. (1984) *Keeping a Personal-Professional Journal*. Deakin University Press, Victoria.

Hulatt, I. (1995) A sad reflection. *Nursing Standard*, **8**(9), 22–24.

Jarvis, P. (1992) Reflective practice and nursing. *Nurse Education Today*, **12**(3), 174–181.

Johns, C. (1994a) Nuances of reflection. *Journal of Clinical Nursing*, **3**, 71–75.

Johns, C. (1994b) Guided reflection. In: *Reflective Practice in Nursing: The Growth of the Professional Practitioner* (eds A. Palmer, S. Burns & C. Bulman), pp. 110–129. Blackwell Scientific, Oxford.

Johns, C. (1995) Framing learning through reflection within Carper's fundamental ways of knowing in nursing. *Journal of Advanced Nursing*, **22**, 226–234.

Kemmis, S. & McTaggart, R. (1988) *The Action Research Planner*, 3rd edn. University Press, Geelong.

Kobert, L.J. (1995) In our own voices: journalling as a teaching/learning technique for nurses. *Journal of Nursing Education*, **34**(3), 140–142.

Landeen, J., Byrne, C. & Brown, B. (1995) Journal keeping as an educational strategy in teaching psychiatric nursing. *Journal of Advanced Nursing*, **17**, 347–355.

Lubinski, J. (1990) Reflective withdrawal through journal writing. In: *Fostering Critical Reflection in Adulthood: A Guide to Transformative and Emancipatory Learning* (ed J. Mezirow), pp. 213–234. Jossey Bass, San Francisco.

McCougherty, D. (1991) The theory-practice gap in nurse education: its causes and possible solutions. Findings from an action research study. *Journal of Advanced Nursing*, **16**, 1055–1061.

Parker, D.L., Webb, J. & D'Souza, B. (1995) The value of critical incident analysis as an educational tool and its relationship to experiential learning. *Nurse Education Today*, **15**(2) 111–116.

Pierson, W. (1998) Reflection and nursing education. *Journal of Advanced Nursing*, **27**, 165–170.

Reid, B. (1993) But we're doing it already! Exploring a response to the concept of reflective practice in order to improve its facilitation. *Nurse Education Today*, **13**, 305–309.

Rolfe, G. (1997) Writing ourselves: creating knowledge in post modern world. *Nurse Education Today*, **17**, 442–448.

Schon, D.A. (1983) *The Reflective Practitioner*. Basic Books, New York.

Schon, D.A. (1987) *Educating the Reflective Practitioner*. Jossey Bass, San Francisco.

Smith, A. & Russell, J. (1991) Using critical incidents in nurse education. *Nurse Education Today*, **11**(4), 284–291.

Smyth, J. (1989) Developing and sustaining critical reflection in teacher education. *Journal of Teacher Education*, **40**(2), 2–9.

Smyth, J. (1992) Teachers' work and the politics of reflection. *American Education Research Journal*, **29**(2), 267–300.

Smyth, J. (1993) Reflective practice in teacher education and other professions. Key address to the *Fifth National Practicum Conference*, Macquarie University, Sydney.

Sorrell, J.M. (1994) Writing as inquiry. In qualitative nursing research: elaborating the web of meaning. In: *Advances in Methods of Inquiry for Nursing* (ed. P. Chinn), pp. 1–12. Gaithersbury, Maryland, Aspen.

Spradley, J.P. (1980) *Participant Observation*. Holt, Rinehart & Winston, New York.

Van Manen, M. (1977) Linking ways of knowing with ways of being. *Curriculum Inquiry*, **6**(3), 205–28.

Van Manen, M. (1990) *The Tact of Teaching: The Meaning of Pedagogical Thoughtfulness*. University of New York Press, New York.

Waterman, H., Webb, C. & Williams, A. (1995) Parallels and contradictions in the theory and practice of action research and nursing. *Journal of Advanced Nursing*, **22**, 779–784.

Wellard, S.J. & Bethune, E. (1996) Reflective journal writing in nurse education: whose interests does it serve? *Journal of Advanced Nursing*, **24**, 1077–1082.

Welty, E. (1984) *One Writer's Beginnings*. Harvard University Press, Cambridge, Massachusetts.

Witherell, C. (1991) The self in narrative: a journey into paradox. In: *Stories Lives Tell* (eds C. Witherell & N. Noddings). Teachers College Press, New York.

Wong, F.K.Y., Kember, D., Chung, L.Y.F. & Yan, L. (1995) Assessing the level of student reflection from reflection journals. *Journal of Advanced Nursing*, **22**, 48–57.

19 Maximising Learning Opportunities and Preparing for Professional Practice

Martin Johnson, Jane Conway
and Margaret McMillan

LEARNING OBJECTIVES

Upon completing this chapter the reader should be able to:

- appreciate the interaction between university-based learning activities and clinical practice;
- consider strategies that maximise learning opportunities in a range of contexts;
- view themselves as autonomous, action-oriented learners;
- appreciate the interaction between lifelong learning and professional development;
- develop strategies to address self development.

KEY WORDS

TRANSITION, GRADUATE, ACCOUNTABILITY, LIFELONG LEARNING, CURRICULUM, CLINICAL EDUCATION, FACILITATOR.

INTRODUCTION

Registered nurses have diverse roles and functions that will vary according to the setting or client group cared for.

Among functions or roles undertaken by nurses are the following:

- clinician;
- care coordinator;
- counsellor;
- health educator;
- patient/client advocate;
- change agent;
- clinical teacher;
- mentor/assessor.

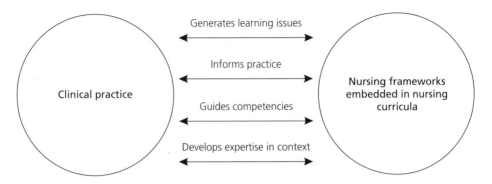

Fig. 19.1   The interrelationship between practice and curriculum in nursing programmes.

In this text Chapters 1 and 13 review key concepts underlying nursing practice and the regulatory and professional framework for nursing. This chapter is based on the belief that the transition from student to graduate and practitioner requires the development of the ability to examine critically our own and others' practice and be accountable for our actions. These abilities are often linked to the idea of being a lifelong learner (Maslin-Prothero 2001; UKCC 1999) and are seen as increasingly important to professional nursing practice in the twenty-first century (Clark *et al.* 1997). We recognise that, for many student nurses, clinical practice is the goal of nursing education. However, as we will show, the principles that underpin learning in the clinical area and in the university setting are transferable across contexts.

The role of the professional nurse has changed from being a person who practised modified medicine to a person who appreciates the dynamic and evolving nature of nursing and is able to use the skills of inquiry, critical thinking, problem solving and reflective practice. Clinical practice provides the stimulus for students and practitioners alike to use these skills in order to recognise best practice and, if necessary, enhance and modify existing practice. This chapter is designed to encourage students to view clinical and on-campus learning as one entity. Figure 19.1 depicts the interrelationship between clinical practice and the nursing-specific frameworks embedded in nursing curricula and indicates that clinical activity and on-campus learning are interdependent.

WHAT IS CLINICAL PRACTICE?

Clinical practice is the part of the student's learning where she or he experiences, usually with the help of a mentor or clinical educator, the 'real' world of nursing practice. The role of the student ranges from being observer of others' practice to demonstrating competence and confidence in professional practice situations.

Nursing programmes globally recognise that the clinical area is an important, if not the most important, area for practice professions such as nursing (Melia 1987; UKCC 1999), and the value of clinical experience to nursing practice, and hence to nursing students, cannot be over-emphasised. Definitions of clinical teaching and learning invariably include some notion that clinical practice is the place where students apply theory in practice (White & Ewan 1991), or where contradictions between theory and practice, and nursing and educational values, are highlighted (Melia 1987). It is, in fact, where students begin to develop professional identities as nurses.

In writing about the development of registered nurses, Benner (1984) has identified that the ability to integrate theory and practice to the point of being able to generalise is essential to development from novice (newly qualified nurse) to later and more advanced levels of nursing. However, Benner also acknowledges that there are particular challenges in being able to transfer concepts across contexts. Effective clinicians are aware that *context* is the crucial moderator in nursing practice, and have developed mechanisms for managing situations contextually rather than seeking to manage all situations in the same way. Such ability to transfer core concepts across situations and modify actions according to context is an indication of 'expert' nursing practice (Benner 1984). Clinical learning experiences provide nursing students with the opportunity to begin to develop the skills of identifying general principles of practice, transferring these across contexts, and modifying actions based on principles of management.

The Peach Report (UKCC 1999) argued that education programmes in the UK, although generally sound, did not provide enough opportunity to integrate classroom theory into 'real life' practice situations. As a result newly registered nurses and their employers felt that a greater emphasis on early practical experiences linked directly to theory would render newly qualified nurses more 'fit for purpose'. A good deal of work has been undertaken adjusting programmes and increasing the early exposure of students to practice to 'make a difference'. From the students' point of view this should reduce the stress of feeling insufficiently skilled to offer a useful contribution to the clinical setting.

Experiential knowledge is not merely being exposed to an experience. It is that which emerges when the experience is structured to achieve learning as an outcome of the experience. Therefore, students should use the theoretical base developed from university-based activities to frame the clinical experience so that learning, rather than merely experiencing, occurs. Students should ask themselves 'What is it that I want to achieve from this learning experience and how does this relate to my ability to practise nursing?'

I WANT TO NURSE … WHY DO I NEED ALL THIS THEORY?

While clinical experience clearly is a powerful motivator for students to learn *how to* nurse, the literature suggests that clinical experiences are an important part of the transfer of learning from the classroom to the practice setting (Seed 1994; White & Ewan 1991). Thus, *how* we think about nursing practice shapes *what* we learn from practice.

Being a nurse requires the ability to integrate the knowledge, skills and attitudes of nursing into who we are and how we practise (Thorne & Hayes 1997).

Clinical educators, university lecturers and clinicians often declare that they have a shared goal of ensuring quality education for nursing students. However, each of these sectors of the nursing community have what, at times, may seem to students to be very different definitions of nursing.

Much of this perceived lack of alignment between the education and health service sectors in relation to the goals of nursing education has been put down to what students and clinicians may hear described as the theory/practice gap. Nursing education has the important goal to assist people to *be* nurses. Being a nurse requires the ability to do nursing activity, to think about nursing, and to communicate that thinking to others.

There is an essential tension in nursing education between what practice is and what practice could be. Benner put this quite well as follows: "'knowing *that*" and "knowing *how*" are two different kinds of knowledge'. By this she seems to mean that in an applied discipline like nursing, knowledge development consists of extending practical knowledge (know-how) through theory-based scientific investigations (Benner 1984 p. 2–3). As both the guardians and visionaries of nursing's future, it is important that students be given the opportunity to develop the skills to evaluate critically existing nursing practice and to create and consider alternatives to this from the increasing evidence base of research-based knowledge.

The overarching structure of all nursing courses is the nursing curriculum, which determines both the content, the outcomes that should be achieved and the processes by which this should be achieved. Nursing education programmes in the UK and Europe provide students with opportunities to practise the skills of nursing, to develop and demonstrate their knowledge base about nursing, and to acquire academic skills that support communication of their thinking about nursing.

The curriculum should cause students to think about what they do as nurses, why they do what they do, and how they might do it differently. For this reason it is important that the nursing curriculum raises theory-related questions like: 'What is nursing?', 'What does it mean to nurse?', 'Whom do nurses nurse?', 'Where do nurses nurse?', 'Is nursing the same as caring?' and so on, as well as helping students to learn the task-oriented content of how to nurse.

Thinking about nursing needs to both direct and emerge from practice, and it is not our intention to give the impression that qualified nurses should think only about nursing. The goal of nursing programmes is to develop registered nurses who can apply concepts to practice, manage complex nursing situations, and accept accountability for practice. Of course, this demands skills in doing nursing activities. However, we believe that students should be aware that nursing is about the ability to analyse situations and respond appropriately. How we interpret and analyse situations depends upon how we think about them. As our thinking about nursing develops, the meaning we give to situations changes and learning occurs. We then take this learning with us to the next situation and create new meanings and new knowledge. Figure 19.2 demonstrates the continual process of situation deconstruction, analysis and reconstruction essential to professional practice and the development of knowledge.

HOW CAN I BEST DEVELOP NEW KNOWLEDGE?

In order to learn we need to develop the process skills for lifelong learning (Maslin-Prothero 2001). These process skills are the basis of learning and are transferable across disciplines. In the case of nursing, nursing knowledge provides specific

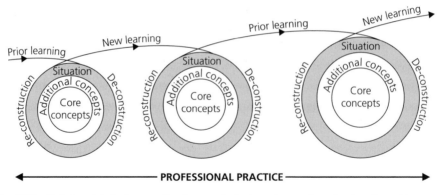

Fig. 19.2 Relationship between situation analysis, learning and professional practice.

content which, when processed, results in nursing action. That is to say, when we become nurses we have developed general learning skills and we demonstrate our use of these through being able to 'think and act like a nurse'. In order to be lifelong learners in relation to nursing practice, we need to become what has been termed 'reflective practitioners'. We need to reflect about what we do as nurses, how we respond as nurses and individuals, and what we would do again in a similar situation. We then need to act when a similar situation occurs. The skills of reflective practice unite university and clinical learning.

In Fig. 19.3 Gibbs (1988) provides a useful framework for situation analysis that is both thought- and action-oriented.

Classroom-based learning activity provides us with the opportunity to explore safely what we know, what we do and how we are as nurses so that we are more prepared for professional practice situations. Clinical learning activity provides us with the opportunity both to test out what we have learnt in practice and to confront new situations from which we can further our learning. However, we can only learn

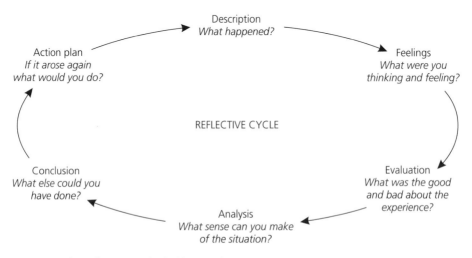

Fig. 19.3 The reflective cycle (Gibbs 1988).

if we are prepared to do so. It is important that we value learning as much as we value what we have learnt. It is our ability to question ourselves and our practice that enhances our professional development.

Little (1996) has developed a framework of questions that are applicable in both classroom and clinical learning situations. These questions provide a useful guide to developing lifelong learning skills, yet are equally important questions for clinical decision making. The framework recognises that learning is inherently a personal experience and places emphasis on the subjective nature of learning. In order to be accountable for their practice, nurses need to become subjectively engaged in that practice.

Little's approach consists of the following questions.

About situation/analysis or decision making

- What information do I have?
- What further information do I need?
- What options/alternatives do I have?
- What should I prioritise?
- What action/s should I take?
  - Why?
- Can I justify this action (lawfully, ethically, effectively, theoretically, etc.)?

About the learning process

- What do I already know?
- How do I know it?
- What do I need to know?
- Where will I find it?
- What resources can I use?
- How will I know I know?
- Why should I learn it?

About perceptions

- What are my feelings?
- What are my beliefs about the situation?
- What are my assumptions?
- How have I derived these beliefs/assumptions?
- How do my feelings/beliefs
  - affect my interpretation?
  - affect my response?
  - relate to espoused professional values?
- Why do I hold this belief/assumption?
- What are alternative beliefs/assumptions?

About my learning

- What is the validity of my source?
  - Legislation
  - Data based on research
  - Opinion

- Practice
- Expertise
- Experience
- What is the currency of the knowledge, skills, behaviour?
- What is the support for this view?
  - Political/ideological
  - Cultural
- What other ideas/concepts/skills does it relate to?
- How does it relate to my view of the world (current understanding)?

About the situation revisited
- How does my learning relate to/apply in this situation?
- How does my learning relate to/affect my original ideas?
- What gaps/misconceptions did my learning identify?
- What ideas/skills did my learning confirm?
- What response would I give now in the situation?

About reflection
- On situation analysis:
  - How well did I use the data?
  - How well did I define the situation in need of a response?
  - How comprehensive were my alternatives?
  - How well can I justify my response?
- On the learning process:
  - How valid/relevant were my sources?
  - How comprehensive were my sources?
  - How effective was my learning?
- On group process:
  - How well did I contribute?
  - What was my role in the group?
  - How effective was each member's contribution?
  - Did the group remain on task?
  - Did the group attend to process, i.e. how people were feeling/responding/behaving, etc.?

This framework of questions is useful because it encourages us to look at situations in context and to appreciate that, as learners and professionals who make sound clinical judgments, we are required to interact effectively with others, provide reasoning and support for our actions and decisions, and be aware that we are accountable for our own learning and practice actions.

Whilst both Gibbs' and Little's frameworks are relevant to a number of practice disciplines, including nursing, there is potential for nurses selectively to utilise the 'learning' components of models such as these and to overlook the critical elements related to action. Ultimately, professional accountability is related to actions, not a capacity to generate ideas. Although theory is important, because it provides a framework for the work nurses do, it is of little consequence unless it results in effective nursing actions. Conversely, practice can become meaningless unless we seek to

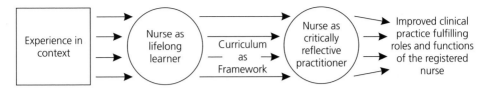

Fig. 19.4   An educational equation for improved nursing practice.

understand it through theories. Such integration of theory and practice leads to our moving beyond *becoming* nurses to *being* nurses who integrate our knowing, doing and being to produce what is known as praxis. Being reflective practitioners means that we are, both personally and professionally, constantly transformed and emancipated from our previous ways of thinking and acting (Freire 1972; Mezirow 1985).

We agree that the goal of nursing education is to prepare nurses:

> to be more responsive to societal needs, more successful in humanizing the highly technological milieus of health care, more caring and compassionate, more insightful about ethical and moral issues, more creative, more capable of critical thinking and better able to bring scholarly approaches to client problems and issues and to advocate ethical positions on behalf of clients
>
> Bevis & Watson (1989:1)

and are concerned that the attitude that clinical and classroom learning are separate entities may result in the mistaken perception that there is an insurmountable division between the theoretical and practical aspects of nursing. Students of nursing need to be encouraged to develop skills in reflective practice and situation analysis, not for the purpose of intellectualising or rationalising nursing practice but for the purpose of identifying and maintaining excellence in clinical practice and meeting the goals of nursing identified above by Bevis and Watson.

Figure 19.4 represents what we perceive to be the relationships between context and lifelong learning processes and curriculum and improved practice.

GAINING THE MOST FROM CLINICAL AND CLASSROOM LEARNING

Commonly, when nursing students, qualified nurses and their employers are asked to evaluate nursing education, they feel that the time in clinical placements was inadequate and suggest that there needs to be an increase in clinical time (UKCC 1999). However, it may well be that an increase in *quality* of the clinical experience is preferable to an increase in *quantity* of clinical placements (Barnard & Dunn 1994). We believe that while clinical educators, lecturers and unit staff share in structuring the clinical experience, students are also accountable for ensuring that they gain a quality clinical experience. This accountability for self-learning links closely with the principles of adult learning and ongoing professional development (Maslin-Prothero 2001).

Chun-Heung and French (1997) report that, despite the emphasis on skills such as critical thinking, problem solving and reflective practice in on-campus learning experiences, in clinical settings students are encouraged to operate routinely and are not challenged to reflect upon their practice in a way that creates intellectual challenge. Each student has a responsibility to integrate on-campus learning and clinical experiences, and should seek intellectual challenge. A useful framework for this can be reflective practice models discussed earlier.

In order to gain the most out of learning experiences it is important that each experience be approached as a way of linking theory and practice, and as an opportunity for further learning and generation of new perspectives. The role of the registered nurse is increasingly one of health care facilitator/manager as well as direct caregiver. Andersen's model identifies a number of nursing roles that students should explore while in the clinical setting. At the very least, students need to think about how these roles and functions that registered nurses perform have shaped, and been shaped by, the situation.

Nursing students should explore roles other than direct caregiver during university learning and clinical placements. In Europe nursing programmes are required to include a range of clinical settings (e.g. mental health, obstetrics, acute care and the community). However, it is unclear whether students are encouraged to explore a range of nursing roles and functions while in those settings. In order to prepare for the diversity of practice, students themselves should analyse each situation and try to determine what nursing roles and competencies are applicable.

Figure 19.5 presents an adaptation of Andersen's (1991) roles and functions model, which delineates the domain of registered nurse (RN) practice from enrolled nurse (EN) and health care support worker (HCSW) or auxiliary nurse roles and functions.

WHO CAN ASSIST ME IN MY PERSONAL AND PROFESSIONAL DEVELOPMENT?

To maintain effectiveness as clinicians, nurses need to learn continually from a range of situations. In order to achieve this, it is essential that someone facilitate their learning towards *nursing* outcomes. Learners often seek, indeed need, external support, guidance and assessment (Brennan & Hunt 2001, Maslin-Prothero 2001). Thus the clinical educator, the university lecturing staff and other personnel can provide feedback and support to students or peers.

Gaining the most from clinical practice

The nurse lecturer in the practice setting and the clinical educator have been reported to fulfil many roles which seemingly mirror the roles of nurses including practitioner, administrator, teacher, counsellor, problem solver, manager, assessor, advocate, guide and facilitator (White & Ewan 1991, Maslin-Prothero & Owen 2001).

The current trend in education to view educators as 'facilitators' rather than 'givers' of learning has been well recognised in nursing education literature. It implies that nurses as educators are increasingly adopting a more student-centred, collaborative

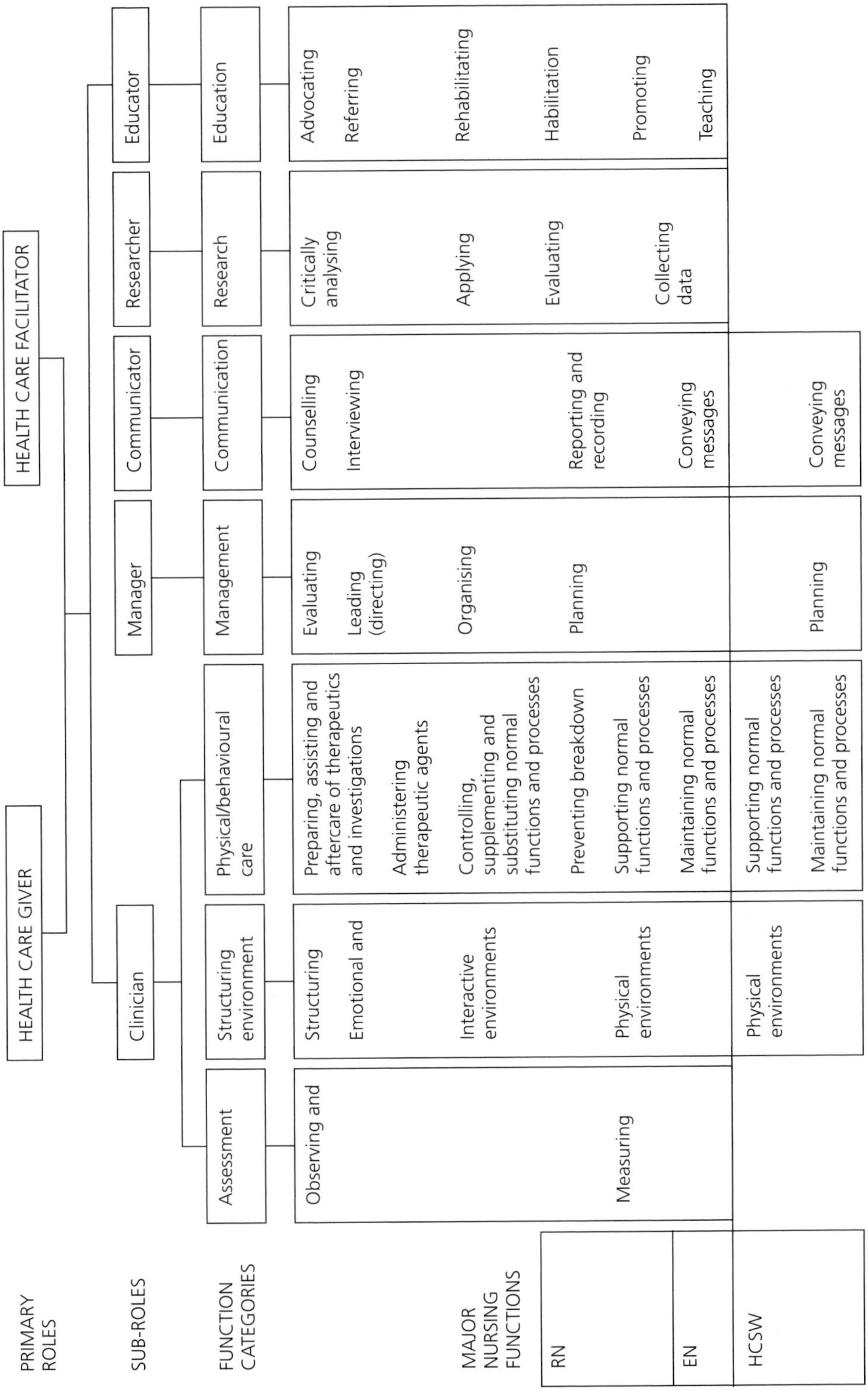

PRIMARY ROLES

- HEALTH CARE GIVER
- HEALTH CARE FACILITATOR

SUB-ROLES

- Clinician
- Manager
- Communicator
- Researcher
- Educator

FUNCTION CATEGORIES

- Assessment
- Structuring environment
- Physical/behavioural care
- Management
- Communication
- Research
- Education

Assessment
- Observing and
- Measuring

Structuring environment
- Structuring Emotional and
- Interactive environments
- Physical environments
- Physical environments

Physical/behavioural care
- Preparing, assisting and aftercare of therapeutics and investigations
- Administering therapeutic agents
- Controlling, supplementing and substituting normal functions and processes
- Preventing breakdown
- Supporting normal functions and processes
- Maintaining normal functions and processes
- Supporting normal functions and processes
- Maintaining normal functions and processes

Management
- Evaluating
- Leading (directing)
- Organising
- Planning
- Planning

Communication
- Counselling
- Interviewing
- Reporting and recording
- Conveying messages
- Conveying messages

Research
- Critically analysing
- Applying
- Evaluating
- Collecting data

Education
- Advocating
- Referring
- Rehabilitating
- Habilitation
- Promoting
- Teaching

MAJOR NURSING FUNCTIONS

- RN
- EN
- HCSW

Fig. 19.5 Nursing roles and functions model.

model of education which views nursing as a client-centred mutual interaction. More-over, the nurse as educator needs to model the way students or peers are expected to approach learning, as well as modelling exemplary nursing practice.

Clinical experiences provide the opportunity for students to observe and par-ticipate in nursing practice. Inherent in the notion of effective practice is the ability to make sound clinical judgments based on assessments and reassessments, to col-laborate with others, to provide meaningful feedback to colleagues about perform-ances, and to establish and maintain professional relationships. Clinical experiences acclimatise students to the real world of practice and its culture. Not all these experi-ences may seem positive and it important to be prepared to cope with difficult staff as well as 'difficult' patients.

For example, Seed (1994) undertook a longitudinal study of the experiences of one cohort of 'general' student nurses. She worked with each student at least once on each placement. Although the students gained much from experience in practice, not all of this was easy learning. Sometimes they felt, as Melia (1987) had also noted in her interviews with 40 students a decade or so earlier, that qualified staff often kept information about patients to themselves, which made caring for individuals more difficult and stressful.

One of Seed's respondents was a student nurse (Lillian) who said:

> Well, the trained staff keep it to themselves. At first I thought I didn't know because I was ignorant, then I thought they weren't teaching me the right things in school. But really it's that people like to keep things to themselves. It doesn't make my job very easy.
>
> Seed (1994:742)

Despite a good deal of change over the years in the design and location of courses, studies have consistently found that nursing programmes can seem like a series of obstacles to be overcome. Nursing can be hard. On the lighter side, however, col-leagues, senior staff and the patients themselves can ease the strain by balancing professionalism with humour. During her research, Seed found a 'lot of laughing and joking going on' (p. 743) which is explained by student nurse Chris, who has been preparing a female patient for a gynaecological operation: 'We use it to relieve the tension I suppose. There's something about gynae patients, perhaps because you're all women and they tend to be younger … I would say there's more camaraderie.'

Humour is just one of the more informal strategies used to deal with the 'emotional labour' of caring. Smith and Gray (2001), updating earlier work Smith had done into the concept of emotional labour experienced by students, focus on the students' relationship with their 'mentor' as a way of learning constructively from clinical ex-perience. Strategies of this kind include 'frequent high quality liaison between the student nurse, mentor, link lecturer and other members of staff'. Others might include sharing experiences with peers and maintaining a life unrelated to day-to-day nurs-ing experiences to retreat to.

As Seed, Melia and others have found, there sometimes remains a tension be-tween the students' need to learn and the need to provide care. Specifically, we have observed that students and clinicians in the clinical setting are often confused about when students should be observing another's practice and when they should be actively participating in the provision of client care. Understandably, students and clinicians alike want to seize what they perceive to be limited practice learning opportunities and may, with the very best of intentions, place themselves and the client at risk. Our advice would be for the student to be sure of the core objectives and concepts of the clinical placement, to determine the relationship between these goals and the activity to be performed, and to seek advice from the clinical educator or link lecturer about the scope of the student's practice while in the clinical setting. When students are invited to perform care that they do not feel comfortable with, they might tell the qualified nurse that they are too busy or have other things to do. Sometimes the nurse, who has made an effort to give the student a meaningful learning experience, may interpret this response as uninterest in nursing. In situations such as these, we would suggest that students recognise the nurse's offer as being meant to enhance their learning. The student should explain their situation to the senior nurse on duty, confirm that the qualified nurse is ultimately responsible for the client's care and engage in the activity as far as possible.

Gaining the most from on-campus learning

We have already made substantial reference to the necessity to use university-based learning to frame clinical learning, and *vice versa*. Classroom learning provides opportunities to explore options and alternatives, to justify thinking and to learn from examples drawn from practice. It also gives students opportunities to develop the 'scholarly approaches' referred to by Bevis and Watson (1989:1).

In our experience, it is essential to be able to access, retrieve and use information from reputable sources, to draw conclusions about implications of ideas for nursing practice, and to communicate these in writing. Increasingly nursing programmes are integrating these skills into the core nursing programme and instructing students in information literacy and writing skills.

Universities provide what have been termed 'learning skills units' to provide additional support to all students. These units provide generic assistance to students in a number of ways, ranging from short courses to individual consultations. Most universities offer a variety of courses to assist in essay writing, including analysing and interpreting questions, planning, structuring and writing essays, referencing; and assistance with mathematics for drug calculations. Students also benefit from spending time with the librarian, learning how to use the library effectively, to conduct literature searches, and use databases to access resources.

While we encourage the use of these support services, we would caution students that they do not provide discipline-specific information. That is to say, staff of these units can assist you in structuring your writing, ensure your grammar and punctuation are correct and inform you about referencing, but they cannot provide the ideas for your work because they do not 'think and act like nurses'. It is important that students seek assistance from lecturing and library staff who are aware of current issues and debates in nursing, to clarify questions and check their understanding of aspects of nursing.

Of particular value is working through one of the better 'study skills' books such as that by Maslin-Prothero (2001), which gives excellent practical advice on all aspects of learning from clinical practice, reading, doing projects, writing essays and other coursework. The important thing is to be systematic in what you do and to give your learning the proper amount of time. Putting a couple of hours aside on most days to refresh your notes, read new work or prepare coursework ahead of deadlines will pay dividends.

Perhaps the most effective strategy we have seen students use during on-campus learning is the peer learning group, which provides students with a forum for discussion and clarification of their ideas, mutual assistance and support. We would encourage all students to participate in such a learning group. Your nursing department may already provide a web-based support service (such as 'Blackboard' or 'Web CT') which perhaps you can ask about. This need not necessarily be on campus. The internet has made it possible to access a number of resources, including other students via the world wide web. Of course, users should be cautious about disclosing personal information and should check the validity of any information obtained via 'the net'.

CONCLUSION

Nursing has not fully appreciated the integration of thinking and doing to create informed action, and has historically tended to 'compartmentalise thinking from doing' (Pearson 1992:219). Discussion of the separation of thinking and doing does little to promote integration of on-campus and clinical learning activity. Students should view their learning to be nurses as occurring in two distinct yet interdependent contexts, the university and the clinical setting.

While there is increasing emphasis on the development of cognitive abilities in nursing students as well as the nature of contemporary practice, this should not lead to what has been labelled as a dichotomy between clinical skills and theoretical knowledge. Despite claims made by some authors that emphasis on theoretical knowledge in nursing results in a devaluing of clinical skills and, consequently, a devaluation of clinical practice (Bjork 1995, 1997; Elzubier 1995), practical and theoretical nursing knowledge are inevitably and infinitely intertwined.

Recent decades have provided evidence that there is a paradigm shift in education, which now views learning as the construction of meaning in context rather than what to learn and how to do things (Townsend 1994). Nurse education is about the ability – indeed flexibility – to examine situations, deconstruct them from a number of perspectives, and reconstruct them around core concepts essential to nursing practice.

Nursing is emerging as a distinct entity with curricula that emphasise nursing as a discipline distinguished from others (Greenwood 1996). Contemporary nursing curricula include discipline-specific knowledge, and integrate knowledge from other disciplines to inform the practice of nursing. This differs from previous practices of modifying knowledge from other disciplines to suit nursing situations. Thus nursing education serves both an epistemological and political purpose and students should be able to articulate and conceptualise the nature of their discipline and apply their thinking to actual practice. Contemporary nursing education challenges nurses to question and justify practice, and emphasises the ability to think about nursing as well as the ability to perform nursing actions to best manage nursing situations. The challenge for students is to develop an integrated approach to practice which values thoughtful, highly skilled and efficient action, and to continue with lifelong learning and professional development.

REFLECTIVE QUESTIONS

(1) How can you become more responsible and accountable for your own learning?
(2) How can you plan and evaluate your ongoing professional development?
(3) Who can assist you with meeting these needs?

RECOMMENDED READING

Andersen, B.M. (1991) Mapping the terrain of the discipline. In: *Towards a Discipline of Nursing* (eds G. Gray & R. Pratt). Churchill Livingstone, Melbourne.

Fairbairn, G.J. & Fairbairn, S.A. (2001) *Reading at University: A Guide for Students.* Open University Press, Buckingham.

Maslin-Prothero, S. (2001) *Baillière's Study Skills for Nurses.* Baillière Tindall, London.

Palmer, A.M., Burns, S. & Bulman, C. (1994) *Reflective Practice in Nursing: The Growth of the Professional Practitioner.* Blackwell, Oxford.

United Kingdom Central Council for Nursing, Midwifery and Health Visiting (1993) *Code of Professional Conduct,* 3rd edn. UKCC, London.

REFERENCES

Andersen, B.M. (1991) Mapping the terrain of the discipline. In: *Towards a Discipline of Nursing* (eds G. Gray & R. Pratt), pp. 95–123. Churchill Livingstone, Melbourne.

Barnard, A.G. & Dunn, S.V. (1994) Issues in the organization and structure of clinical education for undergraduate nursing programs. *Journal of Nursing Education,* **33**(9), 420–422.

Benner, P. (1984) *From Novice to Expert: Excellence and Power in Clinical Nursing Practice.* Addison Wesley, Menlo Park.

Bevis, E.O. & Watson, J. (1989) *Toward a Caring Curriculum: A New Pedagogy for Nursing.* National League for Nursing, New York.

Bjork, I.T. (1995) Neglected conflicts in the discipline of nursing: Perceptions of the importance and value of practical skill. *Journal of Advanced Nursing,* **22**, 6–12.

Bjork, I.T. (1997) Changing conceptions of practical skill and skill acquisition in nursing education. *Nursing Inquiry,* **4**(3), 184–195.

Brennan, A.M. & Hunt, R. (2001) The challenges and conflicts of facilitating learning in practice: the experiences of two clinical nurse educators. *Nurse Education in Practice,* **1**(4), 181–188.

Chun-Heung, L. & French, P. (1997) Education in the practicum: A study of the ward learning climate in Hong Kong. *Journal of Advanced Nursing,* **26**(3), 455–462.

Clark, J., Maben, J. & Jones, K. (1997) Project 2000: perceptions of the philosophy and practice of nursing: shifting perceptions – a new practitioner? *Journal of Advanced Nursing*, **26**(1), 161–168.

Elzubier, M. (1995) Education and debate: Nursing skills and practice. *British Journal of Nursing*, **4**(18), 1087–1092.

Freire, P. (1972) *The Pedagogy of Oppression*. Penguin, Harmondsworth.

Gibbs, G. (1988) *Learning by Doing: A Guide to Teaching and Learning Methods*. Further Education Unit, Oxford Polytechnic, Oxford.

Greenwood, J. (ed.) (1996) *Nursing Theory in Australia: Development and Application*. Harper Educational, Sydney.

Little, P. (1996) *Questions For Learning*. Unpublished workshop material. PROBLARC. University of Newcastle.

Maslin-Prothero, S. (2001) *Baillière's Study Skills for Nurses*. Baillière Tindall, London.

Maslin-Prothero, S. & Owen, S. (2001) Enhancing your clinical links and credibility: The role of nurse lecturers and teachers in clinical practice. *Nurse Education in Practice*, **1**(4), 189–195.

Melia, K. (1987) *Learning and Working*. Tavistock, London.

Mezirow, J. (1985) A critical theory of self directed learning. *New Directions for Continuing Education*, **25** 17–30.

Pearson, A. (1992) Knowing nursing: Emerging paradigms in nursing. In: *Knowledge for Nursing Practice* (eds K. Robinson & B. Vaughan), pp. 213–226. Butterworth Heinemann, Oxford.

Seed, A. (1994) Patients to people. *Journal of Advanced Nursing*, **19**(4), 738–748.

Smith, P. & Gray, B. (2001) Reassessing the concept of emotional labour in student nurse education: role of link lecturers and mentors in a time of change. *Nurse Education Today*, **21**(3), 230–237.

Thorne, S.E. & Hayes, V.E. (eds) (1997) *Nursing Praxis: Knowledge and Action*. Sage, Thousand Oaks, California.

Townsend, J. (1994) Challenge models for learning and knowing. In: *Reflections on Contemporary Nursing Practice* (eds M. McMillan & J. Townsend). Butterworth, Sydney.

United Kingdom Central Council for Nursing, Midwifery and Health Visiting (1999) *Fitness for Practice: The UKCC Commission for Nursing and Midwifery Education, Chair: Sir Leonard Peach*. UKCC, London.

White, R. & Ewan, C. (1991) *Clinical Teaching in Nursing*. Chapman and Hall, London.

Glossary

Acceptability   The test applied to a premise or reason. In order to have a sound argument, premises must be acceptable to the person evaluating the argument.

Acculturation   The incorporation into one's own culture, of values and norms of the host culture.

Aesthetic   A term defined in the *Australian Concise Oxford Dictionary* (1987) as 'belonging to the appreciation of the beautiful; having such appreciation; in accordance with principles of good taste … philosophy of the beautiful or of art … set of principles of good taste and appreciation of beauty'. An abstract notion used in discussing the artistic aspect of nursing (and its creative expression). In this context it relates broadly to theoretical and practical aspects of nursing art.

Affective   'Pertaining to the affections … being affected, mental state, emotions … mental disposition, good will, kindly feeling, love' (*Australian Concise Oxford Dictionary* 1987).

Altruism   'Regard for others as a principle for action; unselfishness' (*Australian Concise Oxford Dictionary* 1987).

Argument   A conclusion that is supported by a set of reasons intended to provide grounds for the acceptability of the conclusion.

Assimilation   The attempt by the host culture to engender its values, norms and lifestyles within its migrant communities by encouraging them to believe that holding on to their cultural identities would be detrimental to them.

Asylum seeker   A person who has applied to the Immigration and Nationality department of a host country, to be recognised as a refugee but who has not yet received a decision, or is in the process of appealing against an initial rejection of a claim for asylum.

Autonomy   'Personal freedom; freedom of the will' (*Australian Concise Oxford Dictionary* 1987). Right to self-determination.

Binary   Comprised of two parts. See also **dichotomy**.

Bioethics   An interdisciplinary field of inquiry characterised by a systematic and critical examination of the moral dimensions of health care and other associated fields (for example, the life sciences) from the standpoint of various ethical perspectives.

Biologism   A particular form of essentialism (see below) in which (women's essence) is defined in terms of their biological capacities.

Concepts   The building blocks of theory. Ideas, mental images or generalisations formed in mind (Chinn & Kramer 1995; Keck 1994).

Conceptual framework   A developing theoretical model that has little empirical support.

Congruency   'Agreement or consistency' (*Australian Concise Oxford Dictionary* 1987). For example, in examining two or more theoretical views one may find that there are areas of agreement across the same ground, hence there is evidence of congruency.

Construct   'A type of highly abstract and complex concept whose reality base can only be inferred. Constructs are formed from multiple less abstract or more empirical concepts' (Chinn & Jacobs 1983:200). For example 'pain' is a construct while 'pain intensity' is a concept (Dulock & Holzemer 1991).

Cultural essentialism   The belief that cultural groups have a set of essential (or fixed) characteristics which are then used to explain people's ill health and lifestyles without much consideration being given to other underlying factors such as poverty, discrimination, communication barriers, the process of ageing and so on.

Cultural/transcultural competence   The capacity to provide effective health care taking into consideration people's cultural beliefs, behaviours and needs.

Culture   The learned, shared, and transmitted values, beliefs, norms and lifeways of a particular group that guides their thinking, decisions and actions in patterned ways.

Deductive reasoning   The process of inferring particulars from general laws or principles.

Dialectic   Defined in the *Australian Concise Oxford Dictionary* (1987) as (the) 'art of investigating the truth of opinions, testing of truth by discussion (or) logical disputation or criticism dealing with metaphysical contradictions and their solutions; existence or action of opposing forces'.

Dialectical   A process or perspective involving a dialectic. For example, in theory development using a dialectical approach to generation of knowledge, the process could involve debate with presentation of an argument (thesis) which is considered critically and challenged by a counter-argument (antithesis), which is considered critically in relation to the thesis and other knowledge, possibly leading to new areas of agreement and understanding (synthesis).

Dichotomy   'A division (esp. sharply defined) into two; result of such division; binary classification …' according to the *Australian Concise Oxford Dictionary* (1987). The term can be used to indicate a divide between two theoretical positions that are polarised or incompatible.

Discourse   An abstract notion used to label a collection of theoretical perspectives within an academic discipline. This may comprise theses or arguments representing knowledge in the discipline including areas of agreement and disagreement, fundamental assumptions, values and beliefs, etc., expressed in disciplinary language and symbols. The notion reflects the idea of a conversation using language within these boundaries.

Empiricist/logical positivist model   An approach grounded in the belief that the world can be viewed as a machine and that the task of science was to discover the laws by which the machine operated; emphasis on predictability, measurement, and the quantification of observable data.

Epistemology   The theory of knowledge; the origins, nature, methods and limits of human knowledge.

Essentialism   The attribution of a fixed essence (to women); that there are given, universal characteristics (of women) including biological, psychological, and social characteristics which are not readily amenable to change.

Ethical principalism   The view that moral decisions are best guided by appealing to sound universal moral principles, such as the principles of autonomy, beneficence, nonmaleficence and justice. Ethical principalism is one of the most popular approaches used to examine ethical issues in health care.

Ethical universalism   The view that there exists one set of universal values/standards that is applicable to all people throughout space and time regardless of their histories and/or cultural backgrounds (contexts).

Ethics   A branch of philosophic inquiry concerned with understanding and examining the moral life. It seeks rational clarification and justification of basic assumptions and beliefs that people hold about what constitutes right or wrong/good or bad conduct. Can also be defined as a system of action guiding rules and principles that function by specifying that certain types of conduct are either required, prohibited or permitted. The term ethics/ethical may be used interchangeably with the term morality/moral.

Etiquette   A set of behavioural action guides concerned with the maintenance of style and decorum in social settings; often, although mistakenly, confused with ethics/morality.

Existentialism   'A school of thought or theory in philosophy. Existentialism takes human existence as its basic focus, including personal experience (Sarter 1988). It is a philosophical perspective or theory that focuses on individual existence. Major beliefs from this perspective are that human beings are subjects, not objects, that the individual is free up to a point, chooses meaning in life and is responsible for choices. Existentialism also places emphasis on open examination of the experiences that individuals have in life, including what may be regarded as tragic. This requires consideration of personal meaning in living through human experiences, life suffering, grief, loss and hope. A number of major thinkers in philosophy contributed to the development of this theory, including Nietzsche, Kierkegaard, Sartre, Merleau-Ponty, Heidegger, Tillich and Camus (Sarter 1988)' (Daly & Watson 1996:198).

Existential-phenomenology 'A combination of ideas from existentialism and phenomenology. Existential-phenomenology is concerned with phenomena encountered in living and the meaning of human existence including interpretation of experiences in life. This requires exploration of subjective, individual experiences in life. In this view, it is accepted that valid knowledge can be developed through advances in understanding of lived human experiences, such as suffering, grief or hope' (Daly & Watson 1996:197–198).

Feminisms The variety of theoretical approaches to the advocacy of equal rights for women, accompanied by a commitment to improve the position of women in society; includes liberal feminism, socialist feminism, radical feminism, post-modern feminism, and so on.

Gender A social construction which expresses the many areas of social life, as distinguished from biological sex; the socially learned behaviours and expectations that are associated with the two sexes.

Generic A characteristic which is 'general, not specific or special' (*Australian Concise Oxford Dictionary* 1987).

Grounded theory A research process designed to lead to generation of theory through study of a particular human situation or context. This involves a 'search for social processes present in human interaction' (Hutchinson 1993:181).

Grounds The degree to which a set of reasons supports a conclusion.

Hermeneutics A process of interpretive analysis that is concerned with uncovering meaning and a technique for interrogating text. Van Manen states that 'Hermeneutics is the theory and practice of interpretation. The word derives from the Greek god Hermes whose task it was to communicate messages from Zeus and other gods to the ordinary mortals' (Van Manen 1990:179). Hermeneutics was originally a technique used to interpret religious text, which has made a transition into research activity in the social sciences and humanities. **Hermeneutical** refers to a process or perspective involving hermeneutics.

Holism A perspective in which people are seen as made up of biological, psychological, social, and spiritual components that are indivisible.

Hypotheses Tentative statements of relationships between two or more variables, which have little empirical support. The repeated confirmation of hypotheses changes their status to empirical generalisations (statements with moderate empirical support) and thence to law (statements with overwhelming empirical support).

Iconography   'Illustration of subject by drawings or figures; book whose essence is pictures; treatise on pictures or statuary; study of portraits esp. of an individual …' (*Australian Concise Oxford Dictionary* 1987).

Ideology   A set of discourses, images and myths that establish an imaginary (imaged) relationship between the individual and the world (where 'imaginary' does not mean non-existent or false since people do indeed live their lives according to these 'imaginary' relationships with the world) (Zavarzadeh & Morton 1991, after Althusser).

Inductive reasoning   The process of inferring a general law or principle from the observation of particular instances.

Masculinist   Pertaining to the masculine; the male gender characteristics derived from social construction and expectation.

Meaning   A concept that is not easily defined particularly if one is seeking to develop an agreed definition! It can be defined as the 'whatness' of a situation (Parse 1992), or the essence, trend intention, significance of a situation, etc. (Parse 1998). 'Meaning refers to the linguistic and imagined content of something and the interpretation that one gives to something' (Parse 1998:29). In the human science worldview, as underpinned by existential-phenomenology, meaning is said to occur on two levels: the ultimate meaning of life, and meaning in moments of living – which constantly changes.

Meta   A prefix commonly encountered in theoretical literature. In this context it means 'beyond or higher order' (*Australian Concise Oxford Dictionary* 1987). For example, metatheory is 'theory about the nature of theory and the processes for its development' (Chinn & Jacobs 1983:203).

Model   A schematic representation of some aspect of reality which may be empirical or theoretical. Empirical models are replicas of observed realities, e.g. a plastic model of the ear. Theoretical models represent the world in language or mathematical symbols e.g. nursing's 'grand theories'.

Moral duty   An act that a person is bound to perform for moral reasons.

Moral obligation   An act that a person is bound to perform for moral reasons; is generally regarded as being weaker than a moral duty and may be overridden by stronger moral duties.

Moral principles   General standards of conduct that make up an ethical system of action guides and which carry particular imperatives (e.g. 'Do no harm').

Moral right   A special interest that a person has and that ought to be protected for moral reasons (e.g. the right to life) (contrast with legal right, e.g. a special interest that a person has and that ought to be protected for legal reasons).

Moral rules   Derived from principles and prescribed particular standards of conduct (e.g. 'Always tell the truth'). Rules have less scope than principles; they also do not have the same force as and can be overridden by principles.

Moral/morality   See ethics above.

Naturalism   A form of essentialism in which a fixed nature is assumed (for women) not readily amenable to change.

Nursing diagnosis   'The patient problem identified by the nurse for nursing intervention by analysis of assessment findings in comparison with what is considered to be normal' (*Taber's Cyclopedic Medical Dictionary* 1997).

Nursing ethics   The examination of all kinds of ethical and bioethical issues from the perspective of nursing theory and practice which, in turn, rest on the agreed core concepts of nursing, i.e. person, culture, care, health, healing, environment and nursing itself.

Nursing process   The nursing process reflects a problem-solving approach to nursing care (O'Connell 1996). It comprises five interconnected stages (dynamic and continuous rather than linear) that structure how nursing care is determined, delivered, communicated and documented.

Occam's razor   The principle that the simplest explanation is most likely to be the right one.

Ontology   A term from metaphysics, which is a branch of philosophy. Ontology 'deals with the nature of being' (*Australian Concise Oxford Dictionary* 1987). Central to this is consideration of the relationship between the human being and the world. The term 'world view' is commonly used in nursing knowledge to capture how this relationship may be conceptualised. World views are concerned with 'philosophic claims about the nature of human beings and the human-environment relationship' (Fawcett 1992:56). A world view may be called an 'ontological perspective', because it is based on ontological assumptions, which are beliefs about the nature of human beings and the human-environment relationship (Daly & Watson 1996:198–199).

Paradigm   'A paradigm is a theoretical construction which is comprised of values and beliefs about the nature of reality, which organises a number of theoretical views into a coherent whole' (Chinn & Jacobs 1983:204), and specifies ways of conducting inquiry to develop new knowledge in a discipline. Attributes of a paradigm serve to synthesise shared aspects of the theories included therein (Chinn & Jacobs 1983). A paradigm in nursing can also provide broad guidelines for nursing practice' (Daly in press).

Patriarchy   The social system in which men dominate, oppress and exploit women, including reproduction, sexuality, violence, work, culture and the state.

Phenomenology   'May be defined as 'the study of phenomena as they unfold' (Parse 1981: 178). The term 'phenomena' may be defined as circumstances or events that capture our attention. Husserl, a German philosopher, is credited with creating phenomenology. His focus was 'on the nature of human consciousness, which he characterised as exhibiting intentionality, or objective reference, in other words the mind is always actively encountering the world' (Sarter 1988:57). Intentionality is a state where the mind exhibits directedness-to-objects (Urmson & Ree 1991). Husserl was interested in the way in which objects are constituted in consciousness. The most profound insight of phenomenology is that consciousness is always consciousness-of-something. Thus, there is always a link between subject and object' (Daly & Watson 1996:199). In a phenomenological research study the focus is on the meaning of the phenomenon under investigation for the research participants who participate in the study.

Philanthropic   'Loving one's fellow men, benevolent, humane' (*Australian Concise Oxford Dictionary* 1987).

Philosophy (alternative view)   'A way of reflecting not so much on what is true and false but on our relationship to the truth' (Foucault 1989).

Philosophy/philosophic inquiry (conventional view)   An argumentative intellectual discipline concerned with the discovery of 'truth' and meaning. Unlike science, which seeks answers to questions that can only be answered by empirical evidence, philosophy seeks answers to questions that cannot be answered by empirical evidence.

Postmodernism   Relates to the critique of modern, capitalist, industrialised society; new political and social strategies which embrace pluralism and diversity of cultures and values.

Poststructuralism   Refers to a range of theoretical positions in which the mode of knowledge production uses particular theories of language, subjectivity, social processes and institutions to understand existing power relations and to identify areas and strategies for change.

Praxis   Praxis can be seen as the link between reflection and action. Freire (1972) defines praxis as 'reflection and action upon the world in order to transform it' (Cox *et al.* 1991: 385).

Premise   A reason offered in support of a conclusion.

Preventive ethics   The study and practice of ethics (including ethic education) aimed at preventing (as opposed to remedying) moral problems.

Racism   A doctrine or ideology or dogma characterised by the behaviour of individuals and institutions based on concepts of racial difference (Fernando 1991), and the belief that some races are superior to others.

Rationalism   A philosophical position that argues that there is (or can be) knowledge which does not depend for its justification on experience and yet is still substantially informative and not merely verbal or analytic in character (which makes it roughly the opposite of **empiricism**) (Bullock *et al.* 1988).

Reductive   From reduction 'in reducing or being reduced; amount by which prices, etc. are reduced; reduced copy of picture, map, etc., … to absurdity … so reductive' (*Australian Concise Oxford Dictionary* 1987).

Refugee   Anyone who, owing to a well-founded fear of being persecuted for reasons of race, religion, nationality, membership of a particular social group or political opinion, is unable, or, owing to such fear, is unwilling to return to the country of her/his nationality or former habitual residence (United Nations Convention 1951).

Relevance   A test applied to a premise or reason. If a premise or reason is relevant, it helps to support the conclusion of the argument.

Sound   An argument is **sound** when the premises are acceptable and provide adequate grounds for accepting the conclusion.

Theory   A logically consistent set of propositions that presents a systematic view of some aspect of reality.

Transcultural nursing   A humanistic and scientific area of formal study and practice in nursing that is focused upon the comparative study of cultures with regard to differences and similarities in care, health, and illness patterns, based upon cultural values, beliefs, and practices of different cultures in the world, and the use of this knowledge to provide culturally-specific and/or universal nursing care to people (Leininger 1984). Transcultural nursing is also concerned with the impact of societal structures on the health of cultural groups.

Universalism   Refers to the attributions of functions, social categories, activities to which (women of) all cultures are assigned; asserts what is shared in common by all (women).

Validity   An argument is **valid** when the premises that are offered provide adequate grounds for acceptance of the conclusion.

Xenophobia   A Greek word derived from 'xenos' meaning stranger, and 'phobia' meaning fear.

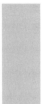

Bibliography

Abel, E. (1994) Productivity versus quality of care: Ethical implications for clinical practice during health care reform. *Nurse Practitioner Forum*, **5**(4), 238–242.

Acheson, Sir Donald (Chair) (1998) *Independent Inquiry into Inequalities in Health.* The Stationery Office, London.

Ahmad, W.I.U. (1993) Making black people sick: race, ideology and health research. In: *'Race' and Health in Contemporary Britain* (ed. W.I.U. Ahmad). Open University Press, Buckingham.

Ahmad, W.I.U. (1996) The trouble with culture. In: *Researching Cultural Differences in Health* (eds D. Kelleher & S. Hillier). Routledge, London.

Allen, D.G., Allman, K.K.M. & Powers, P. (1991) Feminist nursing research without gender. *Advances in Nursing Science*, **13**(3), 49–58.

Allmark, P. (1995) Uncertainties in the teaching of ethics to students of nursing. *Journal of Advanced Nursing*, **22**, 374–378.

Alspach, G. (1993) Editorial: Nurses as victims of violence. *Critical Care Nurse*, **13**(5), 13–14, 17.

Amin, K. & Oppenheim, C. (1992) *Poverty in Black and White Deprivation and Ethnic Minorities.* Child Poverty Action Group, London.

Andersen, B.M. (1991) Mapping the terrain of the discipline. In: *Towards a Discipline of Nursing* (eds G. Gray & R. Pratt), pp. 95–123. Churchill Livingstone, Melbourne.

Anderson, J.R. (1995) *Cognitive Psychology and its Implications*, 4th edn. Freeman, New York.

Andrews, M. (1996) Using reflection to develop clinical expertise. *British Journal of Nursing*, **5**(8), 508–513.

Andrews, S. & Hutchinson, S. (1981) Teaching nursing ethics: A practical approach. *Journal of Nursing Education*, **20**(1), 6–11.

Appleby, F. & Sayer, L. (2001) Public health nursing–health visiting. In: *Community Healthcare Nursing* (eds D. Sines, F. Appleby & E. Raymond). Blackwell Science, Oxford.

Appleton, J. & Clemerson, J. (1999) Family based interventions with children in need. *Community Practitioner*, **72**(5), 134–136.

Applin, L. (1991) *Health and Nursing in the United Kingdom.* Royal College of Nursing, London.

Argyris, C. & Schön, D. (1977) *Theory in practice.* Jossey Bass, San Francisco.

Argyris, C., Putman, R. & Smith, D.M. (1985) *Action Science.* Jossey Bass, San Francisco.

Armitage, S. & Kavanagh, K. (1996) Hospital nurses' perceptions of discharge planning for medical patients. *Australian Journal of Advanced Nursing*, **14**(2), 16–23.

Astrom, G., Norberg, A. & Hallberg, I.R. (1995) Skilled nurses' experience of caring. *Journal of Professional Nursing*, **11**(2), 110–118.

Australian Nursing Council Inc (1998) *ANCI National Competency Standards for the Registered Nurse* 2nd edn. ANCI, Dickson ACT.

Australian Nursing Council Inc (1993) *Code of Ethics for Nurses in Australia*. ANCI, Canberra.

Baldwin, J.H., Conger, C., Abegglen, J. & Hill, E. (1998) Population-focused and community-based nursing – moving toward clarification of concepts. *Public Health Nursing*, **15**(1), 12–18.

Bandman, E.L. & Bandman, B. (1985) *Nursing Ethics in the Life Span*. Appleton, Century, Crofts, Norwalk, Connecticut.

Barnard, A.G. & Dunn, S.V. (1994) Issues in the organization and structure of clinical education for undergraduate nursing programs. *Journal of Nursing Education*, **33**(9), 420–422.

Barnum, B.S. (1998) Leadership: can it be holistic? In: *Contemporary Leadership Behaviour: Selected Readings* (ed. E.C. Hein), 5th edn. Lippincott, New York.

Bashford, A. (1997) Starch on the collar and sweat on the brow: Self sacrifice and the status of work for nurses. *Journal of Australian Studies*, **67**, 74.

Bass, B. & Avolio, J. (1994) *Improving Organisational Effectiveness through Transformational Leadership*. Sage, London.

Bassett, C. (1993) Socialisation of student nurses into the qualified nurse role. *British Journal of Nursing*, **2**(3), 179–182.

Baum, F., Fry, D. & Lennie, I. (eds) (1992) *Community Health Policy and Practice in Australia*. Pluto Press, Sydney.

Beare, P. & Meyers, J. (1994) *Principles and Practice of Adult Health Nursing*, Mosby, St Louis.

Begany, T. (1994) Your image is brighter than ever. *RN*, **57**, 28.

Benierakis, C.E. (1995) The function of the multidisciplinary team in child psychiatry – clinical and educational aspects. *Canadian Journal of Psychiatry*, **40**, 348–353.

Benner, P. (1984) *From Novice to Expert: Excellence and Power in Clinical Nursing*. Addison-Wesley Publishing Company, Menlo Park, California.

Benner, P. (1991) The role of experience, narrative, and community in skilled ethical comportment. *Advances in Nursing Science*, **14**(2), 1–21.

Benner, P. (ed.) (1994) *Interpretive Phenomenology: Embodiment, Caring, and Ethics in Health and Illness*. Sage, Thousand Oaks, California.

Benner, P., Hooper-Kyriakidis, P. & Stannard, D. (1999) *Clinical Wisdom and Interventions in Critical Care: A Thinking-in-Action Approach*. WB Saunders, Philadelphia.

Benner, P. & Wrubel, J. (1989) *The Primacy of Caring: Stress and Coping in Health and Illness*. Addison-Wesley, Menlo Park California.

Benoliel, J. (1983) Ethics in nursing practice and education. *Nursing Outlook*, **31**(4), 210–215.

Bent, K.N. (1993) Perspectives on critical and feminist theory in developing nursing praxis. *Journal of Professional Nursing*, **9**(5), 296–303.

Bernard, M. (1998) Back to the future? Reflections on women, ageing and nursing. *Journal of Advanced Nursing*, **27**(3), 633–640.

Berriot-Salvadore, E. (1993) The discourse of medicine and science. In: *A History of Women in the West: Vol. 3 Renaissance and Enlightenment Paradoxes* (eds N.Z. Davis & A. Farge). The Belknap Press of Harvard University Press, Cambridge, Massachusetts.

Berry, D.C. & Dienes, Z. (1993) *Implicit Learning: Theoretical and Empirical Issues*. Lawrence Erlbaum Associates Ltd, Hove, Sussex.

Bevis, E. (1978) *Curriculum Building in Nursing*. Mosby, St Louis.

Bevis, E.O. & Watson, J. (1989) *Toward a Caring Curriculum: A New Pedagogy for Nursing*. National League for Nursing, New York.

Bishop, A. & Scudder, J. (1990) *The Practical, Moral, and Personal Sense of Nursing: A Phenomenological Philosophy of Practice.* State University of New York Press, Albany.

Bishop, N.J. & Goldie, S. (1962) *A Bio-bibliography of Florence Nightingale.* International Council of Nurses, London.

Bjork, I.T. (1995) Neglected conflicts in the discipline of nursing: Perceptions of the importance and value of practical skill. *Journal of Advanced Nursing,* **22**, 6–12.

Bjork, I.T. (1997) Changing conceptions of practical skill and skill acquisition in nursing education. *Nursing Inquiry,* **4**(3), 184–195.

Black, F. (ed.) (1992) *Primary Nursing: An Introductory Guide.* King's Fund Centre, London.

Bolton, S.C. (2000) Who cares? Offering emotion work as a 'gift' in the nursing labour process. *Journal of Advanced Nursing,* **32**(3), 580–586.

Bond, M. & Holland, S. (1998) *Skills of Clinical Supervision for Nurses: A Practical Guide for Supervisees, Clinical Supervisors and Managers.* Open University Press, Buckingham.

Boorse, C. (1975) On the distinction between disease and illness. *Philosophy and Public Affair,* **5**(1), 49–68.

Borbasi, S.-A. (1996) Living the experience of being nursed: A phenomenological text. *International Journal of Nursing Practice,* **2**(4), 222–228.

Bordens, K.S. & Abbott, B.B. (1996) *Research Design and Methods: A Process Approach.* Mayfield, Mountain View, California.

Boud, D., Keogh, R. & Walker, D. (1985) Promoting reflection in learning: a model. In: *Reflection: Turning Experience into Learning* (eds D. Boud, R. Keogh & D. Walker), pp. 18–40. Kogan Page, London.

Bowers, L. (1989) The significance of primary nursing. *Journal of Advanced Nursing,* **14**, 13–19.

Boyd, E.M. & Fales, A.W. (1983) Reflective learning: a key to learning from experience. *Journal of Humanistic Psychology,* **23**(2), 99–117.

Brennan, A.M. & Hunt, R. (2001) The challenges and conflicts of facilitating learning in practice: the experiences of two clinical nurse educators. *Nurse Education in Practice,* **1**(4), 181–188.

Briggs, A. (1972) *Report of the Committee on Nursing,* Cmnd 5115. HMSO, London.

Briles, J. (1994) *The Briles Report on Women in Healthcare. Changing conflict to collaboration in a toxic workplace.* Jossey-Bass, San Francisco.

Brink, P.J. & Wood, M.J. (1993) *Basic Steps in Planning Nursing Research.* Jones and Bartlett, Boston.

British Council (2000) *Health Insight,* March 2000- http://www.britishcouncil.org/health

Brown, J. (1992) Nurses or technicians? The impact of technology on oncology nursing. *Canadian Oncology Nursing Journal,* **2**(1), 12–17.

Brykczynska, G. (ed.) (1997) *Caring: The Compassion and Wisdom of Nursing.* Arnold, London.

Buchanan, T. (1997) Nursing our narratives: Towards a dynamic understanding of nurses in literary texts. *Nursing Inquiry,* **4**(2), 80–87.

Buchanan, T. (1999) Nightingalism: Haunting nursing history. *Collegian,* **6**(2), 28–33.

Bullock, A., Stallybrass, O. & Trombley, S. (1988) *The Fontana Dictionary of Modern Thought.* Fontana Press, London.

Bunkers, S., Michaels, C. & Ethridge, P. (1997) Advanced practice nursing in community: Nursing's opportunity. *Advanced Practice Nursing Quarterly,* **2**(4), 79–84.

Buresh, B. & Gordon, S. (1995) Taking on the TV shows. *American Journal of Nursing,* **95**(11), 18–20.

Burnell, S. (1995) Case management and multidisciplinary teams. In: *Managed Care, Case Management and Nursing in Australia* (ed. P. Wilkinson). Australian Nursing Federation, Melbourne.

Burns, N. & Grove, S.K. (1998) *The Practice of Nursing Research: Conduct, Critique, and Utilization*, 3ʳᵈ edn. Saunders, Philadelphia.

Burrows, D.E. (1995) The nurse teacher's role in the promotion of reflective practice. *Nurse Education Today,* **15**(5), 346–350.

Caffrey, R. & Caffrey, P. (1994) Nursing: Caring or codependent? *Nursing Forum,* **29**(1), 12–17.

Callery, P. (1990) Moral learning in nursing education: A discussion of the usefulness of cognitive-developmental and social learning theories. *Journal of Advanced Nursing,* **15**, 324–328.

Cameron, J. & MacWilliams, J. (1995) Health care needs of homeless people. In: *Issues in Australian Nursing: The Nurse as Clinician* (eds G. Gray & R. Pratt). Churchill Livingstone, Melbourne.

Campinha-Bacote, J. (ed.) (1991) *The Process of Cultural Competence: A Culturally Competent Model of Care*, 2ⁿᵈ edn. Transcultural C.A.R.E. Associates, Ohio.

Caplan, G. & Brown, A. (1997) Post acute care: Can hospitals do better with less? *Australian Health Review,* **20**(2), 43–52.

Capra, F. (1982) *The Turning Point: Science, Society and the Rising Culture.* Simon & Schuster, New York.

Carpenter, M. (1977) The new managerialism and professionalism in nursing, In: *Health and the Division of Labour* (eds M. Stacey, M. Reid, C. Heath & R. Dingwall), pp. 165–191. Croom Helm, London.

Carper, B.A. (1978) Fundamental patterns of knowing in nursing. *Advances in Nursing Science,* **1**(1), 13–23.

Cartwright, T., Davson-Galle, P. & Holden, R. (1992) Moral philosophy and nursing curricula: Indoctrination of the new breed. *Journal of Nursing Education,* **31**(5), 225–228.

Cassells, J. & Redman, B. (1989) Preparing students to be moral agents in clinical nursing practice: Report on a national study. *Nursing Clinics of North America,* **24**(2), 463–473.

Cheek, J. (1995) Nurses, nursing and representations: An exploration of the effect of viewing positions on the textual portrayal of nursing. *Nursing Inquiry,* **2**, 235–240.

Cheek, J. & Rudge, T. (1995) Only connect … feminism and nursing. In: *Scholarship in the Discipline of Nursing* (eds G. Gray & R. Pratt). Churchill Livingstone, Melbourne.

Chiarella, M. (1995) Regulating mechanisms and standards: nurses' friends or foes? In: *Issues in Australian Nursing IV* (eds G. Gray & R. Pratt), pp. 61–74. Churchill Livingstone, London.

Chinn, P.L. (1989) Awake, awake. *Advances in Nursing Science,* **11**(2), 1.

Chinn, P.L. & Jacobs, M.K. (1983) *Theory and nursing: A systematic approach.* Mosby, St Louis.

Chinn, P.L. & Kramer, M.K. (1995) *Theory and Nursing: A Systematic Approach,* 4ᵗʰ edn. Mosby, St Louis.

Chinn, P.L., Maeve, M.K. & Bostick, C. (1997) Aesthetic inquiry and the art of nursing. *Scholarly Inquiry for Nursing Practice,* **11**(2), 83–100.

Chinn, P.L. & Watson, J. (eds) (1994) *Art and Aesthetics in Nursing*. National League for Nursing, New York.

Chun-Heung, L. & French, P. (1997) Education in the practicum: A study of the ward learning climate in Hong Kong. *Journal of Advanced Nursing*, **26**(3), 455–462.

Clark, G. (1989) To be or not to be – it's time to market nursing's image. In: *Issues in Australian Nursing 2* (eds G. Gray & R. Pratt), pp. 175–192. Churchill Livingstone, Melbourne.

Clark, J., Maben, J. & Jones, K. (1997) Project 2000: perceptions of the philosophy and practice of nursing: shifting perceptions – a new practitioner? *Journal of Advanced Nursing*, **26**(1), 161–168.

Clayton, L. (1995) Hospital at home: Offering customer choice for post acute care. In: *Issues in Australian Nursing: The Nurse as Clinician* (eds G. Gray & R. Pratt). Churchill Livingstone, Melbourne.

Cochrane, A.L. (1972) *Effectiveness and Efficiency: Random Reflections on Health Services*. Nuffield Provincial Hospitals Trust, London.

Cohen, J.S. (1991) Two portraits of caring: A comparison of the artists, Leininger and Watson. *Journal of Advanced Nursing*, **16**, 899–909.

Community Practitioner and Health Visitor Association (1997) A month in the life of a health visitor: *CPHVA Omnibus, 1997*. CPHVA, London.

Conway, J. (1994) Reflection, the art and science of nursing and the theory-practice gap. *British Journal of Nursing*, **3**(3), 114–118.

Coope, C.M. (1996) Does teaching by cases mislead us about morality? *Journal of Medical Ethics*, **22**(1), 46ff.

Cooper, J.E. (1991) Telling our own stories: the reading and writing of journals or diaries. In: *Stories Lives Tell* (eds C. Witherell & N. Noddings), pp. 96–112. Teachers College Press, New York.

Corbett, N.A. (1997) *Writing a Journal: A Strategy for Lifelong Learning as a Reflective Practitioner*. Proceedings of the 1st International Conference on Correcting Conversations: Nursing Scholarship and Practice, Reykjavik, Iceland, 20–22 June 1995.

Cotroneo, M., Outlaw, F., King, J. & Brince, J. (1997) Integrated primary health care: Opportunities for psychiatric-mental health nurses in a reforming health care system. *Journal of Psychosocial Nursing and Mental Health Services*, **35**(10), 21–27, 41–42.

Cowley, S., Buttigieg, M. & Houston, A. (2000) *A first steps project to scope the current and future regulatory issues for health visiting*. Report prepared for the UKCC. UKCC, London.

Cox, H., Hickson, P. & Taylor, B. (1991) Exploring reflection: Knowing and constructing practice. In: *Issues in Australian Nursing: The Nurse as Clinician* (eds G. Gray & R. Pratt). Churchill Livingstone, Melbourne.

Coxon, T. (1990) Ritualised repression. *Nursing Times*, **86**(31), 35–36.

Crookes, P.A. (1992) The politics of health care. In: *Health: Perspectives and Practices* (eds J. Boddy & V. Rice), 2nd edn. pp. 216–232. The Dunmore Press, Palmerston North, New Zealand.

Crookes, P.A. & Davies, S. (eds) (1998) *Research into Practice: Essential Skills for Reading and Applying Research in Nursing and Health Care*. Baillière Tindall, Edinburgh.

D'Antonio, P. (1997) Toward a history of research in nursing. *Nursing Research*, **46**(2), 105–110.

Dahlgren, G. & Whitehead, M. (1991) *Policies and Strategies to Promote Equity in Health*. Institute for Future Studies, Stockholm.

Dalrymple, J. & Burke, B. (1995) *Anti-oppressive Practice: Social Care and the Law.* Open University Press, Buckingham.

Daly, J. & Watson, J. (1996) Parse's human-becoming theory of nursing. In: *Nursing Theory in Australia: Development and Application* (ed. J. Greenwood), pp. 177–200. Harper Educational, Sydney.

Darbyshire, P. (1985) Bedpans or broomsticks? *Nursing Times*, **81**, 44–45.

Darbyshire, P. (1994) Understanding the life of illness: Learning through the art of Frida Kahlo. *Advances in Nursing Science*, **17**(1), 51–59.

Darbyshire, P. (1994) Understanding caring through arts and humanities: A medical/nursing humanities approach to promoting alternate experiences of thinking and learning. *Journal of Advanced Nursing*, **19**(5), 856–863.

Darbyshire, P. (1995) Reclaiming 'Big Nurse': A feminist critique of Ken Kesey's portrayal of Nurse Ratched in One Flew Over the Cuckoo's Nest. *Nursing Inquiry*, **2**, 198–202.

David, B.A. (2000) Nursing's gender politics: Reformulating the footnotes. *Advances in Nursing Science*, **23**(1), 83–94.

Davies, C. (1995) *Gender and the Professional Predicament in Nursing.* Open University Press, Buckingham.

Davis, A. & Slater, P. (1988) Ethics in nursing: implications for education and practice. *The Australian Nurses Journal*, **17**(8), 18–20.

Dean, D.J. (1992) *Royal College of Nursing of the United Kingdom – Working: Policy and Practice.* Royal College of Nursing, London.

Delacour, S. (1991) The construction of nursing: Ideology, discourse and representation. In: *Towards a Discipline of Nursing* (eds G. Gray & R. Pratt), pp. 413–433. Churchill Livingstone, Melbourne.

Delbridge, A., Bernard, J., Blair, D., Peters, P. & Butler, S. (eds) (1991) *The Macquarie Dictionary*, 2nd edn. The Macquarie Library, Macquarie University, Sydney.

Demerouti, E., Bakker, A.B., Nachreiner, F. & Schaufeli, W.B. (2000) A model of burnout and life satisfaction amongst nurses. *Journal of Advanced Nursing*, **32**(2), 454–464.

Denzin, N.K. & Lincoln, Y.S. (1994) Introduction: Entering the field of qualitative research. In: *Handbook of Qualitative Research* (eds N.K. Denzin & Y.S. Lincoln). Sage, Thousand Oaks, California.

Department of Health (1990) *The NHS and Community Care Act.* HMSO, London.

Department of Health (1991) *Research for Health: A Research and Development Strategy for the National Health Service.* HMSO, London.

Department of Health (1993) *Report of the Taskforce on the Strategy for Research in Nursing, Midwifery and Health Visiting.* Department of Health, Leeds.

Department of Health (1998) *The New NHS: Modern and Dependable: A National Framework for Assessing Performance.* The Stationery Office, London

Department of Health (1998) *Chief Medical Officers project to strengthen the public health function in England: A report of emerging findings.* HMSO, London.

Department of Health (1999) *Reducing Health Inequalities: An Action Report.* Department of Health, London.

Department of Health (1999) *Making a Difference: Strengthening the Nursing, Midwifery and Health Visiting Contribution to Health and Healthcare.* Department of Health, London.

Department of Health (1999) *Saving Lives: Our Healthier Nation.* HMSO, London.

Department of Health (2000) *Towards a Strategy for Nursing Research and Development.* Department of Health, London.

Department of Health (2000) *The NHS Plan: A Plan for Investment, a Plan for Reform*. HMSO, London.

Department of Health (2001) *Shifting the Balance*. Department of Health, London.

Department of Health (2001) *National Statistics Summary Information for 2000–01, England* – http://www.doh.gov.uk/public/kc560001/index.htm

Department of Health (2001) *Research Governance Framework for Health and Social Care*. Department of Health, London.

Department of Human Services and Health (1994) *Nursing Education in Australian Universities*: Report of the national review of nurse education in the higher education sector, 1994 and beyond. AGPS, Canberra.

Dewey, J. (1993) *How we Think*. Regnery, Chicago.

Deyo, R.A. & Carter, W.B. (1992) Strategies for improving and expanding the application of health status measures in clinical settings: A researcher-developer viewpoint. *Medical Care*, **30**(5 suppl.), 176–186.

Dickens, C. (1910) *Martin Chuzzlewit*. McMillan Co, New York.

Dickoff, J. & James, P. (1968) Theory in practice discipline: Part I. *Nursing Research*, **17**(5), 415–35.

Doering, L. (1992) Power and knowledge in nursing: A feminist poststructuralist view. *Advances in Nursing Science*, **14**(4), 24–33.

Dolan, B. (1990) Project 2000: The gender mender? *Nursing Standard*, **4**, 52–53.

Donahue, P. (1996) *Nursing: The Finest Art*. Mosby, St Louis.

Droogan, J. & Cullum, N. (1998) Systematic reviews in nursing. *International Journal of Nursing Studies*, **35**, 13–22.

Duffield, C. & Lumby, J. (1994) Caring nurses: The dilemma of balancing costs and quality. *Australian Health Review*, **17**(2), 72–83.

Dulock, H. & Holzemer, W. (1991) Substruction: Improving the linkage from theory to method. *Nursing Science Quarterly*, **4**(2), 83–87.

Dunlop, M. (1986) Is a science of caring possible? *Journal of Advanced Nursing*, **11**(3), 661–670.

Dunn, A. (1985) Images of nursing in the nursing and popular press. *Bulletin of the Royal College of Nursing (UK) History of Nursing Group*, **6**, 2–8.

Durgahee, T. (1996) Reflective practice: linking theory and practice in palliative care nursing. *International Journal of Palliative Nursing*, **2**(1), 22–25.

Dyson, J. (1996) Nurses' conceptualizations of caring attitudes and behaviours. *Journal of Advanced Nursing*, **23**, 1263–1269.

Edwards, S.D. (1999) The idea of nursing science. *Journal of Advanced Nursing*, **29**(3), 563–569.

Ehrenreich, B. & English, D. (1979) *For Her Own Good: 150 years of experts' advice to women*. Pluto, London.

Ekstrom, D.N. (1999) Gender and perceived nurse caring in nurse-patient dyads. *Journal of Advanced Nursing*, **29**(6), 1393–1401.

Elzubier, M. (1995) Education and debate: Nursing skills and practice. *British Journal of Nursing*, **4**(18), 1087–1092.

Emden, C. (1991) Becoming a reflective practitioner. In: *Issues in Australian Nursing: The Nurse as Clinician* (eds G. Gray & R. Pratt). Churchill Livingstone, Melbourne.

Emden, C. (1991) Becoming a reflective practitioner. In: *Towards a Discipline of Nursing* (eds G. Gray & R. Pratt), pp. 335–54. Churchill Livingstone, Melbourne.

Errser, S. & Tutton, S. (eds) (1991) *Primary Nursing in Perspective*. Scutari Press, London.

Estes, C. & Binney, E. (1989) The biomedicalisation of ageing: Dangers and dilemmas. *The Gerontologist*, **29**(5), 587–596.

European Commission (1997) Advisory committee on training in nursing. *Document XV/E/9432/7/96*. European Commission, Brussels.

Evans, M. (1997) *Introducing Contemporary Feminist Thought*. Blackwell Publishers, Oxford.

Fagin, C. & Diers, D. (1983) Nursing as a metaphor. *The New England Journal of Medicine*, **309**, 116–117.

Falk Rafael, A. (1996) Power and caring: A dialectic in nursing. *Advances in Nursing Science*, **19**(1), 3–17.

Falk Rafael, A. (1998) Nurses who run with the wolves: The power and caring dialectic revisited. *Advances in Nursing Science*, **21**(1), 29–42.

Fargason, C.A. & Haddock, C.C. (1992) Cross-functional, integrative team decision making: Essential for QI in health care. *Quality Review Bulletin*, **May**, 157–163.

Farmer, B. (1993) The use and abuse of power in nursing. *Nursing Standard*, **7**(23), 33–36.

Farrington, D. (1995) Intensive health visiting and the prevention of juvenile crime. *Health Visitor*, **68**(3), 100–102.

Fawcett, J. (1984) The metaparadigm of nursing: Present status and future refinements. *Image: The Journal of Nursing Scholarship*, **16**(3), 84–89.

Fawcett, J. (1992) From a plethora of paradigms to parsimony in worldviews. *Nursing Science Quarterly*, **6**(2), 56–58.

Fawcett, J. & Downs, F. (1986) *The Relationship of Theory and Research*. Appleton-Century-Crofts, Norwalk, Connecticut.

Fenton, M. (1986) Development of a scale of humanistic nursing behaviours. *Nursing Research*, **39**(2), 82–87.

Fernando, S. (1991) *Mental Health, Race and Culture*. Macmillan and Mind Publications, London.

Feyerabend, P. (1975) *Against Method*. Verso, London.

Fiedler, L. (1988) Images of the nurse in fiction and popular cultures. In: *Images of Nurses: Perspectives from History, Art, and Literature* (ed. A. Jones), pp. 100–112. University of Pennsylvania Press, Pennsylvania.

Field, J. & FitzGerald, M. (1989) Therapeutic nursing: emerging imperatives for nursing curricula. In: *Nursing as Therapy* (eds R. McMahon & A. Pearson), pp. 93–111. Stanley Thornes, Cheltenham.

Fisher, M. (1988) Hospice nursing. *Nursing*, **3**(32), 8–10.

FitzGerald, M. (1991) Change in the ward, making things happen. *Nursing Times*, **87**(30), 25–27.

FitzGerald, M. (1994) Lecturer practitioners: Creating the environment. In: *Unifying Nursing Theory And Practice* (eds J. Lathlean & B. Vaughan), pp. 55–70. Butterworth Heinemann, Oxford.

Flaherty, B. (1995) Advanced practice nursing: What's all the fuss? *Journal of Nursing Law*, **2**(3), 7–25.

Flaskerud, J.H. & Halloran, E.J. (1980) Areas of agreement in nursing theory development. *Advances in Nursing Science*, **3**(1), 1–7.

Forester, S. (2002) UKCC Consultation on standards for health visitor education. *Community Practitioner and Health Visitors Association*, **75**(1), 14–15.

Foster, J. & Greenwood, J. (1998) A challenging innovation for nurses. *Contemporary Nurse*, **7**, 165–172.

Foucault, M. (1989) *Foucault Live* (ed. S. Lotringer). Semiotext(e), New York.

Freire, P. (1972) *The Pedagogy of Oppression*. Penguin, Harmondsworth.

Fromer, M. (1980) Teaching ethics by case analysis. *Nursing Outlook*, **October**, 604–609.

Fry, S. (1989) Teaching ethics in nursing curricula. Traditional and contemporary models. *Nursing Clinics of North America*, **24**(2), 485–497.

Fulford, K.W.M. (1989) *Moral theory and medical practice*. Cambridge University Press, Cambridge.

Gallagher, R. (1995) Team building. In: *Leading and Managing in Nursing* (ed. P.S. Yoder Wise), pp. 275–299. Mosby, St Louis.

Gamarnikow, E. (1978) Sexual division of labour: The case of nursing. In: *Feminism and Materialism* (eds A. Kuhn & A.M. Wolpe). Routledge and Kegan Paul, London.

Garnham, A. & Oakhill, J. (1994) *Thinking and Reasoning*. Blackwell Publishers, Oxford.

Gattuso, S. & Bevan, C. (2000) Mother, daughter, patient, nurse: women's emotion work in aged care. *Journal of Advanced Nursing*, **31**(4), 892–899.

Gaul, A. (1989) Ethics content in baccalaureate degree curricula. *Nursing Clinics of North America*, **24**(2), 475–483.

Gaze, H. (1987) Man appeal. *Nursing Times*, **83**(20), 24–27.

Germain, C.P. (1993) Ethnography: The method. In: *Nursing Research: a Qualitative Perspective* (eds P.L. Munhall & C. Oiler Boyd), 2nd edn, pp. 237–268. National League for Nursing, New York.

Gerrish, K. & Papadopoulos, I. (1999) Transcultural competence: The challenge for nurse education. *British Journal of Nursing*, **8**(21), 1453–1457.

Gibbs, G. (1988) *Learning by Doing: A Guide to Teaching and Learning Methods*. Further Education Unit, Oxford Polytechnic, Oxford.

Glover, S., Gott, C., Loizillon, A. *et al.* (2001) *Migration: An economic and social analysis*. RDS Occasional Paper No 67. Home Office, London.

Gold, C., Chambers, J. & Dvorak, E. (1995) Ethical dilemmas in the lived experience of nursing practice. *Nursing Ethics*, **2**(2), 131–141.

Goltz, K. & Bruni, N. (1995) Health promotion discourse: Language of change? In: *The Politics of Health. The Australian experience* (ed. H. Gardner), 2nd edn, pp. 510–546. Churchill Livingstone, Melbourne.

Gortner, S.R. (1983) The history and philosophy of nursing science and research. *Advances in Nursing Science*, **5**(2), 1–8.

Govier, T. (1992) *A Practical Study of Argument*, 3rd edn. Wadsworth Publishing Company, Belmont, California.

Gray, J, & Forsstrum, S. (1991) Generating theory from practice: the reflective technique. In: *Towards a Discipline of Nursing* (eds G. Gray & R. Pratt), pp. 355–372. Churchill Livingstone, Melbourne.

Green, L. & Kreuter, M. (1991) *Health Promotion Planning. An Educational and Environmental Approach*, 2nd edn. Mayfield Publishing, Mountain View, California.

Greenhalgh, J., Vanhanen, L. & Kyngas, H. (1998) Nurse caring behaviours. *Journal of Advanced Nursing*, **27**(5), 927–932.

Greenhalgh, P. (1997) *How to read a paper*. BMJ Publishing, London.

Greenwood, J. (1993) Reflective practice: A critique of the work of Argyris and Schon. *Journal of Advanced Nursing*, **19**, 1183–1187.

Greenwood, J. (1993) The apparent desensitisation of student nurses during their professional socialisation: a cognitive perspective. *Journal of Advanced Nursing*, **18**, 1471–1479.

Greenwood, J. (1994) Action research: A few details, a caution and something new. *Journal of Advanced Nursing*, **20**(1), 13–18.

Greenwood, J. (1996) Nursing research and nursing theory. In: *Nursing Theory in Australia: Development and Application* (ed. J. Greenwood), pp. 16–30. Harper Educational, Sydney.

Greenwood, J. (1996) Nursing theories: An introduction to their development and application. In: *Nursing Theory in Australia: Development and Application* (ed. J. Greenwood), pp. 1–14. Harper Educational, Sydney.

Greenwood, J. (ed.) (1996) *Nursing Theory in Australia: Development and Application*. Harper Educational, Sydney.

Greenwood, J. (1998) The role of reflection in single- and double-loop learning. *Journal of Advanced Nursing*, **27**, 1048–1053.

Greenwood, J. (1998) The write advice, or how to get a journal article published. *Contemporary Nurse*, **7**(2), 81–90.

Griffiths, R. (1996) Australian reactions to the DCCT: Existing practices and new initiatives. *Practical Diabetes International*, **13**(2), 41–42.

Grosz, E. (1990) Conclusion: A note on essentialism and difference. In: *Feminist Knowledge: Critique and Construct* (ed. S. Gunew). Routledge, London.

Guyatt, G. & Rennie, D. (eds) (2002) *Users' Guides to the Medical Literature: A Manual for Evidence-based Clinical Practice*. AMA Press, Chicago.

Hadfield, L. (1991) Guest Editorial: Violence in the accident and emergency department: Differences across the Atlantic. *Journal of Emergency Nursing*, **15**(5), 269–270.

Hagell, E.I. (1989) Nursing knowledge: Women's knowledge. A sociological perspective. *Journal of Advanced Nursing*, **14**, 226–233.

Hagland, M.R. (1998) Reflection: a reflex action. *Intensive and Critical Care Nursing*, **3**, 96–100.

Hallam, J. (1998) From angels to handmaidens: Changing constructions of nursing's public image in post-war Britain. *Nursing Inquiry*, **5**, 32–42.

Halpern, D.F. (1998) *Critical Thinking Across the Curriculum: A Brief Edition of Thought and Knowledge*. Lawrence Erlbaum Associates, Mahweh, New Jersey.

Hardy, M.E. (1974) Theories: Components, development, evaluation. *Nursing Research*, **23**, 100–107.

Harris, M.R. & Warren, J.J. (1995) Patient outcomes: Assessment for the CNS. *Clinical Nurse Specialist*, **9**(2), 82–86.

Heath, H. (1998) Keeping a reflective practice diary: a practice guide. *Nurse Education Today*, **18**, 592–598.

Hein, E.C. (ed.) (1998) *Contemporary Leadership Behaviour: Selected Readings*, 5th edn. Lippincott, New York.

Hektor, L. (1994) Florence Nightingale and the women's movement: Friend or foe? *Nursing Inquiry*, **1**, 38–45.

Henderson, A. (2001) Emotional labour and nursing: An under-appreciated aspect of caring work. *Nursing Inquiry*, **8**(2), 130–138.

Henderson, V. (1964) The nature of nursing. *American Journal of Nursing*, **64**(8), 62.

Henderson, V. (1966) *The Nature of Nursing*. Collier Macmillan, London.

Hicks, C. (1997) The research-practice gap: Individual responsibility or corporate culture? *Nursing Times,* **93**(39), 38–39.

Hicks, C. (1999) Incompatible skills and ideologies: The impediment of gender attributions on nursing research. *Journal of Advanced Nursing,* **30**(1), 129–139.

Hill, M.N. & Becker, D.M. (1995) Roles of nurses and health workers in cardiovascular health promotion. *The American Journal of the Medical Sciences,* **310**(Suppl.), S123–S126.

Hockey, L. (1986) The nature and purpose of research. In: *The Research Process in Nursing* (ed. D.F.S. Cormack), pp. 3–13. Blackwell Scientific, Oxford.

Hodge, B. (1993) Uncovering the ethic of care. *Nursing Praxis in New Zealand,* **8**(2), 13–22.

Hodges, F. (1996) Journal writing as a mode of thinking for RN-BSN students: a leveled approach to learning to listen to self and others. *Journal of Nursing Education,* **35**(3), 137–141.

Holden, R.J. (1991) In defence of Cartesian dualism and the hermeneutic horizon. *Journal of Advanced Nursing,* **16**(11), 1375–1381.

Holloway, I. & Wheeler, S. (1996) *Qualitative Research for Nurses.* Blackwell Science, Oxford.

Holly, M. (1984) *Keeping a Personal-Professional Journal.* Deakin University Press, Victoria.

Holmes, C. (1997) Why we should wash our hands of medical soaps. *Nursing Inquiry,* **4**, 135–137.

Home Office (1998) *Supporting Families: A consultation Document.* HMSO, London. http://www.northdevon.gov.uk/dris/main-mnu.html

Hoskins, P.L., Fowler, P.M., Constantino, M., Forrest. J., Yue, D.K. & Turtle, J.R. (1993) Sharing the care of diabetic patients between hospital and general practitioners: Does it work? *Diabetic Medicine,* **10**, 81–86.

Howard, R.W. (1987) *Concepts and Schemata: An Introduction.* Cassell Education, London.

Hulatt, I. (1995) A sad reflection. *Nursing Standard,* **8**(9), 22–24.

Hull, R.T. (1980) Codes or no codes. *Kansas Nurse,* **55**(10), 8, 18–19, 21.

Hull, R.T. (1981) The function of professional codes of ethics. *Westminster Institute Review,* **1**(3), 12–14.

Hunter, K. (1988) Nurses: the satiric image and the translocated ideal. In: *Images of Nurses: Perspectives from History, Art, and Literature* (ed. A. Jones), pp. 113–127. University of Pennsylvania Press, Pennsylvania.

Huntington, A. (1996) Nursing research reframed by the inescapable reality of practice: A personal encounter. *Nursing Inquiry,* **3**(3), 167–171.

Hussey, T. (1990) Nursing ethics and project 2000. *Journal of Advanced Nursing,* **15**, 1377–1382.

Hutchinson, S.A. (1993) Grounded theory: The method. In: *Nursing Research: a Qualitative Perspective* (eds P.L. Munhall & C. Oiler Boyd), 2ⁿᵈ edn, pp. 180–212. National League for Nursing, New York.

Hyde, V. (1995) Community nursing: A unified discipline? In: *Community Nursing: Dimensions and Dilemmas* (eds P. Cain, V. Hyde & E. Howkins), pp. 1–26. Arnold, London.

Ivancevich, J.M. & Matteson, M.T. (1993) *Organisational Behaviour and Management,* 3ʳᵈ edn. Irwin, Boston.

Jackson, D. (1995) Constructing nursing practice: Country of origin, culture and competency. *International Journal of Nursing Practice,* **1**(1), 32–36.

Jackson, D. (1997) Feminism: a path to clinical knowledge development. *Contemporary Nurse*, **6**(2), 85–91.

Jackson, D. & Raftos, M. (1997) In uncharted waters: Confronting the culture of silence in a residential care institution. *International Journal of Nursing Practice*, **3**(1), 34–39.

Jacobs, P.M., Ott, B., Sullivan, B., Ulrich, Y. & Short, L. (1997) An approach to defining and operationalizing critical thinking. *Journal of Nursing Education*, **36**(1), 19–22.

Jamieson, M., Griffiths, R. & Jayasuriya, R. (1998) Developing outcomes for community nursing: the nominal group technique. *Australian Journal of Advanced Nursing*, **16**(1), 14–19.

Jarvis, P. (1992) Reflective practice and nursing. *Nurse Education Today*, **12**(3), 174–181.

Jenkins, E. (1989) Nurses' control over nursing. In: *Issues in Australian Nursing 2* (eds G. Gray & R. Pratt). Churchill Livingstone, Melbourne.

Jennings, B.M. (1986) Nursing science: More promise than threat. *Journal of Advanced Nursing*, **11**(5), 505–511.

Johns, C. (1994) Nuances of reflection. *Journal of Clinical Nursing*, **3**, 71–75.

Johns, C. (1994) Guided reflection. In: *Reflective Practice in Nursing: The Growth of the Professional Practitioner* (eds A. Palmer, S. Burns & C. Bulman), pp. 110–129. Blackwell Scientific, Oxford.

Johns, C. (1995) Framing learning through reflection within Carper's fundamental ways of knowing in nursing. *Journal of Advanced Nursing*, **22**, 226–234.

Johnson, D.E. (1980) The behavioural system model for nursing. In: *Conceptual Models for Nursing Practice* (eds J.P. Riehl & C. Roy), 2nd edn. Appleton-Century-Crofts, New York.

Johnson, J.L. (1994) A dialectical examination of nursing art. *Advances in Nursing Science*, **1**(1), 1–14.

Johnson, J.L. (1996) The perceptual aspect of nursing art: Sources of accord and discord. *Scholarly Inquiry for Nursing Practice: An International Journal*, **10**(4), 307–327.

Johnson, J.L. (1996) The art of nursing. *Image: Journal of Nursing Scholarship*, **28**, 169–175.

Johnston, C. & Cooper, P. (1997) Patient-focused care: What is it? *Holistic Nursing Practice*, **11**(3), 1–7.

Johnston, T. (1980) Moral education for nursing. *Nursing Forum*, **19**(3), 284–299.

Johnstone, M. (1998) *Determining and responding effectively to ethical professional misconduct: A report to the Nurses Board of Victoria*. Melbourne.

Johnstone, M. (1999) *Bioethics: A Nursing Perspective*, 3rd edn. Harcourt/Saunders, Sydney.

Johnstone, M.J. (1994) *Nursing and the Injustices of the Law*. WB Saunders/Baillière Tindall, London.

Jones, A. (1988) *Images of Nurses: Perspectives from History, Art, and Literature*. University of Pennsylvania Press, Pennsylvania.

Jones, A. (2001) Time to think: temporal considerations in nursing practice and research. *Journal of Advanced Nursing*, **33**(2), 150–158.

Jones, T. (1993) *Britain's Ethnic Minorities*. Policy Studies Institute, London.

Kalisch, B. & Kalisch, P. (1983) An analysis of the impact of authorship on the image of the nurse presented in novels. *Research in Nursing and Health*, **6**, 17–24.

Kalisch, B. & Kalisch, P. (1983) Heroine out of focus: Media images of Florence Nightingale. Part 1: Popular biographies and stage productions. *Nursing & Health Care*, **4**, 181–187.

Kalisch, B. & Kalisch, P. (1984) An analysis of news coverage of maternal-child nurses. *Maternal-Child Nursing Journal*, **13**, 77–90.

Kalisch, B., Kalisch, P. & McHugh, M. (1982) The nurse as a sex object in motion pictures. *Research in Nursing & Health*, **5**, 147–154.

Kalisch, P. & Kalisch, B. (1987) *The Changing Image of the Nurse.* Addison Wesley, Menlo Park, California.

Kalisch, P., Kalisch, B. & Scobey, M. (1983) *Images of Nurses on Television.* Springer, New York.

Kampen, N. (1988) Before Florence Nightingale: A prehistory of nursing in painting and sculpture. In: *Images of Nurses: Perspectives from History, Art, and Literature* (ed. A. Jones), pp. 6–39. University of Pennsylvania Press, Pennsylvania.

Keck, J.F. (1994) Terminology of theory development. In: *Nursing Theorists and their Work* (ed. A. Marriner-Toomey). Mosby, St Louis.

Keegan, F. & Kent, D. (1992) Community health nursing. In: *Community Health Nursing Policy and Practice in Australia* (eds F. Baum, D. Fry & I. Lennie), pp. 156–169. Pluto Press, Sydney.

Keleher, H. (1994) Public health challenges for nursing and allied health. In: *Just Health: Inequalities in Illness, Care and Prevention* (eds C. Waddell & A. Peterson). Churchill Livingstone, London.

Keleher, H. & McInerney, F. (1998) *Nursing Matters: Critical Sociological Perspectives.* Churchill Livingstone, Sydney.

Kelly, A. (1985) The construction of masculine science. *British Journal of Sociology of Education*, **6**, 33–154.

Kelly, K. & Van Vlaenderen, H. (1996) Dynamics of participation in a community health project. *Social Science & Medicine*, **42**, 1235–1246.

Kelly-Thomas, K.J. (1998) *Clinical and Nursing Staff Development: Current Competence, Future Focus*, 2nd edn. Lippincott, New York.

Kelsey, A. & Hollindale, P. (1996) Equal but different: Health visiting and the new curriculum. *Health Visitor*, **69**(11), 457–458.

Kemmis, S. & McTaggart, R. (1988) *The Action Research Planner*, 3rd edn. University Press, Geelong.

Kendrick, K. (1994) Building bridges: Teaching ward-based ethics. *Nursing Ethics*, **1**(1), 35–41.

Kenrick, M. & Luker, K.A. (1996) An exploration of the influence of managerial factors on research utilisation in district nursing practice. *Journal of Advanced Nursing*, **23**(4), 697–704.

Kenway, J. & Watkins, P. (1994) *Nurses, Power Politics and Post-Modernity: A Monograph.* University of New England Press, Armidale.

Kickbush, I. (1997) Think health – what makes a difference? Address given at *WHO 4th International Health Promotion Conference*, Jakarta, July 1997.

Kickbush, I. (1997) Designing the future: Strategic directions for primary health care in economically advanced countries. Paper given at *Centre for Primary Health Care National Conference*, Queensland, Australia, 12–14 March 1997.

Kiger, A. (1993) Accord and discord in students' images of nursing. *Journal of Nursing Education*, **32**, 309–317.

Kikuchi, J.F. & Simmons, H. (eds) (1992) *Philosophic Inquiry in Nursing.* Sage, London.

Kikuchi, J.F. & Simmons, H. (eds) (1994) *Developing a Philosophy of Nursing.* Sage, London.

Kikuchi, J.F., Simmons, H. & Romyn, D. (eds) (1996) *Truth in Nursing Inquiry.* Sage, London.

King, K. & Norsen, L. (1994) The care/cure, nurse/physician dichotomy doesn't do it anymore. *Image: Journal of Nursing Scholarship*, **26**(2), 89.

King, M. (1981) *A Theory for Nursing: Systems, Concepts Process.* Wiley, New York.

Kinkle, S. (1993) Violence in the ED: How to stop it before it starts. *American Journal of Nursing*, **93**(7), 22–24.

Kitson, A.L. (1987) Raising standards of clinical practice – the fundamental issue of effective nursing practice. *Journal of Advanced Nursing*, **12**(3), 321–329.

Kitson, A.L. (1997) Using evidence to demonstrate the value of nursing. *Nursing Standard*, **2**(11), 34–39.

Klaidman, S. & Beauchamp, T.L. (1987) *The Virtuous Journalist.* Oxford University Press, Oxford.

Kobert, L.J. (1995) In our own voices: journalling as a teaching/learning technique for nurses. *Journal of Nursing Education*, **34**(3), 140–142.

Koch, T. & Webb, C. (1996) The biomedical construction of ageing: Implications for nursing care of older people. *Journal of Advanced Nursing*, **23**(5), 954–959.

Kralik, D., Koch, T. & Wootton, K. (1997) Engagement and detachment: Understanding patients' experiences with nursing. *Journal of Advanced Nursing*, **26**(2), 399–407.

Kramer, M. (1974) *Reality Shock.* Mosby, New York.

Kritek, P.B. (1985) Nursing diagnosis in perspective: Response to a critique. *Image: The Journal of Nursing Scholarship*, **17**(1), 3–8.

Kuhn, T.S. (1970) *The Structure of Scientific Revolutions*, 2nd edn. University of Chicago Press, Chicago.

Labonte, R. (1997) Designing the future: Strategic directions for primary health care in economically advanced countries. Paper given at *Centre for Primary Health Care, National Conference*, Queensland, Australia, 12–14 March 1997.

Lafferty, P.M. (1997) Balancing the curriculum: promoting aesthetic knowledge in nursing. *Nurse Education Today*, **17**, 281–286.

Landeen, J., Byrne, C. & Brown, B. (1995) Journal keeping as an educational strategy in teaching psychiatric nursing. *Journal of Advanced Nursing*, **17**, 347–355.

Langford, G. (1973) The concept of education. In: *Essays in the Philosophy of Education* (eds G. Langford & D.J. O'Connor), pp. 3–32. Routledge & Kegan Paul, London.

Larsson, G., Peterson, V., Lampic, C., von Essen, L. & Sjoden, P. (1998) Cancer patients and staff ratings of the importance of caring behaviours and their relations to patient anxiety and depression. *Journal of Advanced Nursing*, **27**(4), 855–864.

Lather, P. (1991) *Feminist Research in Education: Within/Against.* Deakin University Press, Geelong.

Lawler, J. (1991) *Behind the Screens: Nursing, Somology and the Problem of the Body.* Churchill Livingstone, Melbourne.

Lea, A., Watson, R. & Dreary, I. (1998) Caring in nursing: A multivariate analysis. *Journal of Advanced Nursing*, **28**(3), 662–671.

Leftwich, R. (1993) Care and cure as healing processes in nursing. *Nursing Forum*, **28**(3), 13–17.

Leininger, M.M. (1984) Transcultural nursing: An essential knowledge and practice field for today. *Canadian Nurse.* **Dec**, 41–57.

Leininger, M.M (1984) *Care: The Essence of Nursing and Health.* Slack Books, New Jersey.

Leininger, M.M (1986) Care facilitation and resistance factors in the culture of nursing. *Topics in Clinical Nursing*, **8**(2), 1–12.

Leininger, M.M. (1988) Leininger's theory of nursing: Culture care diversity and universality. *Nursing Science Quarterly*, **1**(4), 152–160.

Leininger, M.M. (1995) *Transcultural Nursing: Concepts, Theories, Research and Practices*, 2nd edn. McGraw-Hill, New York.

Lenkman, S. & Gribbins, R. (1994) Multidisciplinary teams in the acute care setting. *Holistic Nursing Practice*, **April**, 81–87.

Levine, M. (1971) Holistic nursing. *Nursing Clinics of North America*, **6**(2), 253–263.

Lifton, R. (1990) Foreword to HM Weinstein. *Psychiatry and the CIA: Victims of mind control*. pp. ix–xiv. American Psychiatric Press, Washington DC and London UK.

Long, L., Hobbs, W. & Mander, T. (1999) *Primary nursing in the haematology ward: Does it make a difference. Research Paper Series No. 1.* University of Adelaide Dept. of Clinical Nursing, Adelaide.

Loveridge, C.E. (1991) Lessons in excellence for nurse administrators. *Nursing Management*, **22**(2), 47.

Lubinski, J. (1990) Reflective withdrawal through journal writing. In: *Fostering Critical Reflection in Adulthood: A Guide to Transformative and Emancipatory Learning* (ed J. Mezirow), pp. 213–234. Jossey Bass, San Francisco.

Macdonald, J. (1993) The caring imperative: A must? *The Australian Journal of Advanced Nursing*, **11**(1), 26–30.

MacGuire, J. (1991) Quality of care assessed: Using the senior monitor index in three wards for the elderly before and after a change to primary nursing. *Journal of Advanced Nursing*, **16**, 511–520.

Mackereth, C. (1997) Health visiting: Is it a nursing matter? *Health Visitor*, **70**(4), 155–157.

Madjar, I., McMillan, M., Sharkey, R. & Cadd, A. (1997) *Project to review and examine expectations of beginning registered nurses in the workforce*. NSW Nurses Registration Board, Sydney.

Magee, B. (1997) *Confessions of a Philosopher*. Phoenix, London.

Malin, N. & Teasdale, K. (1991) Caring versus empowerment: considerations for nursing practice. *Journal of Advanced Nursing*, **16**, 657–662.

Manthey, M. (1980) *The Practice of Primary Nursing*. Blackwell, Boston.

Marriner-Toomey, A. (1994) Introduction to analysis of nursing theory. In: *Nursing Theorists and their Work* (ed. A. Marriner-Toomey), pp. 3–16. Mosby, St Louis.

Martin, C.R. & Thompson, D.R. (2000) *Design and Analysis of Clinical Nursing Research Studies*. Routledge, London.

Maslin-Prothero, S. (2001) *Baillière's Study Skills for Nurses*. Baillière Tindall, London.

Maslin-Prothero, S. & Owen, S. (2001) Enhancing your clinical links and credibility: The role of nurse lecturers and teachers in clinical practice. *Nurse Education in Practice*, **1**(4), 189–195.

Mayer, R. & Goodchild, F. (1995) *The Critical Thinker*, 2nd edn. Brown & Benchmark Publishers, Madison.

McCoppin, B. & Gardner, H. (1994) *Tradition & reality: Nursing and politics in Australia*. Churchill Livingstone, Melbourne.

McCougherty, D. (1991) The theory-practice gap in nurse education: its causes and possible solutions. Findings from an action research study. *Journal of Advanced Nursing*, **16**, 1055–1061.

McDonald, A., Langford, I. & Boldero, N. (1997) The future of community nursing in the United Kingdom: District nursing, health visiting and school nursing. *Journal of Advanced Nursing*, **26**(2), 257–265.

McGee, P. & Ashford, R. (1996) Nurses' perceptions of roles in multidisciplinary teams. *Nursing Standard*, **10**(45), 34–36.

McIntosh, J. (1996) The question of knowledge in district nursing. *International Journal of Nursing Studies*, **33**(3), 316–324.

McMahon, R. (1996) Individual vs collective activity: a primary nursing paradox. *British Journal of Nursing*, **5**(12), 760–763.

McMurray, A. (1993) The political and economic context, Chap. 5. In: *Community Health Nursing: Primary Health Care in Practice*, 2nd edn. Churchill Livingstone, Melbourne.

Meleis, A.I. (1997) *Theoretical Nursing: Development and Progress*. Lippincott, Philadelphia.

Melia, K.M. (1987) *Learning and Working: The Occupational Socialisation of Nurses*. Tavistock, London.

Mezirow, J. (1985) A critical theory of self directed learning. *New Directions for Continuing Education*, **25**, 17–30.

Miles, M.B. & Huberman, A.M. (1994) *Qualitative Data Analysis*, 2nd edn. Sage, Thousand Oaks.

Miller, M.A. & Babcock, D.E. (1996) *Critical Thinking Applied to Nursing*. Mosby, St Louis.

Monahan, B.B. (1996) The nurses media handbook: A reference for nurses planning to meet the media. *Massachusetts Nurse*, **66**(5), 2, 6, 12.

Moodood, T., Berthoud, R., Lakey, J. *et al.* (1997) *Ethnic Minorities in Britain*. Policy Studies Institute, London.

Moore, T. (1991) *Cry of the Damaged Man*. Picador, Sydney.

Morse, J., Solberg, S., Neander, W., Bottorf, J. & Johnson, J. (1990) Concepts of caring and caring as a concept. *Advances in Nursing Science*, **13**(1), 1–14.

Muff, J. (1982) Battle-axe, whore: An exploration into the fantasies, myths and stereotypes about nurses. In: *Socialization, Sexism and Stereotyping: Women's Issues In Nursing* (ed. J. Muff). CV Mosby, St Louis.

Mulhall, A. (1995) Nursing research: What difference does it make? *Journal of Advanced Nursing*, **21**, 576–583.

Munhall, P.L. (1982) Nursing philosophy and nursing research: In apposition or opposition? *Nursing Research*, **31**(3), 176–177, 181.

Munhall, P.L. & Oiler Boyd, C. (1993) *Nursing Research: A Qualitative Perspective*. National League for Nursing Press, New York.

Nakata, J.A. & Saylor, C. (1994) Management style and staff nurse satisfaction in a changing environment. *Nurse Administration Quarterly*, **18**(3), 51–57.

National Health Service Executive (1999) *Primary Care Trusts: Establishing Better Services*. HMSO, London.

Neff, W. (1929) *Victorian Working Women: An Historical and Literary Study of Women in British Industries and Professions 1832–1850*.

Nelson, S. (1995) Humanism in nursing: The emergence of light. *Nursing Inquiry*, **2**(1), 36–43.

Neuman, B. (1995) *The Neuman Systems Model: Application to Nursing Education and Practice*. Appleton-Century-Crofts, New York.

NHS Centre for Reviews and Dissemination (2001) *Undertaking Systematic Reviews of Research on Effectiveness.* CRD's guidance for those carrying out or commissioning reviews. CRD Report No. 4, 2nd edn. NHS Centre for Reviews and Dissemination, York.

Nightingale, F. (1859/1946) *Notes on Nursing.* Harrison Book Company, London.

Nordenfelt, L. (1995) *On the Nature of Health: An Action Theoretic Approach.* Kluwer, Dordrecht.

Nursing and Midwifery Council (2002) *Code of Professional Conduct,* www.nmc-uk.org, London.

O'Connell, B. (1996) Nursing process: A systematic approach to patient care. In: Greenwood, J. (ed.) *Nursing theory in Australia: Development and application.* Sydney: Harper Educational, 49–73.

O'Connor, M. & Parker, E. (1995) *Health Promotion Principles and Practice in the Australian Context.* Allen & Unwin, Sydney.

O'Hagan, K. (2001) *Cultural Competence in the Caring Professions.* Jessica Kingsley, London.

O'Toole, M.T. (ed.) (1997) *Miller-Keane Encyclopedia and Dictionary of Medicine, Nursing and Allied Health.* W.B. Saunders, Philadelphia.

Oakley, A. (2000) *Experiments in Knowing: Gender and Method in the Social Sciences.* Polity Press, Cambridge.

Office of Population Censuses & Surveys (1992) *1991 Census.* HMSO, London.

Oiler Boyd, C. (1993) Philosophical foundations of qualitative research. In: *Nursing Research: a Qualitative Perspective* (eds P.L. Munhall & C. Oiler Boyd), 2nd edn, pp. 66–93. National League for Nursing, New York.

Oldman, C. (1999) An evaluation of health visitor education in England. *Community Practitioner and Health Visitor,* **72**(12), 392–395.

Orem, D.E. (1991) *Nursing: Concepts of Practice,* 4th edn. Mosby, St Louis.

Papadopoulos, I. (2001) Antiracism, multiculturalism and the third way. In: *Managing Diversity and Inequality in Health Care* (ed. C. Baxter). Baillière Tindall, Edinburgh and Royal College of Nursing.

Papadopoulos. I, Tilki, M. & Taylor, G. (1998) *Transcultural Care: A Guide for Health Care Professionals.* Quay Books, Wilts.

Parker, B. & McFarland, J. (1991) Feminist theory and nursing: An empowerment model for research. *Advances in Nursing Science,* **13**(3), 59–67.

Parker, D.L., Webb, J. & D'Souza, B. (1995) The value of critical incident analysis as an educational tool and its relationship to experiential learning. *Nurse Education Today,* 111–116.

Parker, G.M. (1990) Team players and teamwork. In: *Leading and Managing in Nursing* (ed. P.S. Yoder Wise). Mosby, St Louis.

Parker, J.M. (1995) Searching for the body in nursing. In: *Scholarship in the Discipline of Nursing* (eds G. Gray & R. Pratt). Churchill Livingstone, Melbourne.

Parker, J.M. & Gibbs, M. (1998) Truth, virtue and beauty: Midwifery and philosophy. *Nursing Inquiry,* **5**(3), 146–153.

Parker, J.M. & Rickard, G. (1999) Nursing town and nursing gown: Time space and the reinvention of nursing through collaboration. *Clinical Excellence for Nurse Practitioners,* **3**(1), 36–42.

Parker, R. (1990) Nurses stories: The search for a relational ethic of care. *Advances in Nursing Science,* **13**(1), 31–40.

Parkes, R. (1994) *Specialisation in Nursing.* ANF, Melbourne.

Parse, R.R. (1981) *Man-Living-Health: A Theory of Nursing.* Wiley, New York.

Parse, R.R. (1992) Human becoming: Parse's theory of nursing. *Nursing Science Quarterly,* **5**, 35–42.

Parse, R.R. (ed.) (1995) *Illuminations: The human becoming in practice and research.* Pub. No. 15–2670. National League for Nursing, New York.

Parse, R.R. (1998) *The Human Becoming School of Thought: A Perspective for Nurses and other Health Professionals.* Sage, London and Thousand Oaks, California.

Paul, R. (1993) *Critical Thinking: How to prepare students for a rapidly changing world.* Foundation for Critical Thinking, Santa Rosa, California.

Payne, R. (1988) On being accountable. *Health Visitor,* **61**, 173–175.

Peacock, J.W. & Nolan, P.W. (2000) Care under threat in the modern world. *Journal of Advanced Nursing,* **32**(5), 1066–1070.

Pearson, A. (1989) *Primary nursing: Nursing in the Burford and Oxford Nursing Development Units.* Chapman & Hall, London.

Pearson, A. (1991) Taking up the challenge: The future for therapeutic nursing. In: *Nursing as Therapy* (eds R. McMahon & A. Pearson). Chapman & Hall, London.

Pearson, A. (1992) Knowing nursing: Emerging paradigms in nursing. In: *Knowledge for Nursing Practice* (eds K. Robinson & B. Vaughan), pp. 213–226. Butterworth Heinemann, Oxford.

Pearson, A. & Baker, H. (1992) Quality of care: Do contemporary nursing approaches make a difference? *Deakin Institute of Nursing Research, Research Papers No 5,* Deakin University, Geelong.

Pearson, A., Vaughan, B. & FitzGerald, M. (1996) *Nursing Models for Practice,* 2nd edn. Butterworth Heinemann, Oxford.

Pepin, J. (1992) Family caring and caring in nursing. *Image: Journal of Nursing Scholarship,* **24**(2), 127–131.

Peplau, H.E. (1952) *Interpersonal Relations in Nursing.* Putman, New York.

Peplau, H.E. (1988) The art and science of nursing: Similarities, differences, and relations. *Nursing Science Quarterly,* **1**(1), 8–15.

Peter, E. & Gallop, R. (1994) The ethic of care: A comparison of nursing and medical students, *Image: Journal of Nursing Scholarship,* **26**(1), 47–51.

Pfeffer, G.N. & Schnack, J.A. (1995) Nurse practitioners as leaders in a quality health care delivery system. *Advance Practice Nurses Quarterly,* **1**(2), 30–39.

Phaneuf, M. (1976) *The Nursing Audit.* Appleton Century Crofts, New York.

Pierson, W. (1998) Reflection and nursing education. *Journal of Advanced Nursing,* **27**, 165–170.

Polit, D.F. & Hungler, B.P. (1995) *Nursing Research: Principles and Methods,* 5th edn. Lippincott, Philadelphia.

Porter, S. (1991) A participant observation study of power relations between nurses and doctors in a general hospital. *Journal of Advanced Nursing,* **16**, 728–735.

Porter-O'Grady, T. (1995) Five rules of engagement for multidisciplinary teams. *Aspens Advisor for Nurse Executives,* **September**, 8.

Purnell, L.D. & Paulanska, B.J. (1998) *Transcultural Health Care: A Culturally Competent Approach.* F.A. Davies Co, Philadelphia.

Quality Assurance Agency for Higher Education (2001) *Subject Benchmark Statements: Healthcare Programmes.* Quality Assurance Agency for Higher Education, Gloucester.

Quinn, C. (1990) A conceptual approach to the identification of essential ethics content for the undergraduate nursing curriculum. *Journal of Advanced Nursing*, **15**, 726–731.

Rains, J. & Ray, D. (1995) Participatory action research for community health promotion. *Public Health Nursing*, **12**, 256–261.

Rapport, F. & Maggs, C. (1997) Measuring care: The case of district nursing. *Journal of Advanced Nursing*, **25**(4), 673–680.

Rawls, J. (1971) *A Theory of Justice*. Oxford University Press, Oxford.

Rawnsley, M. (1990) Of human bonding: The context of nursing as caring. *Advances in Nursing Science*, **13**(1), 41–48.

Ray, M. (1987) Technological caring: A new model in critical care. *Dimensions in Critical Care Nursing*, **6**(3), 173–179.

Ray, M. (1989) The theory of bureaucratic caring for nursing practice in the organizational structure. *Nursing Science Quarterly*, **13**(2), 31–42.

Redekopp, M. (1997) Clinical nurse specialist role confusion: The need for identity. *Clinical Nurse Specialist*, **11**(2), 87–91.

Reich, W. (1994) The word 'Bioethics': Its birth and the legacies of those who shaped its meaning. *Kennedy Institute of Ethics Journal*, **4**, 319–335.

Reich, W. (1995) The word 'Bioethics': The struggle over its earliest meanings. *Kennedy Institute of Ethics Journal*, **5**, 19–34.

Reid, B. (1993) But we're doing it already! Exploring a response to the concept of reflective practice in order to improve its facilitation. *Nurse Education Today*, **13**, 305–309.

Reihl, J.P. (1974) Application of interaction theory. In: *Conceptual Models for Nursing Practice* (eds J.P. Riehl & C. Roy), 2nd edn. Appleton-Century-Crofts, New York.

Reverby, S. (1987) A caring dilemma: Womanhood and nursing in historical perspective. *Nursing Research*, **36**(1), 5–11.

Richardson, G. & Maltby, H. (1995) Reflection-on-practice: Enhancing student learning. *Journal of Advanced Nursing*, **22**(2), 235–242.

Roberts, I. & Bedford, H. (1996) Does home visiting reduce the risk of childhood accidents? *Health Visitor*, **69**(7), 268–269.

Roberts, K. & Taylor, B. (1998) *Nursing Research Processes: An Australian Perspective*. Nelson ITP, Melbourne.

Roberts, S.J. (1983) Oppressed group behaviour: Implications for nursing. *Advances in Nursing Sciences*, **5**(4), 21–30.

Robinson, J. (1985) Health visiting and health. In: *Political Issues in Nursing: Past, Present and Future* (ed. R. White). John Wiley, London.

Robinson, K. & Vaughan, B. (eds) (1992) *Knowledge for Nursing Practice*. Butterworth-Heinemann, Oxford.

Robinson, V. (2001) *Jewels in the Crown: the Contribution of Ethnic Minorities to Life in Post-War Britain*. Moneygram International, London.

Rogers, M.E. (1970) *An Introduction to the Theoretical Basis of Nursing*. FA Davis, Philadelphia.

Rolfe, G. (1997) Writing ourselves: creating knowledge in post modern world. *Nurse Education Today*, **17**, 442–448.

Roper, N., Logan, W. & Tierney, A. (1990) *The Elements of Nursing*, 3rd edn. Churchill Livingstone, Edinburgh.

Roy, C. (1980) The Roy adaptation model. In: *Conceptual Models for Nursing Practice* (eds J.P. Riehl & C. Roy), 2nd edn. Appleton-Century-Crofts, New York.

Royal College of Nursing (1992) *The Royal College of Nursing of the United Kingdom*. Royal College of Nursing, London.

Royal College of Nursing (1997) *RCN: Assessment Tool for Nursing Older People*. Royal College of Nursing, London.

Royal College of Nursing (1999) *Link Up*. Royal College of Nursing, London.

Ruggiero, V.R. (1998) *The Art of Thinking: A Guide to Critical and Creative Thought*, 5th edn. Longman, New York.

Rule, J. (1995) Nurses may live to regret the 'angel' image era has ended. (News item) *Nursing Management*, **2**(6), 5.

Rumbold, G. (1986) *Ethics in Nursing Practice*. Baillière Tindall, London.

Rutten, A. (1995) The implementation of health promotion: A new structural perspective. *Social Science & Medicine*, **41**(12), 1627–1637.

Sackett, D.L. & Wennberg, J.E. (1997) Choosing the best research design for each question: It's time to stop squabbling over the 'best' methods (editorial). *British Medical Journal*, **315**(7123), 1636.

Salvage, J. (1983) Distorted images. *Nursing Times*, **79**, 13–15.

Salvage, J. (1990) The theory and practice of the 'new' nursing. *Nursing Times*, **86**(4), 42–45.

Salvage, J. & Heijnen, S. (eds) (1997) *Nursing in Europe: A Resource for Better Health*. WHO Regional Publications, European Series, No. 74.

Salvage, J. & Kershaw, B. (eds) (1986) *Models for Nursing*. John Wiley & Sons, Chichester.

Sandelowski, M. (1997) (Ir)reconcilable differences? The debate concerning nursing and technology. *Image: Journal of Nursing Scholarship*, **29**(2), 169–174.

Sarter, B. (1988) Philosophical sources of nursing theory. *Nursing Science Quarterly*, **1**(2), 52–59.

Saul, J. (1997) *The Unconscious Civilization*. Penguin, Ringwood.

Sawyer, L.M. (1989) Nursing code of ethics: An international comparison. *International Nursing Review*, **36**(5), 145.

Schick, T.J., & Vaughn, L. (1995) *How to Think about Weird Things: Critical thinking for a new age*. Mayfield Publishing Company, Mountain View, California.

Schon, D.A. (1983) *The Reflective Practitioner*. Basic Books, New York.

Schon, D.A. (1987) *Educating the Reflective Practitioner*. Jossey Bass, San Francisco.

Scottish Executive (1999) *Towards a Healthier Scotland: A white paper on health (CM4269)*. The Stationery Office, Edinburgh.

Scottish Executive (2001) *Nursing for Health: A Review of the contribution of nurses, midwives and health visitors to improving the public health in Scotland*. Scottish Executive, Edinburgh.

Seed, A. (1994) Patients to people. *Journal of Advanced Nursing*, **19**(4), 738–748.

Seedhouse, D. (1986) *Health: The Foundations for Achievement*. Wiley, Chichester.

Seeley, S., Murray, L. & Cooper, P. (1996) The outcome for mothers and babies of health visitor intervention. *Health Visitor*, **69**(4), 135–138.

Sellman, D. (1996) Why teach ethics to nurses? *Nurse Education Today*, **16**, 440–448.

Selzer, R. (1993) *Raising the dead: A doctor's encounter with his own mortality*. Penguin, Harmondsworth.

Seymer, L. (1986) In: *Florence Nightingale and the Nursing Legacy* (ed. M. Baly). Heinemann, London.

Sharman, E., Short, S. & Black, D. (1996) Why so many? The masculine mystique and men in the nursing higher education workforce in Australia. In: *Changing Society for Women's Health Conference*, Australian National University, Canberra, Australia.

Shay, L., Goldstein, J., Matthews, D., Trail, L. & Edmunds, M. (1996) Guidelines for developing a nurse practitioner practice. *Nurse Practitioner: American Journal of Primary Health Care*, **21**(1), 72, 75–76, 78 passim.

Smith, A. & Russell, J. (1991) Using critical incidents in nurse education. *Nurse Education Today*, **11**(4), 284–291.

Smith, F.B. (1982) *Florence Nightingale, reputation and power*. Croom Helm, London.

Smyth, J. (1989) Developing and sustaining critical reflection in teacher education. *Journal of Teacher Education*, **40**(2), 2–9.

Smyth, J. (1992) Teachers' work and the politics of reflection. *American Education Research Journal*, **29**(2), 267–300.

Smyth, J. (1993) Reflective practice in teacher education and other professions. Key address to the *Fifth National Practicum Conference*, Macquarie University, Sydney.

Snellgrove, S. & Hughes, D. (2000) Interprofessional relations between doctors and nurses: perspectives from South Wales. *Journal of Advanced Nursing*, **31**(3), 661–667.

Snow, C.P. (1964) *The Two Cultures: And a Second Look*. The New American Library, New York.

Solomos, J. (1993) *Race and Racism in Britain*. Macmillan Press, Basingstoke.

Sorrell, J.M. (1994) Writing as inquiry. In qualitative nursing research: elaborating the web of meaning. In: *Advances in Methods of Inquiry for Nursing* (ed. P. Chinn), pp. 1–12. Gaithersbury, Maryland, Aspen.

Spradley, J.P. (1980) *Participant Observation*. Holt, Rinehart & Winston, New York.

Starck, L., Mackey, T.A. & Adams, J. (1995) Nurse managed clinics: A blueprint for success using the Covey framework. *Journal of Professional Nursing*, **11**(2), 71–77.

Staunton, P. (1997) Don't let us stereotype mediocrity. Forty-fifth annual oration, New South Wales College of Nursing, Sydney, NSWCN.

Stedeford, A. (1984) *Facing Death: Patients, Families and Professionals*. W. Heinemann Books Ltd, London.

Stein, L.I., Watts, D.T. & Howell, T. (1990) Sounding board: The doctor-nurse game re-visited. *The Lamp*, **47**(9), 23–26.

Stevens Barnum, B.J. (1994) *Nursing Theory: Analysis, Application, Evaluation*, 4th edn. Lippincott, Philadelphia.

Strachey, L. (1931) *Portraits in Miniature and Other Essays*. Chatto & Windus, London.

Strasen, L. (1992) *The Image of Professional Nursing: Strategies for Action*. Lippincott, Philadelphia.

Street, A. (1995) *Nursing Replay: Researching Nursing Culture Together*. Churchill Livingstone, Melbourne.

Sullivan, J. & Deane, D. (1994) Caring: Reappropriating our tradition. *Nursing Forum*, **29**(2), 5–9.

Summers, A. (1997) Sairey Gamp: Generating fact from fiction. *Nursing Inquiry*, **4**, 14–18.

Summers, A. & McKeown, K. (1996) Health needs assessment in primary care: A role for health visitors. *Health Visitor*, **69**(8), 323–324.

Suppiah, C. (1996) Working in partnership with community mothers. *Health Visitor*, **67**(2), 51–53.

Swanson, J. & Nies, M. (1997) *Community Health Nursing Promoting the Health of Aggregates,* 2nd edn. WB Saunders, Philadelphia.

Swanson, K. (1993) Nursing as informed caring for the well-being of others. *Image: Journal of Nursing Scholarship,* **25**(4), 352–357.

Swider, S., McElmurry, B. & Yarling, R. (1984) Ethical decision making in a bureaucratic context by senior nursing students. *Nursing Research,* **34**(2), 108–112.

Sykes, J. (ed.) (1976) *Concise Oxford English Dictionary.* Oxford University Press, Oxford.

Taylor, B. (1994) *Being Human: Ordinariness in Nursing.* Churchill Livingstone, Melbourne.

Thagard, P. (1998) Ulcers and bacteria I: Discovery and acceptance. *Studies in History, Biology and Biomedical Science,* **29**(1), 107–136.

Thompson, J. & Thompson, H. (1989) Teaching ethics to nursing students. *Nursing Outlook,* **37**(2), 84–88.

Thorne, S.E. & Hayes, V.E. (eds) (1997) *Nursing Praxis: Knowledge and Action.* Sage, Thousand Oaks, California.

Tomlinson, P.D. (1995) *Understanding Mentoring.* Open University Press, Buckingham.

Townsend, J. (1994) Challenge models for learning and knowing. In: *Reflections on Contemporary Nursing Practice* (eds M. McMillan & J. Townsend). Butterworth, Sydney.

Townsend, P. & Davidson, N. (1992) *Inequalities in Health: The Black Report and the Health Divide.* Penguin, London.

Traynor, M. (1996) Looking at discourse in a literature review of nursing texts. *Journal of Advanced Nursing,* **23**(2), 1155–1161.

Treacy, M.P. (1989) Gender prescription in nurse training: Its effects on health provision. In: *Recent Advances in Nursing: Issues in Women's Health* (eds L.K. Hardy & J. Randell). Churchill Livingstone, Edinburgh.

Trembath, R. & Hellier, D. (1987) *All Care and Responsibility: A History of Nursing in Victoria 1850–1934.* Florence Nightingale Committee, Australia.

Tuckman, B.W. & Jensen, M. (1977) Stages of small group development revisited. In: *Organisational Behaviour and Management* (eds J.M. Ivancevich & M.T. Matteson), 3rd edn. Irwin, Boston.

Turner, C. (1991) *The Ethics of Authenticity.* Harvard University Press, Cambridge, Massachusetts.

Turner, T. (1990) Crushed by the system? *Nursing Times,* **86**(49), 19.

Turner, T. (1992) The indomitable Mr Pink. *Nursing Times,* **88**(24), 26–29.

Umiker, W. (1998) Collaborative conflict resolution. In: *Contemporary Leadership Behaviour: Selected Readings* (ed. E.C. Hein), 5th edn. Lippincott, New York.

United Kingdom Central Council for Nursing, Midwifery and Health Visiting (1992) *Code of Conduct.* UKCC, London.

United Kingdom Central Council for Nursing, Midwifery and Health Visiting (1995) *PREP & You.* UKCC, London.

United Kingdom Central Council for Nursing, Midwifery and Health Visiting (1996) *Guidelines for Professional Practice.* UKCC, London.

United Kingdom Central Council for Nursing, Midwifery and Health Visiting (1999) *Fitness for Practice: The UKCC Commission for Nursing and Midwifery Education, Chair: Sir Leonard Peach.* UKCC, London.

United Kingdom Central Council for Nursing, Midwifery and Health Visiting (1999) *How the UKCC Works for You.* UKCC, London.

United Kingdom Central Council for Nursing, Midwifery and Health Visiting (2000) *The Practice Standard: Information for Registered Nurses, Midwives and Health Visitors.* UKCC, London.

United Kingdom Central Council for Nursing, Midwifery and Health Visiting (2001) *The PREP Handbook.* UKCC, London.

United Kingdom Central Council for Nursing, Midwifery and Health Visiting (2001) *Supporting Nurses, Midwives and Health Visitors through Lifelong Learning.* UKCC, London.

United Kingdom Central Council for Nursing, Midwifery and Health Visiting (2001) *Registrar's Letter Relating to Standards for Specialist Practice and Education,* 11/2001.UKCC, London.

United Kingdom Central Council for Nursing, Midwifery and Health Visiting (2001) *Requirements for Registration as a Health Visitor – Consultation Document.* UKCC, London.

Urmson, J.O. & Ree, J. (eds) (1991) *The Concise Encylopedia of Western Philosophy and Philosophers.* Unwin Hyman, London.

Van Manen, M. (1977) Linking ways of knowing with ways of being. *Curriculum Inquiry* **6**(3), 205–228.

Van Manen, M. (1990) *The Tact of Teaching: The Meaning of Pedagogical Thoughtfulness.* University of New York Press, New York.

Visintainer, M.A. (1986) The nature of knowledge and theory in nursing. *Image,* **2**, 32–38.

Vito, K. (1983) Moral development considerations in nursing curricula. *Journal of Nursing Education,* **22**(3), 108–113.

Walker, K. (1995) Courting competency: Nursing and the politics of performance in practice. *Nursing Inquiry,* **2**(2), 90–99.

Walker, L.O. & Avant, K.C. (1988) *Strategies for Theory Construction in Nursing,* 2nd edn. Appleton & Lange, Norwalk, Connecticut.

Walters, A.J. (1994) *Caring as a Theoretical Construct.* University of New England Press, Armidale.

Warelow, P.J. (1996) Nurse-doctor relationships in multidisciplinary teams: Ideal or real? *International Journal of Nursing Practice,* **2**, 33–39.

Wass, A. (1994) Health promotion in context: Primary health care and the new public health movement. In: *Promoting Health: The Primary Health Care Approach* (ed. A. Wass), pp. 5–31, Harcourt Brace, Sydney.

Wass, A. (2000) The Ottawa charter for health promotion Appendix 2. In: *Promoting Health: The Primary Care Approach,* 2nd edn. pp. 267, 272. Harcourt Brace, Sydney.

Waterman, H., Webb, C. & Williams, A. (1995) Parallels and contradictions in the theory and practice of action research and nursing. *Journal of Advanced Nursing,* **22**, 779–784.

Watson, J. (1985) *Nursing: Human Science and Human Care.* Appleton Century Crofts, Norwalk, Connecticut.

Watson, J. (1985) *Nursing: The Philosophy and Science of Caring.* Colorado Associated University Press, Boulder, Colorado.

Watson, J. (1988) *Nursing: Human Science and Human Care: A theory of nursing.* National League for Nursing, New York.

Webb, C. (1996) Caring, curing, coping: Towards an integrated model. *Journal of Advanced Nursing,* **23**, 960–968.

Wellard, S. & Bethune, E. (1996) Reflective journal writing in nurse education: Whose interests does it serve? *Journal of Advanced Nursing,* **24**(5), 1077–1082.

Welty, E. (1984) *One Writer's Beginnings.* Harvard University Press, Cambridge, MA.

White, J. (1995) Patterns of knowing: review, critique and update. *Advances in Nursing Science*, **17**(4), 73–86.

White, R. & Ewan, C. (1991) *Clinical Teaching in Nursing*. Chapman and Hall, London.

Whittemore, R. (1999) Natural science and nursing science: Where do the horizons fuse? *Journal of Advanced Nursing*, **30**(5), 1027–1033.

Wicks, D. (1999) *Nurses and Doctors at Work: Rethinking Professional Boundaries*. Allen & Unwin, London.

Wilkes, L. & Wallis, M. (1993) The five Cs of caring: The lived experience of student nurses. *The Australian Journal of Advanced Nursing*, **11**(1), 19–25.

Williams, C. (1992) The glass escalator: Hidden advantages for men in the 'female' professions. *Social Problems*, **39**(3), 253–267.

Williams, S. (1997) Caring in patient-focused care: The relationship of patients' perceptions of holistic nurse care to their levels of anxiety. *Holistic Nursing Practice*, **11**(3), 61–68.

Witherell, C. (1991) The self in narrative: a journey into paradox. In: *Stories Lives Tell* (eds C. Witherell & N. Noddings). Teachers College Press, New York.

Wolf, Z.R. (1986) The caring concept and nurse identified caring behaviours. *Topics in Clinical Nursing*, **8**(2), 84–93.

Wolf, Z.R., Giardino, E., Osborne, P. & Ambrose, M. (1994) Dimensions of nurse caring. *Image: Journal of Nursing Scholarship*, **26**(2), 107–111.

Wong, F.K.Y., Kember, D., Chung, L.Y.F. & Yan, L. (1995) Assessing the level of student reflection from reflection journals. *Journal of Advanced Nursing*, **22**, 48–57.

World Health Organization (1992) *Targets for Health for All: The Health Policy for Europe*. (Summary of the updated edition September, 1991) WHO Regional Office for Europe, Copenhagen.

Worth, A. (1996) Focus. Identifying need for district nursing: towards a more proactive approach by practitioners. *NT Research*, **1**(4), 260–269.

Wright, B.A. (1993) Behaviour diagnoses by a multidisciplinary team. *Geriatric Nursing*, **January/February**, 30–35.

Wright, S. (1998) *Changing Nursing Practice*, 2nd edn. Arnold, London.

Wuest, J. (1997) Illuminating environmental influences on women's caring. *Journal of Advanced Nursing*, **26**, 49–58.

Yoder Wise, P.S. (1995) *Leading and Managing in Nursing*. Mosby, St Louis.

Zavarzadeh, M. & Morton, D. (1991) *Theory, (Post)Modernity, Opposition: An 'other' introduction to literary and cultural theory*. Maisonneuve Press, Washington DC.

Index

LIBRARY & INFORMATION SERVICE
STRAYSIDE EDUCATION CENTRE
STRAYSIDE WING
HARROGATE DISTRICT HOSPITAL
LANCASTER PARK ROAD
HARROGATE HG2 7SX